Mobilizing the Myofascial System

A clinical guide to assessment and treatment of myofascial dysfunctions

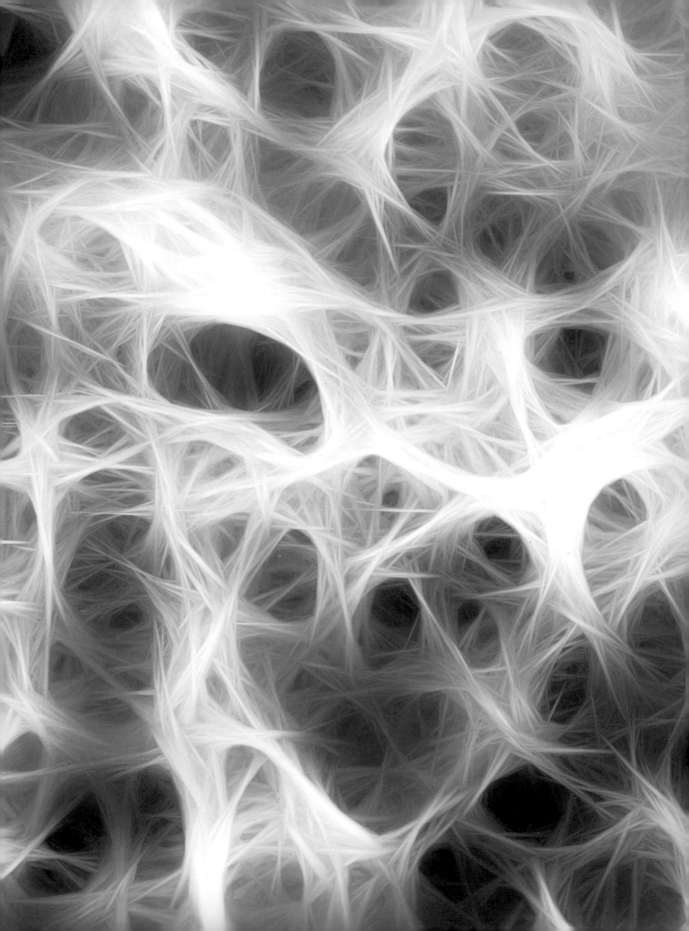

Mobilizing the Myofascial System

A clinical guide to assessment and treatment of myofascial dysfunctions

Doreen Killens BScPT, FCAMPT, CGIMS

Forewords **Diane Lee** BSR, FCAMT, CGIMS
Thomas W Myers BCSI, IASI, FQM
BetsyAnn Baron BCSI, IASI, FQM

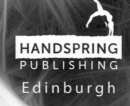

HANDSPRING
PUBLISHING
Edinburgh

HANDSPRING PUBLISHING LIMITED
The Old Manse, Fountainhall,
Pencaitland, East Lothian
EH34 5EY, Scotland
Tel: +44 1875 341 859
Website: www.handspringpublishing.com

First published 2018 in the United Kingdom by Handspring Publishing

Permissions

In addition to the specific permissions given in the captions of figures and tables, the author and publishers are grateful: for permission granted by photographer Michael Slobodian and model Alison McCreary to reproduce the photographs illustrating Chapters 5 to 14; to Elsevier for permission to reproduce Figures 1.2, 1.4, 1.6, 2.9, 6.30, 12.12 and Table 1.1; to Serge Paoletti for Figure 2.15 and for information used in Chapter 1; to the Education Committee of the Orthopaedic Division of the Canadian Therapy Association for permission to use the Contraindications to Manual Therapy list reproduced in Chapter 13; to Hay House Inc., Carlsbad, CA, for permission to quote from *Goddesses Never Age* by Christiane Northrup; and to Tom Myers, specifically for material in Chapter 14 but also in general, for inspiration throughout the book.

ISBN 978-1-909141-90-2
ISBN (Kindle eBook) 978-1-909141-91-9

British Library Cataloguing in Publication Data
A catalogue record for this book is available from the British Library

Library of Congress Cataloguing in Publication Data
A catalog record for this book is available from the Library of Congress

Commissioning Editor Mary Law
Project Manager Stephanie Pickering
Copy-editor Stephanie Pickering
Designer Bruce Hogarth
Indexer Aptara, India
Typesetter DiTech Process Solutions
Printer Melita, Malta

The
Publisher's
policy is to use
paper manufactured
from sustainable forests

CONTENTS

ACKNOWLEDGEMENTS

Gratitude. This is the overall tenet by which I try to live my life, and this book, *Mobilizing the Myofascial System*, provides ample opportunity to express it. An enormous debt of gratitude goes out to a long list of colleagues, friends and family who have, by their support and encouragement, contributed to the book. First and foremost I would like to thank Tom Myers, whose poetic descriptions of fascia in his book *Anatomy Trains* inspired me to think beyond the standard tools used by physiotherapists to treat musculo-skeletal conditions. This book struck a creative spark in me that led to the development of an approach to treatment of the fascial system from the point of view of a physiotherapist, an approach I have called Mobilization of the Myofascial System (MMS). Tom continues to inspire and evolve his work and has touched the lives of many professionals and movement therapists.

I would also like to acknowledge the contribution of Laurie McLaughlin, a colleague, former examiner for the Orthopaedic Division of the Canadian Physiotherapy Association, and soul sister friend. Laurie and I began to discover the world of fascia through the lens of physiotherapy at about the same time (over 20 years ago). Although she lived in Toronto and I in Montreal, when we would get together, we would exchange and explore fascial treatment techniques that we had each separately developed. We were consistently surprised at how similar our approaches were. Our techniques continue to evolve and we each share our fascial treatment approaches with other physiotherapists across the globe.

BetsyAnn Baron has enriched my life with her appreciation for dance and music, as well as her enthusiasm for learning, especially her zest for all things "fascia." A former ballerina with Les Grands Ballets Canadiens, a massage therapist since 1991 and a structural integrator since 2003, she developed an approach to treatment of the fascial system called Structural Myofascial Therapy (SMFT®). Since 2007, BetsyAnn and I have been teaching a series of courses for physiotherapists called Treatment of the Myofascial Body, with Mobilization of the Myofascial System (MMS) and Structural Myofascial Therapy (SMFT®). The course is a combination of MMS, which is based on manual therapy for the articular, muscular and neural systems, and SMFT, which involves techniques that are based in Structural Integration for the muscular system. We have found that these two approaches are mutually complementary. In addition to sharing our passion for fascia, we share a deep friendship, for which I am very grateful. Along with my other soul sisters and brothers, and long-time friends (Margie, Rita, Donna, Gioconda, Sharon, Michèle, Betty, and Ken), I would like to thank you for providing encouragement, love, laughter, and moral support throughout my life.

Elaine Maheu, my friend since our days at McGill University and my business partner for over 27 years – you set the bar high and inspire others to follow you and do the same, whether it be at the clinic, through your teaching around the world, or simply pushing me to do more exercise! My life would not be the same without you in it.

Diane Lee – my mentor, my friend and my inspiration. I have taken countless courses with you and I am always amazed at how you are able to integrate the available science with the art of physiotherapy. You continue to evolve, not only as a professional, sharing your insights with therapists across the globe, but also personally, sharing who you are, with all of your gifts. Thank you for taking the time to discuss and exchange ideas about fascia and how it fits into the world of physiotherapy and thank you for your valuable input into this book. I remain forever grateful.

I would also like to acknowledge my Canadian manual therapy roots and thank my fellow instructors and examiners for sharing their excellent manual therapy and clinical reasoning skills. In addition to the intellectual stimulation, their appreciation for dance and laughter made many orthopedic symposiums and conferences enjoyable and memorable. It was a pleasure to be involved with such an inspiring group for over 30 years.

ACKNOWLEDGEMENTS *continued*

To Eve Sanders, who so generously offered to proofread the text for this book. Her background as a university English professor and her experience in having been the recipient of MMS made her an excellent choice for editing this manuscript. As much as she appreciated the value of MMS techniques and the contribution it brought to her physical well-being, I came to appreciate her gifts as a wordsmith. The reader will no doubt value her input.

To Michael Slobodian, my friend and photographer, who so skillfully produced the photos in this book – I am grateful for your eye for detail and your artistic gifts that depict "beautiful lines" and yet still manage to illustrate the MMS techniques accurately. I couldn't have asked for a better collaborator on this project.

To Joanna Abbatt, a Pilates and Gyrotonics certified massage therapist, who works with dancers, circus performers, and "regular folk" to empower them to move conscientiously. Thank you for your input into the exercise chapter. Your keen eyes don't miss a thing!

Thank you to the team at Handspring Publishing, in particular Mary Law and Andrew Stevenson, who started this project off and guided it through its many phases, as well as Stephanie Pickering (copy-editor), Morven Dean (project manager), and Bruce Hogarth (art design). Your hard work and patient responses to my endless questions and clarifications were much appreciated. You made my first experience as an author a very enjoyable process.

To my husband George, whose unconditional love and support is unparalleled. He, along with my daughter Kelly and my son Michael, has tolerated my fascination with the world of fascia, which often led me far from home and took up a great deal of time. Thanks for waiting so patiently for me to come back into the fold and take more time to "play."

To my mother, Thérèse, who is now a 91-year-old matriarch of an extended family. You have always been ahead of your time and through your example, have encouraged each of your children, grandchildren, and now, great-grandchildren to aspire to be all that we can be. I am glad that my soul chose you to be my mother – I couldn't have asked for a better role model. And finally, to my extended family, including my siblings, in-laws and "out-laws," step-kids and grandkids. Your love defines me.

Thank you to my students, who continue to ask probing questions and push me to clarify in words what my hands are feeling. To my patients, especially the challenging ones, who push me to think beyond "the usual" and sort out "what else could this be." Thank you for sharing your stories and for allowing me to contribute to your healing journeys.

And finally, thank you to my spiritual guides (yes, I dare say such a thing!). I feel your presence in my treatment room and appreciate your input. I have learned to get myself "out of the way," so that I can be open to receiving your guidance. Thank you to my spiritual guide and mentor, Doreen Mary Bray, for teaching me how to connect with "Essence" and whose input changed the trajectory of my life, both personally and professionally. Gratitude. Gratitude.

Doreen Killens

Montréal, Québec, Canada
March 2018

FOREWORD by Diane Lee

I am delighted, and honored, to be asked to write a foreword for Doreen's new book *Mobilization of the Myofascial System – a Clinical Guide to Assessment and Treatment of Myofascial Dysfunctions.* You may be wondering why Handspring Publishing has agreed to produce another book on fascia when their company represents several authors on the topic already. This is the first book to be written on fascia by a physiotherapist with expertise in manual and manipulative therapy.

I have known Doreen Killens for more than thirty-five years and over this time we have witnessed each other's interests and teaching evolve in conjunction with our clinical expertise and the research evidence. We were both instructors and chief examiners for the Canadian Academy of Manipulative Physiotherapy (CAMPT), a division of the Canadian Physiotherapy Association and an IFOMPT accredited program. In the 1980s, the curriculum of courses was primarily focused on the articular system, as were most manual therapy programs world-wide, and while the program is still strongly based in the articular system, it has evolved to include more neuromyofascial concepts for manual therapy. However, what appears to still be missing is an evidence-informed, clinically reasoned approach for the assessment and treatment of fascial dysfunction.

Physiotherapists facilitate posture and movement training by addressing the underlying system impairments (articular, myofascial, neural, visceral) that compromise mobility and/or control of the joints of the skeleton. This perspective differs from many other disciplines and is one that requires a diverse tool box for both assessment and treatment of the whole person that is inclusive of all body regions and systems. For example, is the lack of joint mobility due to:

- a stiff joint that requires a specific articular mobilization technique

- an over-active muscle that requires a technique to reduce the neural drive to the muscle

- lack of visceral mobility that requires a specific visceral release technique, or

- the inability of the fascial system to permit the elongation required for the joint to move?

Is the lack of joint control due to:

- loss of passive integrity of the joint (articular instability)

- altered neuromuscular recruitment strategies (motor control deficits)

- reduced neuromuscular capacity (strength, endurance), or

- loss of anatomical integrity of the fascial sling required for the transference of load?

What is the relationship between impaired body regions? Is one compensating or causal for the other?

Physiotherapists are not specialists in one system, rather they understand the integration and relationships between and within the body regions and systems and have a diverse set of tools (assessment and treatment) to address the specific combination of impairments of the individual patient. The goal is to restore better strategies for function and performance. While evidence-informed, most experienced clinicians will tell you that their clinical expertise is equally important for well-reasoned treatment decisions. The patient's goals are centermost in treatment planning.

This landmark new book, *Mobilization of the Myofascial System*, is the culmination of over twenty years of Doreen's interest, clinical expertise, and understanding of the evidence as it pertains to fascia for physiotherapists with manual therapy training. The book is divided into three sections. The first begins with an introduction to all things fascia: what is it (definition), its anatomy (macroscopic and microscopic), the function and pathophysiology of fascial dysfunction. Chapter 2 outlines the theories of Tom Myers and his fascial Anatomy Trains which were a starting point for Doreen's approach to the fascial lines from a physiotherapy perspective for mobilization of the myofascial system (MMS). The physiotherapy assessment that integrates the fascial system with all others (articular, neural, visceral) is presented in Chapter 3 followed by Chapter 4 which outlines the principles of MMS treatment and describes how, and when, MMS techniques can be integrated with other manual therapies for impairments involving multiple, and different, systems. The manual physiotherapist will find the concepts here align well with the principles of manual therapy treatment. The second section is descriptive and illustrative of a wide variety of MMS techniques for the various regions of the body and the third section completes the text with a discussion on additional topics to consider in treatment for best outcomes (movement, nutrition, hydration, hormones, etc.).

Doreen closes her book with a very personal story about her journey as a mother, physiotherapist, and embodied spirit and shares many experiences that have shaped her as a clinician. This information is rarely shared and reflects what a therapeutic relationship with Doreen would be like. It is truly special, as is she. With heartfelt gratitude, I extend my congratulations to her on the completion of this text for physiotherapists with special training in manual therapy for ways to mobilize the myofascial system, and more.

Diane Lee, BSR, FCAMT, CGIMS

Adjunct Professor, Physical Therapy
Faculty of Medicine, UBC
Clinical Specialist Women's Health, CPA
Surrey, BC, Canada
July 2018

FOREWORD By Tom Myers

All over the world, manual therapists and movement professionals are busy forging a new synthesis of how we are held together and how we move. This over-arching point of view is arising from new knowledge and research on the brain's control of movement combined with new knowledge and research on auto-regulation in the fascial system.

The alembic for this new synthesis, without which it cannot happen, is the willingness of disparate professions to work with each other and learn from each other. The insights from movement systems like Pilates and strength and conditioning training bring new life to physiotherapy. The intrinsic physiological movements employed in osteopathy are being incorporated into work with developmental delay. Movement instruction, touch cueing, and manual therapeutic approaches are all blending and mixing into a single theorctical basis for learning, enhancing, and repairing the human movement function.

This is a happy convocation, where new developments are being shared from one profession to another, and old barriers are breaking down to produce a common language in which all the "spatial medicine" practitioners will eventually converse.

Doreen Killens is one of those synthetic practitioners able to incorporate various methods into a single, coherent whole. Of course I am happy to see another application of the Anatomy Trains map, and doubly so to see it done accurately. But I am especially pleased to see manual therapy and movement so confidently combined. Work with the musculoskeletal frame can never return to the linear, one-to-one correspondences that were the grail of the previous generation. Fractal mathematics, systems theory, and the dawning recognition that everything is related all lead us away from the temptation to isolate particular joints, muscles, or movements. Our bodies just do not work that way.

The approach in this book is sound, enjoyable, and opens the door to a lifetime career that is both challenging and satisfying by turns. Working in a world where everything is connected and interacts can be frustrating to those who need a guide for every step, a defined answer to every problem. But for the artist – see the last chapter for a fine summary of the proper attitude to being a therapist – this book offers a way forward that is at once effective and engaging.

Tom Myers

Clarks Cove, Maine USA
July 2018

FOREWORD By BetsyAnn Baron

I met Doreen Killens in the early 1980s when she was a young physiotherapist and I was still a professional ballet dancer – and her patient. Indeed, I happened to be first in her treatment schedule after she had taken one of her very early postgraduate courses, Muscle Energy. The techniques she learned just happened to be what my injured body needed. This was the beginning of what is now nearly a 40-year relationship.

After I hung up my pointe shoes, I studied massage therapy. I practiced on Doreen to get her professional input. She began referring patients to me that needed more attention to muscular tension than she had time for. Thanks to her referrals, my practice blossomed with a clientele searching for specific therapeutic massage.

We soon began monthly treatment exchanges, not only for our own well-being, but importantly, to share techniques and discoveries. We each took a variety of courses and swapped the information we had learned.

Entering the 21st century, we both began exploring the fascia and the myofascial system, guided by sources that were both similar and different. Our exchanges became more and more fascially focused, often erupting in gales of laughter as we explored body positioning in order to find and treat the line of tension we were searching for.

In the earlier part of her career, during treatment, Doreen would say to me: "Hey Bets, I learned some really cool stuff! This will be perfect for you!" This has evolved into: "Hey Bets, let me *show* you what I've been playing with this week," as she delves into exploring and working with the myofascial system.

In 2007, Doreen and I began teaching a continuing education curriculum we designed for physiotherapists titled "Treating the Myofascial Body." We created a kind of jigsaw puzzle in which the pieces of her work and mine fit into a fascinating myofascial whole that we have been able to pass on to others.

Now Doreen's groundbreaking myofascial techniques are the subject of her first book, *Mobilizing the Myofascial System*. I have been privileged to witness Doreen's growth both in the treatment room and in the classroom, and I am thrilled that she is transmitting her knowledge to you. It is truly outstanding hands-on work that will add another dimension to your understanding of what manual therapy can achieve.

BetsyAnn Baron

Board Certified Structural Integrator, IASI, FQM
Montréal, Québec, Canada
March 2018

PREFACE

Why write this book?

In my 40-year career as an orthopedic physiotherapist, I have amassed many wonderful tools from multiple postgraduate courses that I have taken over the years. I have never believed in only one type of treatment, preferring continually to assess and treat my clients as we explore their healing journey and use "the right tool at the right time" (Diane Lee). Despite this, I too have experienced my fair share of clinical frustrations and this has led me to explore this fascinating world of fascia. This approach to treatment has brought a deeper level of understanding to seemingly complex cases.

As physiotherapists we like to classify dysfunction as much as possible, thinking along the lines of joint dysfunction vs muscle imbalance vs recruitment problems, etc. Therapists may also be experiencing situations where patients are complaining of multiple areas of pain that do not correspond or fit into the paradigms that we are familiar with, even as fully trained manual therapists. Perhaps what is missing is the fascial component, an often overlooked tissue category that may contribute to persistent musculoskeletal pain. Fascia is innervated, making it a potential pain generator, and it has strong mechanical presence that can restrict mobility if not addressed.

The truth is that continuity between tissues does exist. We must be willing to think outside of the box and open up our approach to thinking more globally if we want to move forward with some of our more challenging cases.

The concept of fascia as a contributor to musculoskeletal dysfunction is not a novel one. The osteopathic profession has been writing about fascia for a number of years and Structural Integration has taken its rightful place in the field of rehabilitation. Other professionals are also beginning to explore the world of fascia, as witnessed by the explosion of research in this field and the number of participants from various professions in several International Fascia Research Congresses since 2007. However, most physical therapists are unfamiliar with fascia, aside from the "dead packing material" we had learned to push aside in our dissections in order to visualize the "important stuff" like muscles and nerves. Physiotherapists, with their varied skill-set in manual therapy, are poised to take on this important tissue.

In the world of orthopedic physiotherapy, the use of manual therapy techniques has become increasingly more evidence-based and study after study shows its efficacy along with exercise therapy for the management of the most common orthopedic conditions. However, there has been very little mention of the role of fascia aside from cursory mention of the stabilization role for the thoracolumbar fascia in low back pain. Diane Lee and L. J. Lee have noted the myofascia as one of the impairments in their Integrated Systems Model. Knowledge of fascial connections helps us understand how to direct our approach at the source of the problem (the criminal) and not merely the painful tissue (the victim).

In 2001, Tom Myers, a structural integrator, wrote the first edition of his book *Anatomy Trains: Myofascial Meridians for Manual and Movement Therapists*. This concept of myofascial continuities has helped me understand the multiple ways muscles link and connect to transfer forces and support the body. It is a framework for understanding not only static postural support but dynamic and optimal movement. Inspired by this book and using it as a guideline, along with clinical applications to some of my more challenging cases, I developed an approach to treatment called Mobilization of the Myofascial System (MMS). It is an approach that has its origins in manual physiotherapy for the articular, muscular, and neural systems. This sets it apart from other books written on the myofascia, primarily by structural integrators, who use these concepts to describe techniques that manipulate the fascia around the muscular system with slow and deep maneuvers. Although *Mobilizing the Myofascial System: A Clinical Guide to Assessment and Treatment of Myofascial*

Dysfunctions is primarily intended for physiotherapists who have been trained in manual therapy, it is also valuable for osteopaths, chiropractors, structural integrators, and other body workers who are seeking an alternate way to work with the fascia.

What is the subject of the book?

The techniques described here are taken from the body of work taught in Mobilization of the Myofascial System series of courses taught to physiotherapists across Canada and Europe. The courses present a comprehensive system for working with the whole body and are divided into three courses: Upper Quadrant, Lower Quadrant, and an advanced course entitled Integration of Quadrants. The techniques chosen for this book represent effective tools for some common recurrent dysfunctions encountered in orthopedic manual therapy. This book is intended to be an adjunct to the course notes and it is recommended that this approach to treatment be learned through workshops and courses. However, the book may also be used as a standalone text to guide the therapist in the use of fascial techniques in their practice.

How is the material structured?

My intention was to make the book as user-friendly as possible. It begins with some theory including a historical review of fascial approaches to treatment thus far (Chapter 1), as well as a brief review of Tom Myers's Anatomy Trains fascial lines, upon which the concept of this treatment is developed (Chapter 2). The main emphasis is clinical techniques for various regions of the body (Chapters 5 through 13). The therapist may consult the chapter associated with the cervical spine as an example (Chapter 5) and discover the various fascial approaches to treating this area of the body. However, it is equally important for the clinician to understand how to recognize and diagnose a fascial dysfunction (Chapter 3) as well as being familiar with the basic principles of treatment (Chapter 4).

Dural mobility techniques are described in Chapter 7. This may be an area unfamiliar to many physiotherapists and will give the therapist other tools besides the use of the slump test and single leg raise (SLR) to assess and treat this area of the body. Finally, Chapter 14 will cover how the patient can actively contribute to fascial health via exercises and various types of movement approaches, including yoga therapy. Last, but not least, Chapter 15 discusses ways to optimize therapeutic outcomes, with "out of scope" information that should be considered, such as the effects of nutrition, hydration, and hormone health on fascial tissues. It also covers ways to create an optimal therapeutic environment, not only for the patient but also for the therapist.

I hope that you will be inspired by this book and that it will open up a whole new therapeutic world for you to explore. To quote Robert Schleip, a prominent researcher and author in the field of fascia, "After several decades of severe neglect, this Cinderella of orthopedic science is developing its own identity within medical research." Welcome to the world of fascia!

Doreen Killens, BScPT, FCAMPT, CGIMS

Montréal, Québec, Canada
March 2018

LIST OF ABBREVIATIONS

A/P anteroposterior

AC acromioclavicular

ALL anterior longitudinal ligament

ASIS anterior superior iliac spine

ASLR active straight leg raise

BFL Back Functional Line

C/Thx cervicothoracic

CCFT craniocervical flexion test

CGRP calcitonin gene-related peptide

Cr/V craniovertebral

CTM connective tissue massage

Cx cervical spine

DBAL Deep Back Arm Line

DF dorsiflexion

DFAL Deep Front Arm Line

DFL Deep Front Line

DRA diastasis rectus abdominis

ECM extracellular matrix

EDL extensor digitorum longus

EHL extensor hallucis longus

EO external oblique

ER external rotation

Ev eversion

EZ elastic zone

FABER(E) flexion abduction external rotation (extension)

FADDIR flexion adduction internal rotation

FDA Food and Drug Administration (US)

FFL Front Functional Line

FHL flexor hallucis longus

FLT failed load transfer

GH glenohumeral

IFL Ipsilateral Functional Line

IFOMPT International Federation of Manipulative Physical Therapists

ILA inferior lateral angle

IMS intramuscular stimulation

IO internal oblique

IPT intrapelvic torsion

IR internal rotation

ISGT intra-shoulder girdle torsion

ISM Integrated Systems Model

ITB iliotibial band

LBP low back pain

LHB long head of biceps

LL Lateral Line

Lx lumbar spine

MFB myofibroblasts

MMS Mobilization of the Myofascial System

MTP metatarsophalangeal

mTrP myofascial trigger point

NOI Neuro Orthopaedic Institute

NZ neutral zone

OE obturator externus

OI obturator internus

OLS one leg stand

ABBREVIATIONS *continued*

P/A posteroanterior

PF plantarflexion

PIL postero-inferior-lateral

PIVM passive intervertebral movement

PNF proprioceptive neuromuscular facilitation

PSA postural somatic awareness

PSIS posterior superior iliac spine

QL quadratus lumborum

® right

R1 point in the joint's range where the first resistance to movement is felt

R2 endpoint of joint's range

RA rectus abdominis

ROM range of motion

RWA release with awareness

SAL sitting arm lift

SBAL Superficial Back Arm Line

SBL Superficial Back Line

SC sternoclavicular

SCM sternocleidomastoid

SFAL Superficial Front Arm Line

SFL Superficial Front Line

SIJ sacroiliac joint

SL Spiral Line

SLR straight leg raise

SMFT Structural Myofascial Therapy

SNS sympathetic nervous system

TFGF transforming growth factor

TFL tensor fasciae latae

Th/L thoracolumbar

Thx thoracic spine

TMJ temporomandibular joint

TPR transverse plane rotation

TrA transversus abdominis

UFT upper fibers of trapezius

ULNT upper limb neural tension test

vs versus

WAD whiplash associated disorder

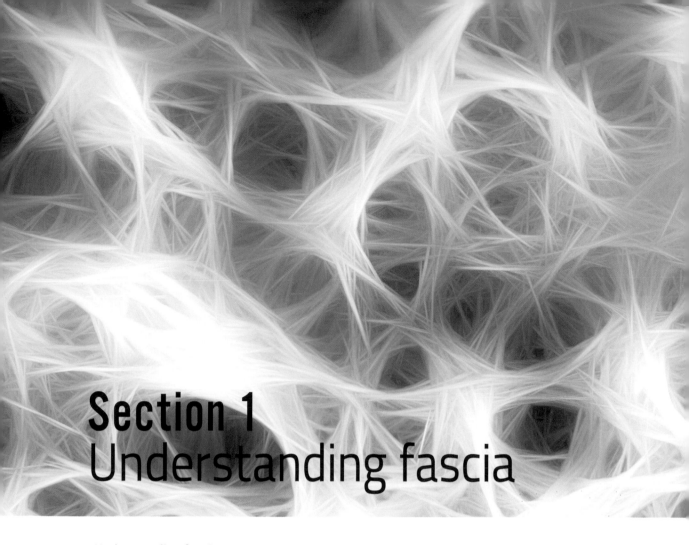

Section 1
Understanding fascia

Understanding fascia

What exactly is fascia? Historically, it has often been ignored as the body has been compartmentalized by the medical profession. The commonly known fascial sheets such as the thoracolumbar fascia and plantar fascia represent only a small portion of a much more extensive system. In fact fasciae are present throughout the entire body, covering not only muscles but also joints, bones, nerves, and organs, all the way down to the cellular level (Oschman 2000).

Fascial continuity can be explained via embryology; connective tissue develops largely from the embryonic mesoderm. Contrary to popular opinion, muscles develop within the fascia as opposed to the other way around. Thus, fascia directs organogenesis (Van der Wal 2009; Scheunke 2015). This generative function implies that fascia is much more than a random three-dimensional packing material that "connects everything." Research indicates that fascia also plays a major role as a body-wide autoregulatory system (Langevin 2006).

How, then, should we define fascia?

Fascia: a definition

Defining fascia remains a work in progress. Terms used to describe the fascial net include "collagenous network," "connective tissue webbing," and "extracellular matrix." In 2015, a group of researchers in the field of fascia came to a consensus about its definition. According to this group, the term fascia denotes: "a sheath, a sheet or any number of other dissectible aggregations of connective tissue that forms beneath the skin to attach, enclose, and separate muscles and other internal organs" (Stecco C. 2015a).

The value of such a "purely anatomical definition," as Stecco explains, is that it enables "everybody to know exactly what we're talking about, to isolate these layers in cadavers and perform histological and morphological analysis, to sample the fasciae during surgery, to evaluate pathological alterations and to study them in living subjects by means of imaging technology." In addition, it helps facilitate "comparison of the results of anatomical studies performed by different researchers."

However, for clinicians concerned more with the function of the fascial net, as, for example, in movement, a strictly anatomical definition of "a fascia" is not always helpful. Such an overly narrow definition may lead towards the exclusion of important tissues, including the interconnections of fascial tissues with joint capsules, aponeuroses, tendons, ligaments, and intramuscular connective tissues (Schleip et al. 2012b). If the purpose of the investigation is to illuminate functional aspects such as force transmission or sensory capacities and wound regulation, then a wider definition of fascia tends to be more helpful (Stecco C. 2015a).

French plastic and hand surgeon Dr Jean-Claude Guimberteau is known for his work documenting living fascia using an endoscope (*in vivo* during surgery). This reveals the surprising complexity of fascial layers that "slide" on each other in a fractal, chaotic manner, accommodating the need for movement and at the same time, the need for maintaining connection. Fascia appears, in his images, as hydrated, frothy fibrils engaged in a dance, forming micro-vacuoles that change shape with movement. This evidence of dynamic movement is in stark contrast to previous descriptions of fascia in cadavers, where the fascia looks like dry fuzz. In his definitive book, *Architecture of Human Living Fascia: The Extracellular Matrix and Cells Revealed Through Endoscopy*, Dr Guimberteau offers a definition more functional in scope: "Fascia is the tensional, continuous fibrillar network within the body, extending from the surface of the skin to the nucleus of the cell. This global network is mobile, adaptable, fractal, and irregular – it constitutes the basic structural architecture of the human body." For Guimberteau, fascia is far more than simple connective tissue. Rather, it is our constitutive tissue (Guimberteau 2015).

Fascial anatomy

Fascia comes in different forms:

- irregular connective tissue found in loose areolar tissue or adipose connective tissue

- regular connective tissue (fibers that orient regularly in response to stresses), commonly found in fascial sheets, aponeuroses, ligaments, and tendons.

Note that some structures in the body have a blend of both regular and irregular connective tissue, such as the linea alba: the posterior third is regularly oriented and the anterior two-thirds of fibers are irregular (Axer et al. 2001a, 2001b).

Myofascia may be defined as a combination of muscle tissue (myo) and its accompanying web of connective tissue (fascia). Although fascia has its own unique characteristics and properties, it functions synergistically with muscle as part of a neuro-musculo-fascial-skeletal system. Thus muscle and fascia are integrated synergistic units and cannot be separated functionally (Myers 2014).

Fascial continuity

The concept that muscles have clear origins and insertions has become outdated in the wake of current research that has shown that there is continuity of fascia throughout the human body tissues. Some have suggested that the separations between muscle/tendon and ligaments were introduced by dissectors themselves, faced with the difficult task of telling where the tissue stops being a tendon and starts being a ligamentous sleeve (Van der Wal 2009). Traditionally, ligaments were seen as being arranged parallel to the muscles, and only really coming into play when fully stretched at the end of joint range. However, research by Jaap Van der Wal, done 30 years ago but disregarded because it did not conform to traditional thought at the time, has put that concept into question. Van der Wal's careful observation of fascial continuities has concluded that the muscles and ligaments are actually arranged in series that reinforce each other. He named this common arrangement a dynament. In other words, muscle contractions, which tense the muscle and its myofasciae (epimysium, perimysium, endomysium, and tendon), also tense associated ligaments; ligaments are activated as well because they are part of this same series of fascia contracted by the muscle, not a separate underlying layer, as we have been taught to believe. Consequently, ligaments, far from being active only at the moment of the greatest elbow extension in a preacher curl, for example, are dynamically active in stabilizing the joint all through the movement, during both concentric and eccentric contraction. These findings redefine our whole concept of functional units within the body (Myers 2011).

Van der Wal was one of the first to use "fascia sparing" techniques in the dissection of cadavers and a number of other researchers have followed suit: Tom Myers of *Anatomy Trains*, Gil Headly, Robert Schleip, and Carla Stecco, to name a few. Thanks to new research and dissection methods, new information about fascial anatomy is being revealed and is slowly filtering down to practitioners. The impact of fascia on the motor control system and its neurophysiological implications cannot be overlooked as we consider the overall function of the patient. It becomes progressively clear that fascia must be viewed as a whole system, leading to different treatment and training strategies.

Musculoskeletal fascia

In the musculoskeletal system, fascia is formed by three fundamental structures: the superficial fascia, the deep fascia, and the epimysium (Stecco L. 2004).

Superficial fascia is composed of subcutaneous loose connective tissue containing a web of collagen, as well as mostly elastic fibers. It blends with the deep fascia at the retinacula of the wrist and ankle and continues with the galea aponeurotica over the scalp. This fascia facilitates the gliding of the skin above the deep fascia and contains fat, cutaneous vessels, and nerves (Stecco L. 2004).

Deep fascia is formed by a connective membrane that sheaths and separates all muscles. It also forms sheaths for the nerves and vessels, envelops various organs and glands and, around the joints, assumes the specialized form of ligaments (Stecco L. 2004).

The ***epimysium*** comprises the fascia that encloses the muscle belly itself and is continuous with the tendons.

The tendons then connect with the periosteum, which envelops the bone. In this context, bone itself may be seen as very dense connective tissue. As Schultz and Feitis explain in their book *The Endless Web*, "muscle does not simply attach to bone. Rather, muscle cells float in a fascial net, their movement pulls on the myofascia, the myofascia blends into the periosteal fascia, and the periosteum pulls on the bone" (Schultz & Feitis 1996).

The concept of fascial continuity also applies on a microscopic level (Figure 1.1). If we look at the muscle itself, deep to the epimysium, the perimysium is a fascia that groups individual muscle fibers into bundles or fascicles. Finally, at the cellular level, the endomysium wraps individual muscle cells and fibrils. This has implications for one of the main roles of fascia – its mechanotransduction function (see roles of fascia below).

Fascia as a mediator between the systems

Fascia is not limited to the musculoskeletal system. It is also present in the fascial envelope layers of the *organs* and in the perineural sheets of the *nervous system*

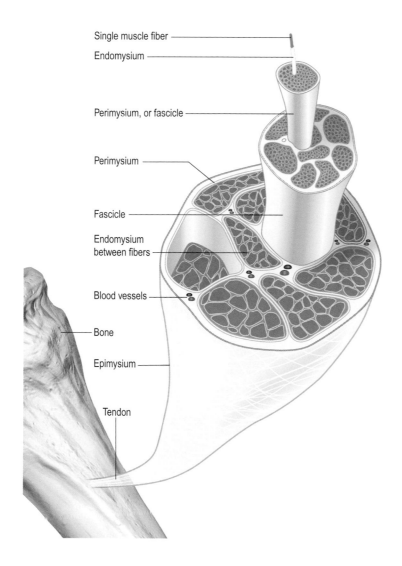

Single muscle fiber

Endomysium

Perimysium, or fascicle

Perimysium

Fascicle

Endomysium between fibers

Blood vessels

Bone

Epimysium

Tendon

Figure 1.1
Fascia of skeletal muscle

5

(Paoletti 2006). Improving mobility in one subsystem will affect mobility in other regions. In its role as a body-wide communication system, fascia serves as "mediator" between the various systems of the organism (Schwind 2006). This concept of a body-wide communication system has interesting implications for the health of the human body. The reader is directed to Scheip et al. (2012a) for further information on this topic.

Composition of fascia

Fascia is composed of cells and extracellular matrix made up of ground substance, collagen, water, and elastin (Paoletti 2006).

1. **Collagen** is the most common protein in body. It predominates in the fascial net and is readily seen in any dissection, or even any cut of meat (Myers 2014). There are around 20 types of collagen fibers and type 1 is by far the most ubiquitous, forming a variety of structures including:

   – transparent cornea of the eye
   – tendons, ligaments
   – lung tissue
   – membranes surrounding the brain.

2. **Fibroblasts** are the most common cell type in connective tissue. They produce the ground substance and precursors for all connective tissue fibers. They secrete enzymes involved in catabolism of macromolecules and play a central role in wound healing and inflammation. They are highly responsive to physical stimuli and are instrumental in constructing and maintaining the collagen matrix. Sustained tension or pressure on fascial tissue will induce local proliferation of fibroblasts and alignment of cells along lines of force due to tension or pressure. If stress is sustained for a long period, the fascia will become more dense (Paoletti 2006). Mechanically stressing fibroblasts leads to increased connective tissue synthesis and decreased production of inflammatory mediators.

3. **Elastin cells** are also common in connective tissue. The proportion of collagen and elastic fibers within any area of fascia depends upon the functional demands placed upon that tissue. Where there are strong tensile forces, the collagen portion predominates – there are fewer elastic fibers. Conversely, there are more elastic fibers where the shape of the segment of body changes repetitively. Due to this adaptive capacity, the fascial system is able to meet the changing functional requirements of the body.

4. **Ground substance** is a viscous transparent substance made up of hydrated proteins (proteoglycans, glycoproteins). It is produced by fibroblasts and mast cells. It is essentially a watery gel – a part of the environment of almost every living cell, the continuous but variable "glue" that holds cells together while allowing substances to be exchanged. It allows for easy distribution of metabolites when sufficiently hydrated and forms part of the immune system barrier, which increases the resistance to spreading of bacteria. In areas that are not moved, the ground substance increases viscosity (like gel) and becomes a repository for metabolites and toxins (Myers 2014).

   Ground substance is thixotropic, a property that enables it to become more liquid and less viscous. Thixotrophy (Juhan 1998) is attained by adding heat or energy to fascial tissue. One way to understand thixotrophy in action is to think of a bottle of ketchup that has been left in the cupboard for a while. Trying to dispense the ketchup in this case may be arduous, as it has become more viscous and less fluid-like with time. The common response is to then shake the bottle of ketchup in order to get it to pour more easily. Adding heat or energy makes the ketchup more liquid-like. Fascia reacts in a very similar way. Manual therapy that is focused on the fascia, as well as certain movement therapies, can help the fascia attain optimal consistency. Activating the thixotropic aspect of fascia facilitates movement and optimizes motor control.

5. **Myofibroblasts** (MFB) are cells found in fascia. They are intermediaries between smooth muscle cells (found in viscera, autonomic nerves) and

traditional fibroblasts (cells that function primarily to build and maintain the collagenous matrix). Fascia is thus able to contract in a smooth muscle-like manner and thereby influence musculoskeletal mechanics (Schleip et al. 2007). Myofibroblasts interpret mechanical signals and set up biochemical responses (concept of mechanotransduction). They are stimulated by either

– mechanical tension going through the tissues, or
– specific cytokines and other pharmacological agents such as nitric oxide (which relaxes MFBs) and histamine (which stimulates contraction of MFBs).

There is a higher density of MFBs in people with Dupuytren's or with past traumatic contractures. In contrast, there is a lower density of MFBs in people with Marfan's syndrome. Within "normal" there is a range of MFB density – the more you have, the stiffer you are (Myers 2014).

It is tempting to deduce that because fascia contains myofibroblasts, this proves that fascia, in and of itself, can "shorten" or "contract" sufficiently to cause significant postural distortion. However, we must remember that fascia and muscle function synergistically and that the myofibroblasts, containing smooth muscle fibers, do not generate near the pulling power of skeletal muscle fibers.

Fascia innervation

The fascial network is one of our richest sensory organs. Fascia is innervated; therefore, it can also be an important pain generator. As such, the contribution of fascia to painful syndromes cannot be underestimated.

Mechanoreceptors

Fascia is densely innervated by mechanoreceptors (Golgi end organs, Pacini corpuscles, Ruffini endings, free nerve endings), which are responsive to manual pressure (Table 1.1).

Schleip (2003) states:

In myofascial manipulation an immediate tissue release is often felt under the working hand. This amazing feature has traditionally been attributed to

mechanical properties of the connective tissue. Yet studies have shown that either much stronger forces or longer durations would be required for a permanent viscoelastic deformation of fascia. A change in attitude in myofascial practitioners from a mechanical perspective toward an inclusion of the self-regulatory dynamics of the nervous system is suggested. (Schleip 2003)

Nociceptors

Fascia contains many nociceptors, mostly A and C fiber nociceptors, which may explain descriptions of fascia pain as "throbbing, stinging and hot." A myriad of tiny unmyelinated free nerve endings are found almost everywhere in fascial tissues, but particularly in periosteum, in endomysial and perimysial layers, and in visceral connective tissues (Mense 2007; Tesarz et al. 2011). Human data indicate that the fascia is more sensitive to pain than either the skin or the muscles (Gibson 2009; Deising et al. 2012).

Proprioceptors

Deep fascia also seems to have a proprioceptive function and so may affect motor control. It is hypothesized that myofascial expansions could guarantee motor coordination among different segments of the body, giving anatomical support to myokinetic chains (Stecco C. 2015a).

Sympathetic fibers

Fascia and the autonomic nervous system appear to be intimately connected. Stimulation of mechanoreceptors leads to a lowering of sympathetic tonus as well as a change in local tissue viscosity. Studies of the anatomy of the thoracolumbar fascia reveal a close relationship between the sympathetic nervous system and the pathophysiology of fascial disorders. Forty percent of thoracolumbar fascia innervation consists of sympathetic fibers, known to have vasoconstrictor effect on blood vessels, which may then lead to ischemia in fascia. This may help explain the phenomenon of increased intensity of pain with psychological stress, which increases activation of the sympathetic nervous system (Willard et al. 2012).

Summary of innervation

Robert Schleip sums up the issue of fascial innervation nicely: "For the sensorial relationship with our own body –

Table 1.1 Mechanoreceptors in fascia.

Reproduced from R. Schleip (2003), Fascial plasticity – a new neurological explanation: Part 1. *Journal of Bodywork and Movement Therapies*. With kind permission from Elsevier.

Receptor type	Preferred location	Responsive to	Known results of stimulation
Golgi Type Ib	Myotendinous junctions Attachment areas of aponeuroses Ligaments of peripheral joints Joint capsules	Golgi tendon organ: To muscular contraction Other Golgi receptors: Probably to strong stretch only	Tonus decrease in related striated motor fibers
Pacini and Paciniform Type II	Myotendinous junctions Deep capsular layers Spinalligaments Investing muscular tissues	Rapid pressure changes and vibrations	Use of proprioceptive feedback for movement control (Sense of kinesthesia)
Ruffini Type II	Ligaments of peripheral joints Dura mater Outer capsular layers Other tissues associated with regular stretching	Like Pacini, yet also to sustained pressure Specially responsive to tangential forces (lateral stretch)	Inhibition of sympathetic activity
Interstitial Type III and IV	Most abundant receptor type. Found almost everywhere, even inside bones. Highest density in periosteum	Rapid as well as sustained pressure changes 50% are high threshold units, and 50% are low threshold units	Changes in vasodilation plus apparently in plasma extravasation

whether it consists of pure proprioception, nociception or the more visceral interoception – fascia provides definitely our most important perceptual organ" (Schleip 2012).

Roles of fascia

Fascia plays several roles in the body:

- maintaining **structural integrity** (Paoletti 2006)
- maintaining **static postural support** (Paoletti 2006)
- **protecting against physical trauma** (think how abdominal fascia are protective to the underlying organs) (Myers 2014)
- functioning as **shock absorber** (Paoletti 2006) and in the **transmission of force** which then has effects on dynamic stability (Huijing & Baan 2003, 2012)
- creating a uniformly smooth/slick surface that essentially lubricates the various tissues that come in contact

with each other during movement. This helps prevent friction injuries and subsequent tissue degeneration and degradation

- allowing muscles to change shape as they are both stretched and shortened

- one of the most important roles of fascia is its **mechanotransduction function**. It transforms mechanical signals into biochemical responses; in other words, turning movement into repair.

According to traditional concepts, cells float next to the extracellular matrix and function autonomously (Figure 1.2A). A more current view, proposed by Oschman, instead posits that the nuclear material, nuclear membrane, and cytoskeleton are mechanically linked via the integrines and laminar proteins to the surrounding extracellular matrix (ECM) (Figure 1.2B) (Oschman 2000; Myers 2014).

Integrins are mechanoreceptors that communicate tension and compression from the cell's surroundings, specifically from the fiber matrix into the cell's interior, even down to the nucleus. These connections act to alter the shape of the cells and their physiological properties. This is the mechanism behind the concept of mechanotransduction, which is the ability of cells to perceive and biochemically interpret mechanical forces generated either within the cytoskeleton or from external sources. The effect of mechanical forces on cell shape is emerging as a key regulatory mechanism at the cellular, tissue, and organ levels. In place of the traditional concepts of fascia as a passive tension transmitter, a new picture is emerging: one of fascia as a dynamically adaptable organ, an important tissue in cell regulation, and a global body-wide communication system:

- Fascia is the "container" through which metabolic, endocrine, and immune exchanges take place in all tissues. It is the conduit through which water, proteins, and immune cells return to the blood via lymphatics. Its role in intercellular communication and cellular exchange processes helps explain how fascia is a major player in the body's **defense and immune system function** (Paoletti 2006).

- Its role in the regulation of the inflammatory response also has implications for cardiac pathologies

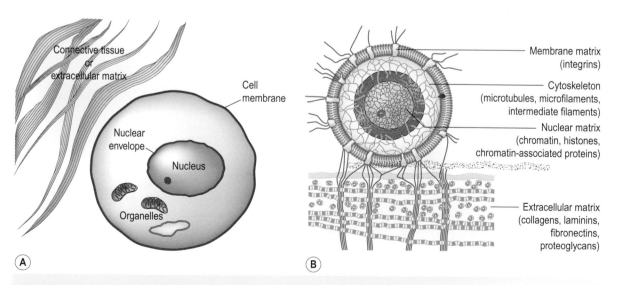

Connective tissue or extracellular matrix

Cell membrane

Nuclear envelope

Nucleus

Organelles

Membrane matrix (integrins)

Cytoskeleton (microtubules, microfilaments, intermediate filaments)

Nuclear matrix (chromatin, histones, chromatin-associated proteins)

Extracellular matrix (collagens, laminins, fibronectins, proteoglycans)

(A)   (B)

Figure 1.2
Reproduced from Tom Myers (2014), *Anatomy Trains: Myofascial Meridians for Manual and Movement Therapists*, 3rd edition. With kind permission from Elsevier

and cancer. Mechanical information combines with chemical signals to tell the cell and cytoskeleton what to do. Very flat cells, with their cytoskeletons over-stretched, sense that more cells are needed to cover the surrounding substrate (as in wound repair) and that cell division is necessary. Alternatively, rounding and pressure indicates that too many cells are competing for space on the matrix and that cells are proliferating too much; some must die to prevent tumor formation. Between those two extremes, normal tissue function is established and maintained. Understanding how this switching occurs could lead to new approaches in cancer therapy (Myers 2014).

How genes in our DNA are expressed as traits within a cell is a complicated mystery with many players, the main suspects being chemical. Each cell in the body has the same DNA, but tissues behave very differently because genes are expressed differently. Cells only have two "senses" with which to interact with their environment. They cannot see or hear, but they can "feel" mechanical forces and "taste" chemical signals. Many studies have detailed chemical signaling pathways, but understanding how the mechanical forces affect the cell is also important. A study by Tajik et al. in 2016 has demonstrated that external mechanical force can directly regulate gene expression. The study also identified the pathway that conveys the force from the outside of the cell into the nucleus, through the fascia (Tajik et al. 2016).

Hélène Langevin and Thomas Findley, in their paper entitled *Connecting Tissues: How Research in Fascia Biology can Impact Integrative Oncology*, state the following:

Recent advances in cancer biology are underscoring the importance of connective tissue in the local tumor environment. Inflammation and fibrosis are well-recognized contributors to cancer, and connective tissue stiffness is emerging as a driving factor in tumor growth. In that sense, cancer can be considered a disease of the collagen. Physical-based therapies have been shown to reduce connective tissue inflammation and fibrosis and thus may have direct beneficial effects on cancer spreading and metastasis. Meanwhile, there is currently little knowledge on potential risks of applying mechanical forces in the vicinity of tumors. Thus, both basic and clinical research is needed to understand the full impact of integrative oncology on cancer biology as well as whole person health. (Langevin et al. 2016)

In summary, the various roles that fascia plays in the human body all point to its importance in maintaining a healthy interstitial fluid environment, metabolic homeostasis, and immune surveillance, all the while allowing the body to move. What a fascinating tissue!

Fascial pathology

There are a number of factors that contribute to fascial pathology. Any number of the following, either singly or in combination, can influence fascial function:

- **trauma**: past or present (falls, contact sports, blows). Inflammation is critical for normal healing processes. However, too much or prolonged inflammation can lead to binding down of fascia and fibrosis (Gautchi 2012)

- **micro-injuries** caused by overloading (over-training, heavy or repetitive jobs) (Gautchi 2012)

- **immobility**: long periods of bed rest or immobilization in a cast (Van den Berg 2007)

- **surgery** (scarring, adhesions): the scars themselves may heal well and have good mobility but their impact on fascial lines is underestimated

- mechanical stress as a result of **poor posture**

- long term systemic chronic tissue inflammation secondary to **diet** (see Chapter 15 for more information)

- **chemical insults**: toxins in the environment (for example, using oil-based paint in an enclosed room for a period of time) can affect the fascia as they may trigger the body's defense and immune system

- **endocrine effects**: patients with diabetes are known to exhibit slow healing responses to injury. It is thought that the changes in the endocrine system may impact the fascia in particular

- **emotional stress**: stress, whether mental, physical, emotional, or spiritual, creates inflammatory chemicals in the brain and body and leads to cellular degeneration. This process may occur in the brain and manifest as memory deterioration. It may also occur in the fascia, where we store all of our traumas, whether physical, mental, or spiritual. These traumas create thickened, dense fascia, which eventually leads to pain and limited range of motion (Northrup 2016).

Whatever the source, these insults may induce biochemical changes in the connective tissue which will, in turn, have effects on its viscoelastic properties. It is proposed that fascial tissue injury causes localized ischemia which leads to localized hypoxia. Cytokines (inflammatory mediators such as bradykinin, substance P, and calcitonin gene-related peptide (CGRP)) are released as well as growth factors and clotting factors. Subsequent oxygen deprivation promotes adhesions of connective tissue (Shah et al. 2005, 2008).

Injury may cause bracing or splinting of the area in question, providing mechanical tension. This reaction stimulates the transition from fibroblast to myofibroblast and helps maintain fascial tension around the injured area. Initially, this process is adaptive but may become maladaptive if sustained.

Ultimately, collagen microfibers form in between adjacent layers of fascia to bind them together. This binding of fascial elements is also called "fibrosis," "adhesion formation," or "scar tissue." Chaitow and Delany, in their book *Clinical Applications of Neuromuscular Techniques*, state "This adhesion formation disrupts the normal 'sliding and gliding' of the tissues. As the fascia thickens, it can disrupt motor patterns, balance and proprioception. This can lead to chronic tissue loading, further injury, and global soft tissue holding patterns" (Chaitow & Delany 2000).

Effects of fibrosis

Fibrosis does not automatically dissipate after the area has healed, and it tends to accumulate over time. Like the cross-links on a net, the more adhesions there are, the stronger the net will be, but the less elastic as well (Schierling 2017). Restricted movement leads to loss of ground substance in connective tissue, loss of lubricating

effect, binding of fascial elements, both microscopic and macroscopic. Nutrition and blood supply to the region are impaired, which in turn promotes the development of fibrotic nodules and myofascial trigger points. Ultimately, joints may become restricted and muscles weak through full range of motion. Such changes may produce changes in self-image/body language and in some cases, bony structural changes.

In addition, as the Steccos stipulate, a stiffer fascia may reduce the contractility of a muscle and cause a chronic compartment syndrome (Stecco C. 2015b).

Connective tissue responds to demand

Both extremes of lifestyle – continuous exertion or "couch potato" – will have an important effect on fascia. Habitual postures will load lines of fascia so that instead of random "spaghetti tubes" that are filled with proteoglycans and fluid, they become "committed" and create vectors that may pull and tug at joints, muscles, organs, or nerves – in fact, any tissue that is surrounded by fascia.

Extracellular elements are altered to meet the demands within the limits imposed by nutrition, age, and protein synthesis. While it is true that in old age, the proportion of elastic fibers decreases and tough collagen fibers predominate, we must keep in mind that the body continuously renews itself in response to how we feed the tissues (hence the importance of good nutrition and hydration) as well as the movement demands we make on the body. My 90-year-old mother, who has always maintained a healthy diet and regularly walks and attends aqua-fitness classes, has had minimal health issues, including those of the musculoskeletal system. Her fascial tissues feel fluid and adaptable. In contrast, I have had some middle-aged patients who do not eat well, hydrate well, or move well and, in these patients, the fascial tissues feel dense and stiff, similar to old dried-up leather. One might argue that perhaps genetics play a role and that some people have familial characteristics of denser fascial tissues. There is some truth to this statement. However, there are factors to consider (see Chapters 14 and 15) that can have positive impacts on the health and function of fascia.

Fascial hydration

Research is pointing to the importance of fascial hydration (Klinger et al. 2004; Reed et al. 2010). The human body is composed of 75 percent water, two-thirds of which is contained in the fascia. It is therefore important to maintain adequate hydration of these tissues for optimal function. It is equally important to move to ensure that water gets into various parts of the fascia. Variability of movement is key here, preferably in patterns differing from usual habits (Myers 2017). Chapter 14 outlines the various movement therapies and exercises that can help maintain optimal health of fascial tissues.

Factors affecting hydration include not only mechanical influences but also pH values, body temperature, and bioactive proteins (notably hormones and growth factors TFGF-β1). In the body, pH levels are regulated by the renal and respiratory systems. An acidic pH in the matrix tends to increase contractility of myofibroblasts, so lends itself to tighter fascia. Activities that produce pH changes such as breathing pattern disorders, emotional distress, or acid-producing foods could induce a general stiffening in the fascial body (Pipelzadeh & Naylor 1998). This impact of pH levels on fascia may explain the recent recommendations (not, as yet, backed by evidence) regarding the effect of an anti-inflammatory alkaline diet for optimal function of the connective tissue matrix.

Fascia as a tensegrity system

Another major concept in fascial anatomy is that of the body as a tensegrity system. This is a system in which compression and tension are dynamically balanced. Looking at Figure 1.3, we may consider the solid elements of the tensegrity array (double lines) represented by the bony architecture of the body, with the elastic element between (single lines) representing the fascia.

When tension or compression is applied to an area in the tensegrity system, there is reaction in the rest of the system. The strain is distributed over the whole structure and not localized in the area being deformed. Therefore, an increase in tension of a tensegrity structure resonates throughout the whole structure, even affecting the opposite side (see the second drawing in Figure 1.3) (Ingber 2003).

As a result, a pull or a push on one corner of the connective tissue framework exerts a force throughout the entire structure, affecting muscles, bone, nerve, blood vessels, glands, and organs (Juhan 1998).

New discoveries highlight how tensional patterns within the fascial matrix communicate instantly and effortlessly what happens throughout the whole system. In his iconic paper, Ingber sums up the process of cellular mechanotransduction: "Very simply, transmission of tension through a tensegrity array provides a means to distribute forces to all interconnected elements, and, at the same time to couple or 'tune' the whole system mechanically as one" (Ingber 2003).

An injury at any given site can be set in motion by long-term strains in other parts of the body. Small kinks in myofascial force transmission such as those provided by scars or adhesions have surprising functional consequences, often at some distance from the site.

Chain reactions in the body

All injuries do not necessarily induce a change in the tensegrity system that may produce a chain reaction. Sometimes a reaction will appear soon after the original trauma; other times, it can take weeks or months. This variation in outcome depends on multiple factors, including:

- the seriousness of the original injury
- the age of the patient
- the capacity of the patient to adapt and compensate.

A lesional chain can start in any part of the body and, from there, spread either up or down (Paoletti 2006). Paoletti cites varied examples of possible chain reactions:

Descending chain reactions

- Epicranial fascia → superficial cervical fascia → scapular girdle → upper thorax→ upper limb.
- Psoas → perineum → short muscles of hip → knee or ankle.

In the first example, the patient may complain of pain in an upper limb, but may get only partial relief with only

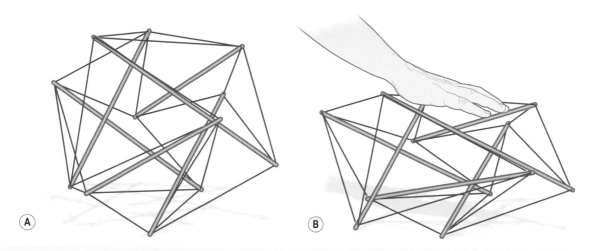

Figure 1.3
Fascia as a tensegrity system

localized treatment to the upper extremity if the fascial chain to the epicranium is not addressed.

Ascending chain reactions

- Ankle sprain → head of fibula → lateral knee → hip/piriformis → sacroiliac joint (SIJ) → thoracolumbar fascia → latissimus dorsi → shoulder → cervical vertebrae → cranium.
- Fall on coccyx → dura mater → intracranial membranes.
- Bladder → round ligament → diaphragm → pericardium → throat symptoms.

In the second example of an ascending reaction, a fall on the coccyx may incur head pain that could persist until mobility of the dura is restored (Paoletti 2006).

Trigger points as a fascia-related disorder

How can we differentiate symptoms arising from increased neural drive vs fascial tension? Are they related to one another and if so, how?

One way to differentiate between these two disorders is via palpation. Palpation of a hypertonic muscle or trigger point frequently feels like "pepperoni stick in the middle of a salami." On the other hand, palpation of a tight fascial line often feels like a "guitar string" that has too much tension (Diane Lee, personal communication).

Symptoms of trigger points may include pain (both local and referred), reflex muscle weakness (caused by pain without atrophy), autonomic and trophic disorders, restricted movement and perfusion disorders (formation of edema). This process may lead to neuromuscular entrapment and/or changes in proprioception; therefore affecting motor output (Gautchi 2012).

Muscle release techniques that work exclusively on the reflexes (e.g., dry needling, Gunn intramuscular stimulation (IMS), positional counterstrain, shockwave therapy) are very effective for treating trigger points. If, however, these trigger points tend to recur despite attempts to normalize muscle balance, control, and strategy, then we must consider another influencing factor – fascia. Gautchi states that muscular pathology in the form of myofascial trigger points (mTrPs) always has a fascial component and can be the cause of fascia dysfunction. Conversely, dysfunctional fascia can provoke or maintain dysfunctions of the muscles (mTrPs) (Figure 1.4)

Because of this interaction, an optimal treatment approach must include consideration of both trigger points *and* fascia. Muscle release techniques that work exclusively on the reflexes

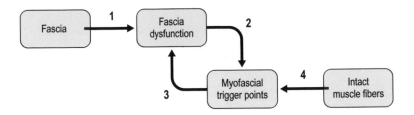

Figure 1.4
Interrelation between fascia dysfunction and myofascial trigger points. 1. Factors which lead to fascia dysfunction.
2. Fascia dysfunction as possible cause of the origin/maintenance of mTrPs. 3. mTrPs as possible cause of the origin/
maintenance of fascia dysfunction. 4. Factors which lead to the origin of mTrPs. Reproduced from R. U. Gautchi, in
R. Schleip et al. (eds) (2012), *Fascia: The Tensional Network of the Human Body* (Chapter 5.7). With kind permission from Elsevier

may indirectly decrease fascial pull. However, these techniques insufficiently affect the fascial aspect. Targeting the connective tissues using manual techniques is necessary in order to address the changed fascial structures (Gautchi 2012).

A historical review of fascial approaches to treatment

The concept of fascia as a contributor to musculoskeletal dysfunction is not a novel idea, nor confined to one country. Several approaches to treatment of the fascial system have emerged over the last century.

Connective tissue massage (Elizabeth Dicke – Germany)

One of the first professionals to consider fascia was a German physiotherapist, Elizabeth Dicke, who in the 1930s developed a technique called connective tissue massage (CTM). This approach to treatment was developed in response to her own frustrations with the system at the time, as she struggled to manage symptoms from a widespread infection of her blood vessels that affected circulation to her right leg and contributed to the development of gangrene. She had also developed angina and gastric, kidney, and liver problems. Too ill for surgery, she was effectively left in a side ward to die. She spent months in bed, studying the anatomy of the autonomic nervous system. Based on her experience and analysis, Dicke developed a

type of massage treatment for the connective tissue that aimed to de-facilitate the autonomic system. Within four months of beginning treatment by a colleague who applied Dicke's own techniques, Dicke was out of hospital and she returned to work within a year. She had normal circulation in her leg and her back pain, angina, kidney and liver problems had all resolved. Dicke and her colleagues then spent the next 10 years investigating this new technique, with the aim of understanding its underlying mechanisms and identifying conditions for which it was effective. They set up a teaching protocol for all physiotherapy students in Germany and incorporated into it the work of J. MacKenzie, who researched changes in muscle tone in relationship to organs. In 1942, Dicke, Kohlrausch, Leube, and MacKenzie published *Massage of Reflex Zones in the Connective Tissue in the Presence of Rheumatic and Internal Diseases*. Many general hospitals and orthopedic hospitals, physical therapists and health spas in Switzerland, Italy, and Germany continue to research and practice CTM (Utting 2013).

My first exposure to this treatment approach was in relation to a case of an elderly lady in a rehabilitation center who, for two years, had not responded to a variety of treatments to deal with an ulcer in her foot. After a 10-session approach with CTM, the wound finally closed. The result propelled me to take a course in CTM (my first postgraduate course). I found this approach to be occasionally useful for my orthopedic clientele at the time.

Rolfing/Structural Integration (Ida Rolf – USA)

Rolfing/Structural Integration was developed by Ida P. Rolf in the 1940s and 1950s. A biochemist and atomic physicist, Rolf sought to experiment with treatments as a result of her own frustrations with the various approaches available at that time to treat her pain (osteopathy, yoga, Alexander technique, Feldenkrais technique). Initially coined Postural Release, her 10-sessions program of myofascial manipulation was developed to help restructure the body. The aim was to improve the body's relationship to gravity, postural integration, and re-educating movement. Her techniques for manipulating the fascia were slow and deep and followed a certain structure or recipe. Initially, this approach was known as Rolfing. Other bodyworkers trained by Ida Rolf soon developed their own interpretation of her approach. For example, Joseph Heller developed *Hellerwork*, Tom Myers developed *Anatomy Trains Structural Integration (ATSI)*, and George Kousaleos developed *CORE*. Ida Rolf was never comfortable with the term Rolfing and in 1990 the approach was renamed Structural Integration. Although it is a type of massage technique, its origins are not in massage therapy.

In 2006, another branch of Structural Integration was developed by BetsyAnn Baron, a massage therapist and structural integrator, with whom I teach Mobilization of the Myofascial System to physiotherapists. Called *Structural Myofascial Therapy (SMFT)*, Baron's technique is less "recipe" than structural integration sessions work (Baron Bodyworks.ca).

SMFT has two key elements:

- postural somatic awareness (PSA), a method of subjective evaluation
- deep, hands-on techniques in the myofascial system.

Osteopathy (USA)

More than 100 years ago, Andrew Taylor Still, MD, founded osteopathic medicine. He was one of the first to describe fascia and he recognized its role in assisting gliding of tissues and fluid flow. Even at that time he realized the link between fascia and the nourishment of all cells of the body, including those of disease and cancer (Findley & Shalwala 2013). Present-day osteopaths use a number of approaches to address imbalances in the body from a whole body perspective, including cranial techniques, visceral manipulation, osteopathic articular techniques, and finally, soft tissue manipulation, which includes fascial techniques to balance the length and tension of the fascia.

Myofascial Release (John Barnes – USA)

Myofascial Release (MFR) is a form of manual therapy that was developed by John F. Barnes, PT. It involves the application of a low load, long duration stretch to the myofascial complex, intended to restore optimal length, decrease pain, and improve function. There is anecdotal evidence that MFR has positive effects as a treatment for various conditions. The approach tends to be localized to a particular area of the body (for example, the diaphragm), but it also encompasses techniques that have some similarities with Structural Integration. What differentiates this approach from MMS (Mobilization of the Myofascial System) is that MFR does not follow the principles of assessment and treatment of the fascial lines as described by Tom Myers in his book *Anatomy Trains*.

Fasciathérapie (Danis Bois – France)

Fasciathérapie is a somatic approach that evolved from Dr Danis Bois's osteopathy and physiotherapy practices in France. With osteopathy, Bois felt he was looking after an organism but that his practice did not address the whole somato-psychic person. He therefore developed another approach, which he called Fasciathérapie. This is a gentle, non-manipulative manual therapy that aims to heighten awareness of the client's relationship to pain, tension, stress, and habitual thought patterns. By using this somatosensory approach, the therapist "dialogues with the body" in order to promote its self-regulating force. In addition to Fasciathérapie, he incorporates a somatic movement practice, called Sensorial Re-education, a meditation practice, called Sensorial Introspection, and a verbal or expressive component that accompanies all of the above (Bois 2013).

This approach is primarily used in western Europe. "Fasciathérapeutes" distinguish themselves from physiotherapists, osteopaths, and "kinésithérapeutes."

Fascial Manipulation (Stecco family – Italy)

The founders of this technique are the Stecco family based in Italy, comprising Luigi Stecco, a physiotherapist, and his children, Carla Stecco, an orthopedic surgeon, and Antonio Stecco, a physiatrist. They are well known for their fascial dissections and their research in this field. The Fascial Manipulation method is based on the concept of myofascial units united in myofascial sequences and involves deep manual friction over specific points (called centers of coordination and centers of fusion) that are located on the deep muscular fascia and retinacula. Although this approach focuses primarily on the fascia around the muscular system, more recently, visceral fascia has been included.

Mobilization of the Myofascial System (Doreen Killens – Canada)

This concept was initially developed by the author and another Canadian physiotherapist, Laurie McLaughlin, both former instructors and chief examiners for the orthopedic division of the Canadian Physiotherapy Association.

Manual therapy in Canada is based on a wide variety of joint mobilization and manipulation approaches taught in the UK (James Cyriax), Norway (Kaltenborn), and Australia (Maitland). As per IFOMPT (International Federation of Manipulative Physical Therapists) standards, the system has evolved to include motor control and muscle imbalance as well as the pain sciences. In addition to this manual therapy background, I have had the opportunity to amass many tools from postgraduate courses taken over the years, such as the Sahrmann approach, Kinetic Control, NOI (Neuro Orthopaedic Institute) courses, craniosacral techniques, Barral Visceral Manipulation, etc. Despite all the tools at my disposal, I too have experienced times of clinical frustration. These moments arose particularly in situations when I was fairly sure that I had a case of primary nociceptive pain on my hands. However, no matter what I tried from my toolkit, it did not bring about the positive effect I was seeking. I also experienced situations in which clients were complaining of multiple areas of pain that did not correspond or fit into the paradigms that physiotherapists had learned, even as fully trained manual therapists. These clinical frustrations led Laurie and myself to explore the role of fascia across multiple musculoskeletal conditions.

Laurie teaches her approach to treatment, which is called Manual Therapy for the Fascia (ProActive Education, Laurie McLaughlin.ca).

The technique that I have developed, called Mobilization of the Myofascial System (MMS), is the one I teach to physiotherapists in Canada and Europe. It is an approach that has its origins in manual therapy for the articular, muscular, and neural systems. This focus on fascia in relation to multiple systems of the body sets it apart from other books written on the myofascia, primarily by structural integrators, who describe techniques for manipulating the fascia around the muscular system. The techniques employed in MMS are the techniques that will be described in this book.

This approach to treatment has brought a deeper level of understanding to seemingly complex cases. Now when I see a chronic injury I ask not only what happened to create the injury but more importantly, why is it not clearing up? When local treatment to the area is insufficient, I question two things:

1. Am I treating a secondary problem and I have not found the driver in the Integrated Systems Model (developed by Diane Lee and Linda-Joy Lee) (www.learnwithdianelee.ca,www.ljlee.ca)?

2. Is this recurrent dysfunction (whether it is articular, muscular, neural, or visceral) connected to something else within fascial system that is maintaining the dysfunction?

The concept of myofascial continuities has become a framework for understanding not only static postural support but dynamic and optimal movement. Knowledge of fascial connections helps us understand how to direct our approach to the source of the problem (the criminal) and not merely to the painful tissue (the victim). I wish to clarify, however, that I am not a "fascia-therapist." I am a physiotherapist with several tools in my toolbox, one of which is the Mobilization of the Myofascial System (MMS). The MMS approach is fully described in Chapters 3 and 4.

Movement re-education approaches

There are a number of movement re-education approaches that encompass the concepts of neuromodulation with functional pattern re-education while at the same time providing valuable input into the fascial system. These include proprioceptive neuromuscular facilitation (PNF) (Knott and Voss), Alexander technique, Feldenkrais and yoga therapy. Chapter 15 will summarize these approaches to treatment as well as exercises to help maintain optimal fascial health.

Where does Mobilization of the Myofascial System (MMS) fit into our paradigms as manual physiotherapists?

As musculoskeletal manual therapists, we are trained to put the patient's subjective complaints in the center of our puzzle, so to speak (Figure 1.5). This approach includes consideration of not only subjective complaints of pain, paresthesia, weakness and so on but also the patient's beliefs about and attitudes toward their experience. Specific functional difficulties are also noted. A good comprehensive subjective exam allows us to choose assessment techniques that guide us to an analysis – that is, a hypothesis as to which factors may be contributing to our client's signs and symptoms.

If our analysis points to a problem that is primarily pain of central origin, then this must be addressed with appropriate education and brain remapping along the lines of *Explain Pain* concepts (Butler & Mosely 2013). If the analysis of the patient points to a problem with heightened sympathetic nervous system (SNS) response, then this must be addressed with techniques to dampen down the SNS, such as breathing techniques and meditation. When dealing with primary nociceptive pain, it is appropriate to consider mechanical pain. Most

physiotherapists consider the contribution of joint dysfunction as well as motor control and stability issues when assessing their clients. Education is also very important, so that the client has tools to self-manage his/her condition and not repeat poor patterns when doing functional activities, such as sitting or bending forward to brush their teeth. However, the missing link in this puzzle is frequently the role of fascia, especially in those with chronic, recurring conditions.

The **Integrated Systems Model** (Lee & Lee 2011), developed by Diane Lee and Linda-Joy Lee, considers the role that underlying system impairments in the articular, neural, visceral, and myofascial systems play in a patient's clinical presentation. The clinical puzzle shown is a reflection tool for charting findings (Figure 1.6). It represents the various vectors that may impact a functional task and directs the therapist to treat those vectors (be it articular, neural, visceral or myofascial).

Their category of myofascial impairment pertains to fascial structures that are overstretched, such as in diastasis rectus abdominis (DRA) or fascia that has become dense, tethered, and resistant to elongation during movement.

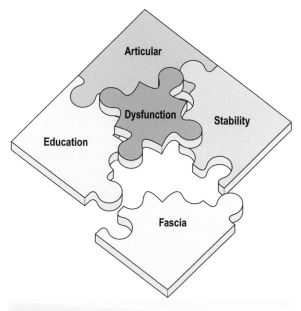

Figure 1.5
The clinical puzzle

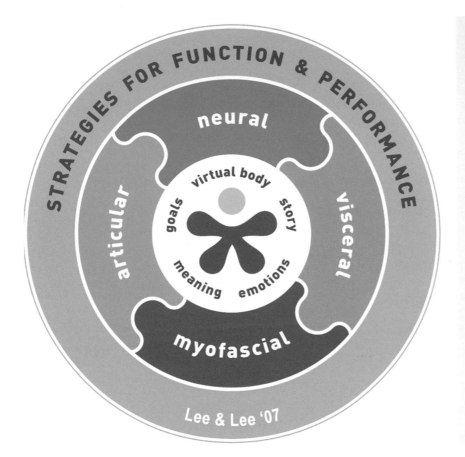

Figure 1.6
Clinical puzzle for the Integrated Systems Model. Reproduced from Lee & Lee (2011), *The Pelvic Girdle: An Integration of Clinical Expertise and Research*, 4th edition. With kind permission from Elsevier

Skilled manual therapists will have multiple tools/techniques to treat all systems; one is not more important than another. MMS is a wonderful tool but it should not be the only one in a manual therapist's toolbox. Even with the same client, what may be appropriate to use at the beginning of treatment may not be so appropriate in later stages. It is important, therefore, to alternate between assessment and treatment and to re-assess the "comparable signs" to determine which tool is best for that client at that particular time. The optimal therapeutic approach is first to test, then to use clinical reasoning to decide which treatment to use (based on the therapist's assessment findings), and re-test to see if there has been a change in the objective signs, including movement patterns. If there is no change, then the therapist should try another approach (another plausible hypothesis, based on clinical findings).

Summary

This chapter is meant to introduce the reader to fascia – its definition, anatomy, composition, and innervation. The various roles that fascia plays in the body have been outlined, as well as the pathophysiology of fascial dysfunctions. Finally, the chapter includes a historical view of the various approaches to treatment that have been developed throughout the world thus far. The next chapter reviews the fascial lines as described by Tom Myers, author of *Anatomy Trains*. Many of the techniques in MMS are developed from these concepts.

A brief summary of Tom Myers's Anatomy Trains fascial lines and clinical implications

Tom Myers, a structural integrator and self-styled "cartographer" of the body, wrote the first edition of his book *Anatomy Trains* in 2001. There have since been two further editions, in which Myers has refined his work as he continues to explore fascial dissections and clinical applications. Drawing on Myers's studies with Ida Rolf and on his published dissections of cadavers, the book maps twelve myofascial meridians that wind through the body, connecting head to toe and core to periphery. Although Myers is not the only person to conceive the idea of myofascial continuities, his writing style and clear descriptions of the functionally integrated fascial webbing makes the concept easy to apply in the clinical situation, no matter what the background of the practitioner is. The beauty of the concept of Anatomy Trains is that it can be easily integrated into the practice of any professional engaged in human structure and movement, be they physiotherapist, chiropractor, osteopath, structural integrator, massage therapist, or yoga or Pilates teacher.

Anatomy Trains was a game changer for me. Despite being a fully trained manual physiotherapist I had had little exposure to the concept of myofascial continuities prior to reading this book in 2001. *Anatomy Trains* has since helped me to understand the multiple ways that muscles link and connect to transfer forces and support the body. Inspired by *Anatomy Trains* and using it as a guide, along with my own clinical experience of particularly challenging cases, I developed an approach to treatment called Mobilization of the Myofascial System (MMS). It is an approach that has its origins in manual physiotherapy for the articular, muscular, and neural systems. Because the concepts in *Anatomy Trains* form the framework for much of my approach to treatment of the myofascial body, I have devoted the whole of this chapter to a summary and review of Tom Myers's twelve fascial lines, in addition to describing the clinical implications for each of them.

Below is a **summary of the twelve fascial lines** or "Anatomy Trains" described by Myers:

- one back line called the Superficial Back Line (SBL)
- two front lines called the Superficial Front Line (SFL) and the Deep Front Line (DFL)
- two Lateral Lines (LL), one on each side of the body
- two Spiral Lines (SL), one beginning on the right side, the other on the left
- three functional lines, termed the Front Functional Line (FFL), the Back Functional Line (BFL), and the Ipsilateral Functional Line (IFL)
- two anterior arm lines, called the Superficial Front Arm Line (SFAL) and the Deep Front Arm Line (DFAL)
- two posterior arm lines, called the Superficial Back Arm Line (SBAL) and the Deep Back Arm Line (DBAL).

Superficial Back Line

The Superficial Back Line (Figure 2.1) involves the following structures:

- scalp fascia, occipital ridge
- erector spinae, lumbosacral fascia
- sacrum, sacrotuberous ligament, hamstrings
- gastrocnemius/Achilles, plantar fascia and short toe flexors.

Clinical implications

- Patients complaining of chronic low back pain frequently also complain of cervical pain and/or headache. The link between these may very well be the SBL.

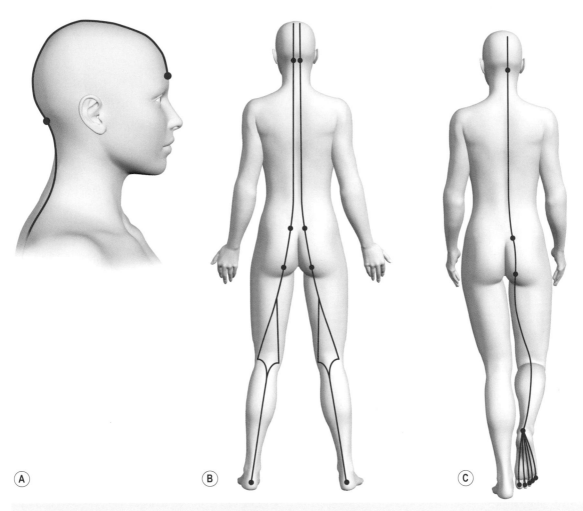

Figure 2.1
A Superficial Back Line upper quadrant; **B** right and left Superficial Back Line – posterior aspect; **C** Superficial Back Line into the foot

- Persistent tension of the *plantar fascia* may be due not only to tightness of the local plantar fascia itself but also tension along the SBL.

- *Tension headaches* felt in the epicranial frontal region may have a fascial component that links to the SBL.

- Persistent *occipital pain* may also be due to SBL issues.

- Persistent *thoracic or low back pain* may also be due to SBL issues.

Superficial Front Line

The Superficial Front Line (Figure 2.2) involves the following structures:

- scalp fascia, sternocleidomastoid muscle, sternochondral fascia

- rectus abdominis, rectus femoris, quadriceps, patellar tendon

- short and long toe extensors, tibialis anterior, anterior crural compartment.

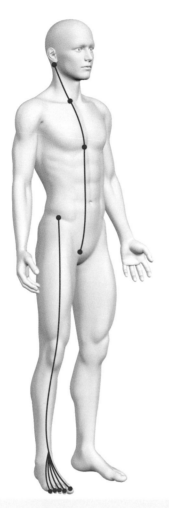

Figure 2.2
Superficial Front Line

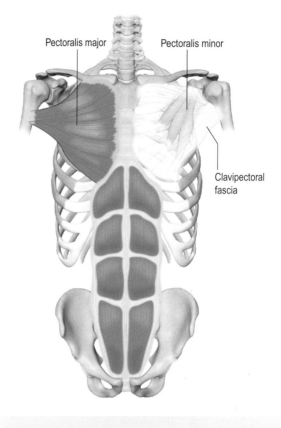

Figure 2.3
Superficial Front Line connections between the rectus abdominis and the pectoral muscles

Clinical implications

- Postural flexion of the trunk, forward head posture, or locked knees are all signs of excessive tension in the SFL (Myers 2014).

- *Tightness of the pectoralis muscles* that contributes to a forward head posture may have fascial connections to the symphysis pubis area or even the quadriceps fascia (Figure 2.3).

- Patients with *hammer toes* tend to have weakness issues in the foot stabilizers (tibialis posterior, foot intrinsics, peroneus longus). Consequently, the toe extensors become overused in the body's attempt to stabilize the foot and the toe extensors are commonly tight. The toe extensors have a fascial connection to the SFL, which may also contribute to the problem of hammer toes.

- *Abdominal scars* may have healed relatively well locally but, if the scar is assessed in relation to the SFL or DFL of fascia, there is commonly tension that may contribute to dysfunction in another part of the body. For example, a tight fascial line between a caesarean section scar and the anterior glenohumeral (GH)/scapular area creates a "holding" that can maintain a forward tilt of the scapula and/or the GH joint, and become a contributing factor to shoulder dysfunction.

21

- The *sternocleidomastoid muscles* are frequently shortened with a forward head posture. The fascial sling connecting both SCM muscles at the occipital region may be a source of occipital pain. The SCMs are part of several fascial lines, so tension in this area may have to be "chased down" to the foot (SFL) or the lateral ribcage (Lateral Line). Tension in this line can also compress the occipitomastoid suture and be a contributing factor to cranial dysfunction. The SCM exerts a strong pull on the temporal bone, which may posteriorly rotate it. This tendency has clinical implications not only for the temporomandibular joint (TMJ) but also for the position of the neck, thorax, and shoulder girdle (Figure 2.4).

Imbalance of the Superficial Back and Superficial Front Lines

According to Tom Myers, myofascial units are often arranged in antagonistic pairs on either side of the skeletal armature. When one side is held chronically short, either muscularly or fascially ("locked short"), the other side is stretched tight ("locked long").

The patient may complain of pain either in the myofascial chain that is locked short (e.g., low back pain) or in the myofascial chain that is under continual strain because it is locked long (e.g., abdominal or sternal pain) (Figure 2.5).

Lateral Line

The Lateral Line (Figure 2.6) involves the following structures:

- splenius capitis, SCM

- external and internal intercostals, ribs, lateral abdominal obliques, iliac crest, anterior and posterior superior iliac spines (ASIS and PSIS)

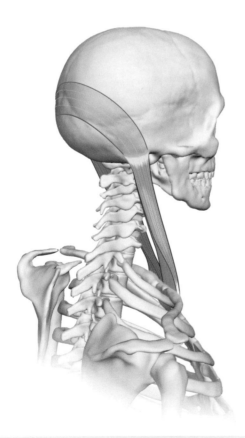

Figure 2.4
Fascial sling between both sternocleidomastoid muscles—connecting the occiput to the Superficial Front Line

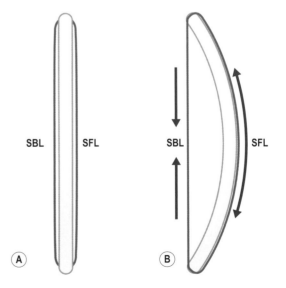

Figure 2.5
A Balanced myofascial tension between the Superficial Front and Back Lines; **B** Superficial Back Line "locked short", Superficial Front Line "locked long"

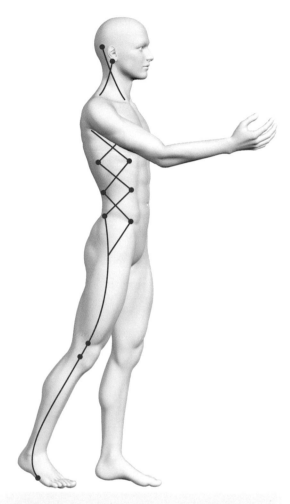

Figure 2.6
Lateral Line

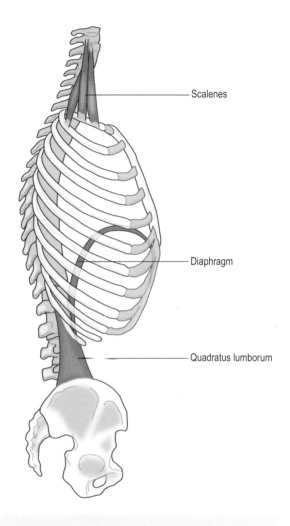

Scalenes

Diaphragm

Quadratus lumborum

Figure 2.7
The scalenes and quadratus lumborum, the deeper components of the Lateral Line

- gluteus maximus, tensor fasciae latae (TFL), iliotibial band (ITB), fibular head, peroneal muscles, lateral crural compartment.

Clinical implications

According to Tom Myers, the Lateral Line operates according to the following characteristics:

- It functions posturally to balance front and back, and bilaterally to balance left and right.

- It also mediates forces along other superficial lines – Superficial Front Line, Superficial Back Line, Arm Lines, and Spiral Line.

- Tightness of the Lateral Line may translate into pain in the area of the *iliac crest*, a frequent site of connective tissue accumulation (see Chapter 9 for MMS technique).

- The scalenes and quadratus lumborum (QL), technically part of the Deep Front Line, are deeper parts of the Lateral Line (Figure 2.7).

My own clinical experience in relation to the Lateral Line of fascia has revealed the following:

- *Recurrent tension in the scalene muscles* may be due to compensation for weakness of the deep neck stabilizers or a faulty breathing pattern. It may also be due to tension in the Lateral Line or in the Deep Front Line (DFL) (see Chapter 5 for MMS technique).

- *Recurrent tension in the QL* may be due to compensation for weak or inhibited lateral hip muscles. QL is often frequently tight in relation to the Lateral Line or the Deep Front Line (DFL) of fascia (see Chapter 9 for MMS technique to release QL in relation to these fascial lines).

- The *iliotibial band (ITB)* syndrome may be frustrating to treat if the therapeutic intervention addresses only the ITB. Clinically, it often presents as "tight", in combination with muscle imbalance issues of the hip, which must also be addressed. From the point of view of the Integrated Systems Model (ISM) (Lee & Lee 2011), the ITB and hip issues may also be the victim of dysfunctions elsewhere in the body, frequently in the thorax, pelvis, or foot. If we have addressed these factors and still feel that the ITB is tight and warrants manual treatment, then we must take into consideration that the ITB is connected to the Lateral Line of fascia. Therefore, treatment should encompass not only the ITB but also the peronei, the intercostal muscles, and the SCM (see Chapter 11, Lower extremity, and Chapter 5, Cervical spine, for MMS techniques).

- The *TMJ muscles* (temporalis and superficial masseter), although technically not part of the lateral line, are frequently tight in relation to this Lateral Line (see Chapter 6 for MMS technique). Release of these fascial lines frequently diminishes the recurrence of myofascial trigger points in these muscles.

Spiral Line

The Spiral Line (Figure 2.8) involves the following structures:

- splenius capitis, splenius cervicis

- spinous processes of C6 to T5, rhomboids major and minor, infraspinatus, serratus anterior, external oblique, internal oblique, ASIS

- tensor fasciae latae, ITB, tibialis anterior, peroneus longus

- biceps femoris, sacrotuberous ligament, sacral fascia, erector spinae.

Clinical implications

According to Tom Myers, the Spiral Line performs a number of important functions:

- It helps maintain balance posturally across all planes.

- It connects foot arches with the pelvic angle.

- It helps determine knee tracking in walking.

- In imbalance, it creates, compensates, and maintains twists, rotations, and lateral shifts in the body.

My own clinical experience in relation to the Spiral Line of fascia has revealed the following:

- *Recurrent tension in the area of the external oblique* region may be due to tension of the spiral line connecting it to the opposite iliacus area (or vice versa) (see Chapter 8 for MMS technique). Such tension may contribute to the maintenance of a thoracic shift. It may also present as pain in the thorax, the lumbar spine, or even the cervical spine (Integrated Systems Model) (Lee & Lee 2011).

- In the right spiral line there is a fascial connection between the right splenius capitis to the spinous processes of the C/Thx area, continuing into the left rhomboid and serratus anterior muscles (rhombo-serratus complex) (Figure 2.9). *Recurrent tension of the right cranioverterbral area* may be due to tension within this part of the right spiral line. Recurrent tension in the area of C2 on the right may also be due to tension this line, especially from the right lamina of C2 (Maitland's unilateral P/A pressures) to the left scapula/thoracic cage (see Chapter 5 for MMS techniques).

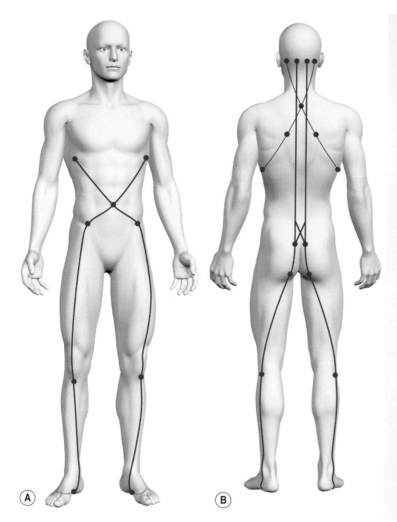

Figure 2.8
A Anterior view of the Spiral Line (right and left); [LD 11:] **B** posterior view of the Spiral Line (right and left)

Deep Front Line

The DFL (Figure 2.10) encompasses the fascia that is **behind** the sternum as opposed to the SFL, which lies anterior to the sternum and is continuous with the rectus abdominis muscle. The DFL connects the entire body at its core. It involves the following structures:

- infrahyoid muscles, suprahyoid muscles, jaw muscles, cranium, and facial bones

- longus colli and capitis, pharyngeal raphe, scalene muscles, parietal pleura, pericardium, posterior diaphragm, central tendon, anterior diaphragm

- psoas, iliacus, quadratus lumborum

- anterior longitudinal ligament, pelvic floor fascia, levator ani, obturator internus fascia, anterior sacral fascia

- pectineus, adductor longus and brevis, adductor magnus and minimus, popliteus, tibialis posterior, long toe flexors.

The anterior sacral fascia unites with the muscles of the pelvic floor to the pubic bone via the pubococcygeus muscle. At the deepest level, this connection wraps around the entire abdomen via the transversus abdominis muscle. The

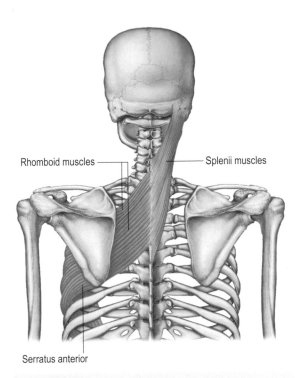

Rhomboid muscles

Splenii muscles

Serratus anterior

Figure 2.9
Upper section right Spiral Line. Reproduced from Tom Myers (2014), *Anatomy Trains: Myofascial Meridians for Manual and Movement Therapists*, 3rd edition. With kind permission from Elsevier

anterior sacral fascia also connects to the anterior longitudinal ligament in front of the lumbar vertebral bodies and then travels cephalically (Figure 2.11). The DFL splits into three portions, anterior to posterior. The anterior portion follows the respiratory diaphragm anteriorly and attaches to the posterior aspect of the sternum and upward to the hyoid muscles. The middle portion follows the crura of the respiratory diaphragm to the pericardium, to the pharyngeal raphe and upward to the scalene muscles. The third and deepest component of the DFL follows the anterior longitudinal ligament all the way to the longus colli and longus capitis muscles (Uridel 2015).

Note that the gastrocnemius muscle is part of the SBL, tibialis anterior is part of the SFL and tibialis posterior

is part of the DFL (Figure 2.12). Although the tibialis posterior is posterior to the tibia, it is considered as part of the DFL of fascia.

Note that the following muscles take part in the following section of the DFL (Figure 2.13):

- diaphragm

- quadratus lumborum

- iliacus

- psoas

- pectineus.

Clinical implications

Functional implications are vast, as the DFL starts (or ends, depending on your viewpoint!) at the top of the head or the bottom of the foot. The involvement of the respiratory diaphragm is an integral part of our core stabilization, and therefore our breath. This also alludes to the core stabilizing function of the hyoid muscles, the core implications of our pharyngeal raphe (throat) and scalene muscles, and lastly the importance of the activation of the longus colli and longus capitis in anterior neck stabilization (Uridel 2015). The DFL is thus a key component to all things core. It is also frequently tight in patients with sedentary jobs that require long periods of time in the sitting position. Unless, of course, they endeavor to offset this excessive time in flexion by doing activities or sports that encourage movement that "opens up" the front lines of the body (see Chapter 14 for more information on movement and fascia).

My own clinical experience in relation to the DFL of fascia has revealed the following:

- The *tibialis posterior* and long toe flexors are at the tail end of this line, so adding a combined movement of ankle dorsiflexion and eversion (dorsiflexion/eversion) to any structure in the DFL will add tension to this line. For example, recurrent tension in the area of the hip flexors may be due to tension of the DFL connecting iliacus to the central tendon of the diaphragm. This part of the DFL may be worked on using the MMS techniques described in Chapter 8.

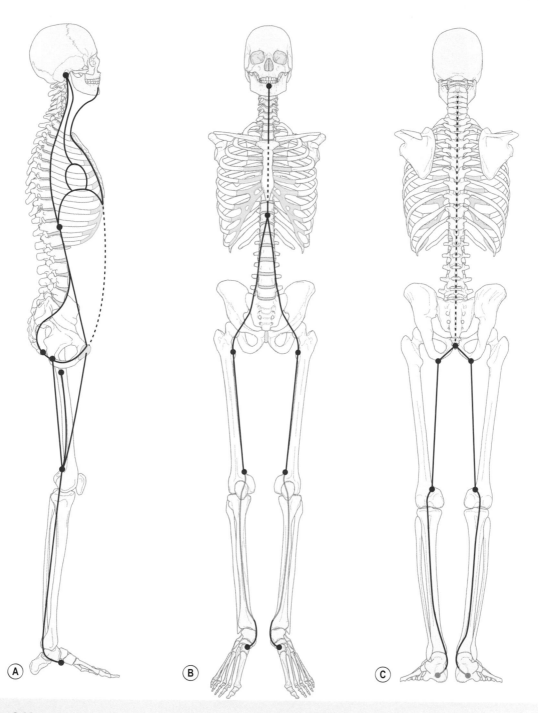

Figure 2.10
A Side view of the Deep Front Line; **B** anterior view of the Deep Front Line (DFL); **C** posterior view of the Deep Front Line

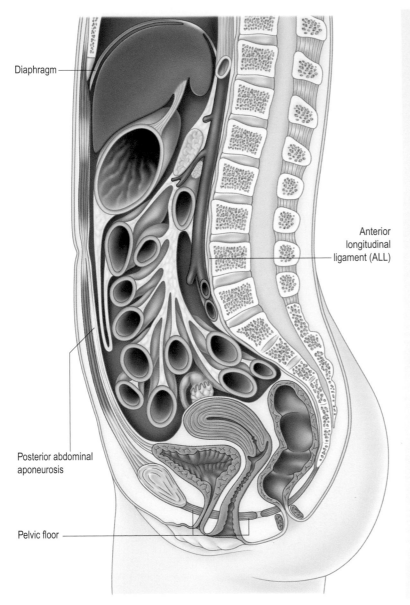

Diaphragm

Anterior longitudinal ligament (ALL)

Posterior abdominal aponeurosis

Pelvic floor

Figure 2.11
The Deep Front Line-pelvic floor fascia connects to the anterior longitudinal ligament, the anterior sacral fascia and the posterior abdominal wall fascia, encompassing both the visceral fascia and the diaphragm

As a progression, the same technique may be repeated, but this time with the feet positioned in combined foot dorsiflexion/eversion, thereby pre-tensing the DFL.

- *Recurrent tension in the quadratus lumborum* may be due to tension of either the lateral line (previously described) or the DFL. Connecting the QL to the ITB will assess the Lateral Line of the lower quadrant (see Chapter 8 for MMS technique). Connecting the QL to the foot by adding active or passive dorsiflexion/eversion will assess the DFL (see Chapter 9 for MMS technique).

- *Pelvic floor pain* is normally the domain of pelvic floor therapists, who specialize in this area of the body.

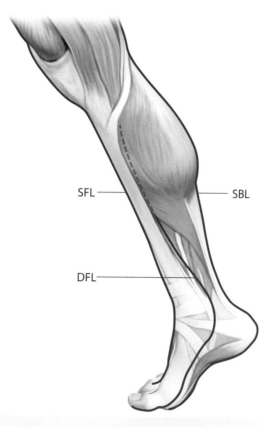

Figure 2.12

Relationship between the Superficial Front Line, Deep Front Line, and Superficial Back Line in the lower leg

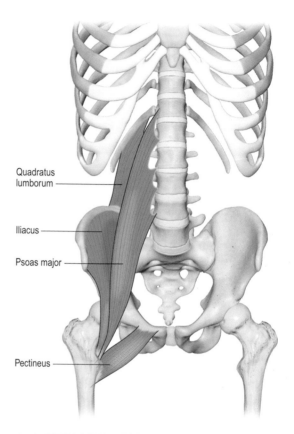

Figure 2.13

Continuity between the diaphragm, quadratus lumborum, psoas, iliacus and pectineus within the Deep Front Line

However, if treatment effects plateau, it would be wise to consider other parts of the body that have a direct or indirect effect on the function of the pelvic floor (such as the thorax in the Integrated Systems Model). Another consideration is that the pelvic floor muscles are part of this DFL of fascia and tension in this area can be traced up to the TMJ muscles and/or down to the toe flexors. Working on releasing the tension of the DFL with clients experiencing pelvic floor pain can be very rewarding. Certain pelvic floor muscles are accessible via external palpation (such as obturator internus and obturator externus), so this may

be a good place to start for physiotherapists who are not trained in internal pelvic floor techniques (see Chapter 10 for MMS technique).

With respect to the *upper quadrant*, the DFL includes several key structures:

- the anterior cervical spine, including scalenes

- the muscles of the TMJ, implicated in TMJ and headache disorders

- the muscles around the hyoid bone (infrahyoid and suprahyoid muscles) (Figure 2.14)

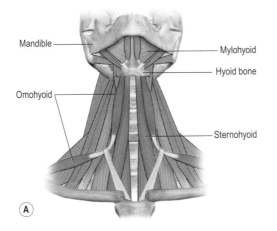

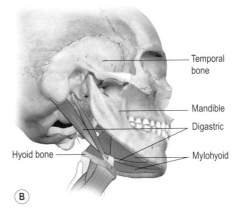

Figure 2.14
A Infrahyoid muscles and fascia within the Deep Front Line; **B** Suprahyoid muscles and fascia within the Deep Front Line

- the pericardial fascia (deep to the sternum)

- the diaphragm, which is an important fascial element separating and connecting the thoracic and abdominal fascial systems (Figure 2.15).

Clinical implications

- Tension in the SFL and/or the SBL can contribute to excessive extension in the craniovertebral area, thus maintaining a forward head posture. The DFL must then provide a counterbalancing flexion to the upper cervical region (Figure 2.16). Patients with chronic neck pain or a history of WAD (whiplash associated disorder) frequently exhibit weakness of the neck stabilizer muscles. This imbalance between the fascial lines exacerbates their condition.

- With a forward head posture, the mid-cervical spine is frequently positioned anteriorly in relation to the upper and lower cervical regions (increased lordosis and/or an exaggerated anterior shear). This anterior pull impacts all of the structures of the mid-cervical region, including the facet joints, the uncovertebral

joints, and the muscles. Tension in the anterior cervical spine may be maintained by excessive tension in the DFL (see Chapter 5 for MMS techniques mid-cervical region in relation to the DFL).

- Patients with complaints of *tightness in the throat* often have issues with the fascial line involving the muscles around the hyoid bone. It is not uncommon to see a history of abdominal or anterior thorax surgery that pre-dates the complaints of tension in the throat. These problems can successfully be treated with attention to the DFL (see Chapter 6 for MMS technique).

- Recurrent tension in the *TMJ muscles* may be due to tension in the DFL, which needs to be addressed in order to achieve optimal results. The temporalis and superficial masseter muscles form a sling on the outside of the head, with the medial pterygoid on the inside (Figure 2.17). Releasing excessive tension between the TMJ muscles and the pericardium, the diaphragm and even down to the tibialis posterior can help alleviate recurrent tension in the TMJ muscles (see Chapter 6 for MMS technique).

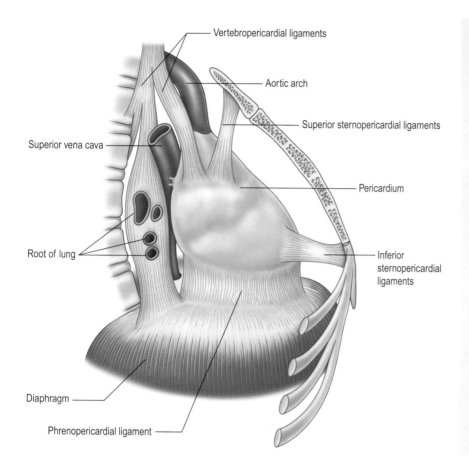

Vertebropericardial ligaments

Aortic arch

Superior sternopericardial ligaments

Superior vena cava

Pericardium

Root of lung

Inferior sternopericardial ligaments

Diaphragm

Phrenopericardial ligament

Figure 2.15
This diagram illustrates the intimate relationship and interconnection between the pericardium, the lung, the diaphragm and the anterior vertebral column. Adapted from *The Fasciae: Anatomy, Dysfunction and Treatment*. With kind permission from Serge Paoletti

Deep and Superficial Front Arm Lines

There are two front arm lines for the upper extremity – a Superficial Front Arm Line (SFAL) and a Deep Front Arm Line (DFAL) (Figure 2.18).

The **Superficial Front Arm Line (SFAL)** involves the following structures:

- pectoralis major, latissimus dorsi, medial intermuscular septum, flexor group of muscles, carpal tunnel.

Clinical implications

- Although the *latissimus dorsi* muscle originates from the back of the body, it is part of the SFL of the trunk owing to its anatomical and functional relationship to the pectoralis major. Its connection to the medial intermuscular septum along the humerus also connects it to the SFAL. It is therefore an important area to consider with patients who have range of motion issues with the shoulder. Decreased flexibility of the latissimus dorsi muscle also affects the lower lumbar spine and sacral area via the thoracolumbar fascia and can be the source of recurring "sacroiliac" pain (see Chapter 9 for MMS technique).

- The SFAL extends above and beyond the territory of the median nerve distribution. In treating problems of mobility for the *median nerve*, we may consider interfaces that include the pectoral muscles in addition to the flexor retinaculum and the anterior cervical spine.

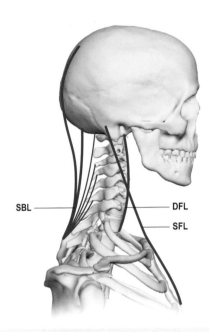

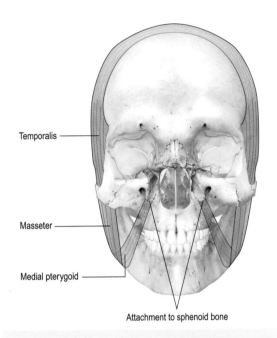

Figure 2.16
Relationship between the Superficial and Deep Front Lines and Superficial Back Line in the cervical spine

Figure 2.17
Temporomandibular joint (TMJ) muscles in relation to the upper part of the Deep Front Line – forming a fascial sling between the medial pterygoid, superficial masseter and temporalis

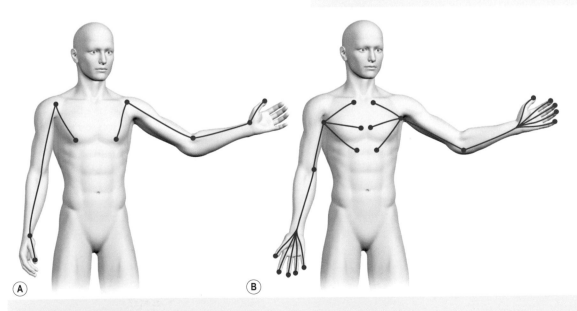

Figure 2.18
A Deep Front Arm Line; **B** Superficial Front Arm Line

- Tension in both the SFAL and the DFAL (below) can maintain a forward head posture, via its action on the position of the shoulder girdle.

- *Dupuytren's contracture* does not simply involve the finger flexor tendons in the hand. There are also strong fascial connections to the SFAL that may contribute to this dysfunction (see Chapter 13 for MMS technique).

The **Deep Front Arm Line (DFAL)** involves the following structures:

- pectoralis minor
- clavipectoral fascia
- biceps
- radial periosteum
- thenar muscles.

Clinical implications

- Adding wrist extension and ulnar deviation can help release the fascial line associated with tightness of *pectoralis minor*, a common dysfunction in those with a forward head posture (see Chapter 13 for MMS technique).

- Releasing *fascia around the clavicle* can have a positive effect on improving shoulder mobility and promoting an axially extended posture (see Chapter 12 for MMS technique).

- If periosteum is to be considered "dense fascia," then (after the appropriate healing time has occurred), the site of a *clavicular fracture* may benefit from fascial release of the clavipectoral fascia in order to minimize the effects of shortening of the clavicle on the upper quadrant (see Chapter 12 for MMS technique).

- Treatment of *De Quervain's tenosynovitis* may extend beyond transverse frictions of the retinaculum with the thumb in Finkelstein position (thumb adduction with wrist ulnar deviation) if we consider this fascial line to include the biceps, clavipectoral fascia and pectoralis minor (see Chapter 13 for MMS technique).

Deep and Superficial Back Arm Lines

There are two back arm lines for the upper extremity – a Superficial Back Arm Line (SBAL) and a Deep Back Arm Line (DBAL).

The **Superficial Back Arm Line (SBAL)** (Figure 2.19) involves the following structures:

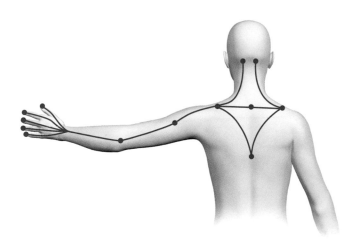

Figure 2.19
Superficial Back Arm Line

- trapezius muscles (upper, middle, and lower), deltoid, brachialis, lateral intermuscular septum, extensor muscles of wrist and fingers.

Clinical implications

- This line extends above and beyond the territory of the radial nerve distribution. In treating problems of mobility for the *radial nerve*, we may consider looking at interfaces that include the trapezii, the deltoid, and the cervicothoracic region in addition to the area of the radial head and the anterior cervical spine.

- *Recurrent tension in the upper fibers of trapezius (UFT)* may be due to tension of the SBAL, which needs to be addressed in order to get optimal results. Adding wrist flexion to a recurrent trigger point in this muscle can help release this line of tension (see Chapter 5 for MMS technique).

- The deltoid, brachialis, and wrist extensor muscle group all have a fascial connection through the SBAL (Figure 2.20). Persistent pain and tension in the lateral elbow area may be due to tension in relation to this line of fascia. Releasing this fascia is frequently helpful with recalcitrant problems of *lateral epicondylosis* (see Chapter 13 for MMS technique).

- Treatment of a *Colles' fracture* post-immobilization can encompass not only the mobility of the wrist joints but also the mobility of the fascia of the distal radius along this Superficial Back Arm Line (see Chapter 13 for MMS technique).

The **Deep Back Arm Line (DBAL)** (Figure 2.21) involves the following structures:

- rectus capitis lateralis, rhomboids, levator scapula, rotator cuff muscles, triceps, ulnar periosteum, hypothenar muscles.

Clinical implications

- This line extends above and beyond the territory of the *ulnar nerve* distribution. In treating problems of mobility for the ulnar nerve, we may consider looking at interfaces that include the rotator cuff and the levator scapula in addition to the area

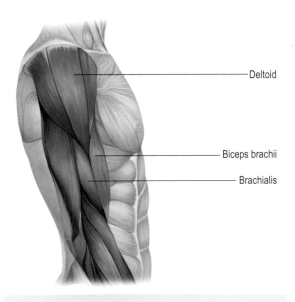

Deltoid

Biceps brachii

Brachialis

Figure 2.20
Brachialis deltoid fascia – connecting the Superficial Back Arm Line and the Deep Front Arm Line

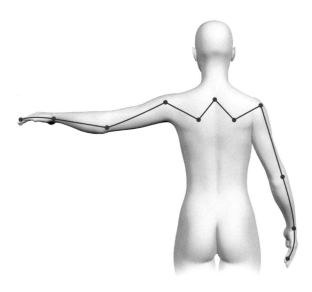

Figure 2.21
Deep Back Arm Line

of the tunnel of Guyon at the wrist and the anterior cervical spine.

- The rhomboid muscles are often "locked long" and are therefore an area where recurring trigger points are common. Releasing the Front Arm Lines helps to achieve balance. These muscles most often need re-education to "shorten" rather than lengthen. However, if the rhomboids are dominant over the trapezii muscles, this may also contribute to a downward rotation position of the scapula, undesirable for optimal function in shoulder elevation.

Functional Lines

Back Functional Line

- This includes latissimus dorsi, thoracolumbar fascia, fascia of the sacrum, gluteus maximus, the posterior margin of the ITB and the patellar tendon (Figure 2.22).

Front Functional Line

- This includes the inferior margin of pectoralis major, the lateral envelope of rectus abdominis, the pubis and the opposite adductor longus (Figure 2.23).

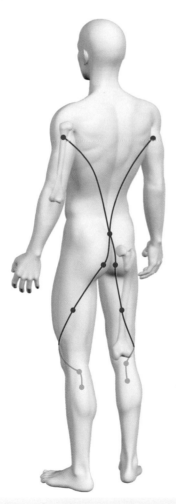

Figure 2.22
Back Functional Line (right and left)

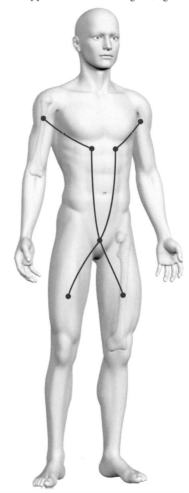

Figure 2.23
Front Functional Line (right and left)

Clinical implications

These lines enable us to give extra power and precision to movement of the limbs by lengthening their lever arm through linking them across the body to the opposite limb in the other girdle. They could be considered as trunk extensions of the Arm Lines (Myers 2014).

Ipsilateral Functional Line

- This includes the lateral portion of the latissimus dorsi, the lower outer ribs, the external oblique over the ASIS and onto the sartorius to the tibial condyle of the knee (Figure 2.24).

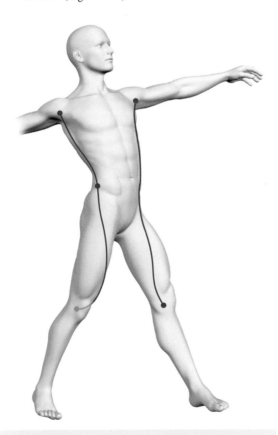

Figure 2.24
Ipsilateral Functional Line (right and left)

Clinical implications

This line is used to stabilize the torso during the pull down of the crawl stroke in swimming (Myers 2014).

Fascial lines and their connection to acupuncture

Fascia is the defining aspect of our body. It sculpts muscles in the arms, the organs in the body, even the walnut textured surface of our brains. Chinese medicine devotes two organs to fascia, the pericardium and the triple burner. The triple burner in particular is the organ with a name, but no form. It is the channel of fascia, the channel of the Tao. Fascia is truly an organ with no form of its own, yet it is everywhere (Keown 2014).

Dr Hélène Langevin, a licensed acupuncturist, is also a renowned researcher in the field of fascia. In 2002 she suggested that meridians follow fascial planes. It is clear if we look at certain meridian lines that there are similarities with Tom Myers's Anatomy Trains fascial lines (see below and Figures 2.25–2.27). In her studies, Langevin found an 80 percent correspondence between sites of acupuncture points and meridians and the location of intermuscular connective tissue planes. One hypothesis is that the needle grasp in acupuncture is due to mechanical coupling between the needle and the connective tissue. Needle manipulation transmits a mechanical signal to connective tissue cells via mechanotransduction. This observation may explain the therapeutic effects of acupuncture (Langevin & Yandow 2002).

Research evidence

What evidence is there for myofascial chains? In 2016, Wilke and colleagues conducted a systematic literature review to evaluate proof for the existence of six myofascial meridians based on anatomic dissection studies. A search for peer-reviewed anatomic dissection studies published between 1900 and 2014, yielded 6584 publications. Next, duplicate articles and articles not pertaining to the research question were removed and exclusion criteria were applied (Wilke et al. 2016). The final review yielded

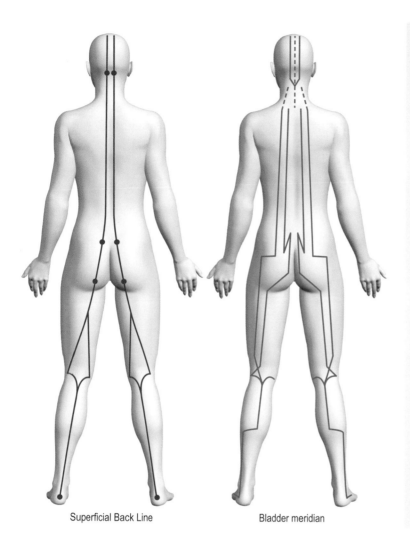

Superficial Back Line

Bladder meridian

Figure 2.25
Similarities between the bladder meridian (Tai Yang) and the Superficial Back Line

62 studies. Of these studies, evidence of each meridian and its transitions were classified as strong, moderate, limited, conflicting, or not existent (Wilke et al. 2016). A transition was considered a myofascial link between two muscles. For example, the gastrocnemius and hamstring are considered to be a transition of the Superficial Back Line.

The results yielded strong evidence for myofascial transitions in three of the six examined myofascial meridians: the Superficial Back Line, Back Functional Line, and Front Functional Line. In the Superficial Back Line, three myofascial transitions (plantar fascia–gastrocnemius; gastrocnemius–hamstrings; hamstrings–lumbar fascia/erector spinae) were verified in 15 studies. In the Back Functional Line, three myofascial transitions (latissimus–lumbar fascia; lumbar fascia–gluteus maximus; gluteus maximus–vastus lateralis) were verified in eight studies. Finally, the Front Functional Line verified strong evidence for two myofascial transitions (pectoralis major–rectus abdominis;

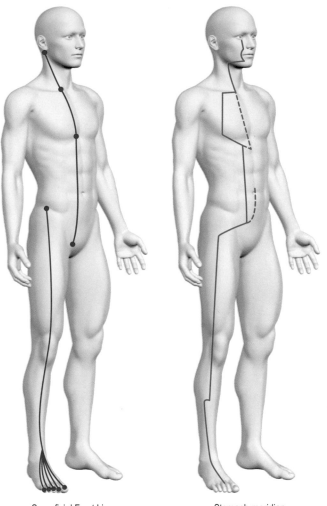

Superficial Front Line   Stomach meridian

Figure 2.26
Similarities between the stomach meridian (Tai Yin) and the Superficial Front Line

rectus abdominis–adductor longus) in six studies. There was moderate evidence for the meridians and transitions of the Spiral Line (five of nine verified transitions, based on 21 studies) and the Lateral Line (two of five verified transitions, based on 10 studies). There was no evidence for the meridians and transitions of the Superficial Front Line, based on seven studies (Wilke et al. 2016).

The researchers suggest that further studies be conducted on the Spiral, Lateral, and Superficial Front Lines to determine if there is stronger evidence to support their existence and begin to explore evidence for the Deep Front Line and Arm Lines. It will be exciting to see the outcomes of future research regarding the Anatomy Train myofascial meridians.

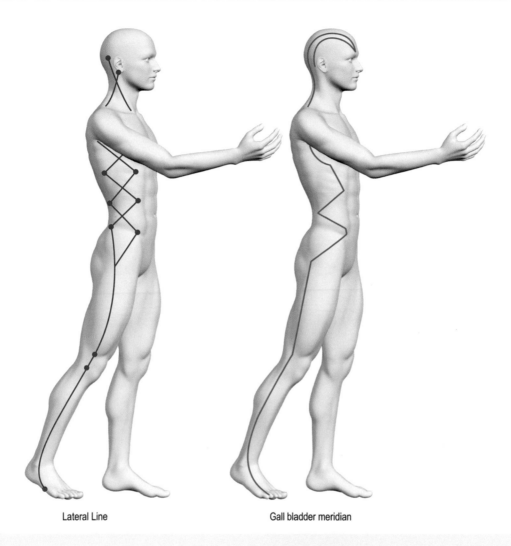

Lateral Line   Gall bladder meridian

Figure 2.27
Similarities between the gall bladder meridian (Jue Yin) and the Lateral Line

Summary

This chapter reviewed the fascial lines as described by Tom Myers in *Anatomy Trains*. Awareness of these fascial lines and their clinical implications will help illuminate the basis for many of the MMS techniques. The next chapter describes the assessment of the fascial system and its relation to the overall physiotherapeutic assessment.

Assessment of fascial dysfunction

How does a patient with fascial dysfunction present?

The subjective exam

Geoffrey Maitland, one of the grandfathers of manual physiotherapy, had a significant global impact on the profession. One of the most important messages he conveyed to physiotherapists was the importance of a thorough subjective evaluation. "Not only will a thorough subjective exam tell you what the problem(s) are," he would say, "but also how to treat them." This is true for all cases of musculoskeletal pain: it is particularly important for cases of fascial dysfunction.

The typical questions asked in a good subjective evaluation include the following topics:

- areas of pain and their relationship to each other
- complaints of paresthesia, numbness, or other neurological symptoms
- previous history of the complaint
- previous medical history, including medications taken
- medical tests performed and their results
- previous treatments tried and their effects
- behavior of pain throughout the day/night
- factors that provoke and ease symptoms
- functional difficulties
- patient's goals for treatment.

A patient with fascial dysfunction may present with the **following additional subjective complaints**:

- "My skin is too small for my muscles."
- "I feel tension in my leg overall, as if I were wearing a twisted pair of pantyhose."

- "I know that other therapists and doctors have told me that my right leg and arm symptoms are separate problems, but that's not how it feels to me."

Other characteristics of myofascial pain include the following symptoms:

- Pain is dull, aching, and often deep.
- Pain may be low-grade to severe in intensity.
- There are frequently many areas of local tenderness.
- There are disturbed sleeping patterns with morning stiffness.
- Pain does not follow dermatomal, myotomal, or sclerotomal patterns.

Does this last category of symptoms not sound suspiciously like fibromyalgia?

Clinically, I have found that clients with this condition tend to manage their symptoms well with a combination of active exercise, dry needling, craniosacral techniques, and fascial techniques as well as appropriate medication such as Lyrica (pregabalin) to tone down the nervous system.

Patients with fascial dysfunction are rarely able to identify specific provocative movements that consistently reproduce their symptoms, unless the activity adds tension to a tight fascial line (e.g., low back pain brought on by walking or standing for a period of time if the Deep Front Line of fascia is restricted). We must, however, rule out other dysfunctions that can reproduce these symptoms such as hypo- or hypermobility of the zygapophysial joints, poor mobility and/or dynamic control of the foot, knee, hip, lumbar spine, pelvis, or thorax that may contribute to the low back pain. Given the connectivity and relationship between body regions, every region of the body can contribute to low back pain.

Other clues that we may be dealing with dysfunction of the fascial system:

- The patient has difficulty maintaining effects of treatment despite good results obtained during treatment.

- The patient has difficulty maintaining effects of treatment despite being diligent in doing recommended flexibility, postural, or stabilization exercises.

- There has been a recent growth spurt in adolescence.

- The patient has difficulty maintaining an optimal posture.

The objective exam

Objectively, the following may be found:

Observation

- Positional faults are noted in observing the patient's posture but testing the accessory movements of the joints only gives a partial explanation for this positional fault. For example, ideally, when assessing the position of the femoral head relative to the pelvis, the therapist is hoping to find a centered femoral head, a key requirement for optimal biomechanics of the hip. An example of a positional fault is one in which the femoral head is positioned anteriorly in relation to the ilium. If the therapist thinks only of articular factors, they will presume that the capsule of the hip joint is the cause of this positional fault. However, optimal biomechanics require not only normal capsular mobility around the hip joint but also balanced activation of all muscle and fascial vectors.

Active range of motion (ROM)

- The area in question may demonstrate normal, or near normal range of motion (ROM), but the range may be decreased if the body is positioned differently. For example, if the SBL of fascia is tight, testing active cervical flexion in sitting may be more restricted than if it is tested in standing.

- Active ROM may or may not produce pain, but the patient frequently reports a sense of "stiffness" or "pulling."

- Testing of individual joint mobility or muscle length is within normal limits (or, at times, hypermobile) but restriction is noted with combined, functional movements.

Muscle length tests

These are often within normal limits. If a muscle is restricted and treatment is targeted to the local muscle, both the patient and the therapist may feel that results from treatment are short-lived and the muscle soon tends to stiffen up again.

Joint mobility (includes both passive physiological movements and passive accessory movements)

Passive physiological movements are movements in which the practitioner produces the motion while supporting the limb or spine. The technique is chosen in order to assess the joint with the muscle in a relaxed position. Accessory or joint play movements are joint movements that cannot be performed by the individual. These accessory movements, including roll, spin, and slide, accompany physiological movements of a joint. Manual therapists have been taught that when assessing passive physiological or passive accessory movements of a joint, attention must be paid to the sensation throughout the whole movement and not simply the end feel of the movement.

All joints have range of motion divided into two zones:

1. A neutral zone (NZ) in which no resistance is felt. The NZ ends once the beginning of the first resistance to movement is perceived (R1).

2. An elastic zone (EZ) in which the first resistance to movement (R1) gradually increases until firm resistance is felt (R2) at the end of range. In a normal joint, it is considered that R2 is due to tension in the ligaments

and capsule of the joint (see Chapter 4 for more information on movement diagrams and grades of passive movement).

A normal accessory movement for a joint, although small in amplitude (usually a few mm of glide or roll), will have a small NZ, where no resistance is felt at the start of the movement, and a gradually increasing EZ until R2 is felt. Training is required in order to determine a normal or abnormal feel for an accessory movement of a joint.

- When there is a myofascial restriction, accessory movements of the joints have a "bouncy" or "rubber-like" end feel as opposed to the end feel of a fibrotic or stiff joint, which is crisper and harder.

- A number of levels in the lumbar spine may exhibit stiffness with PIVM (passive intervertebral movement) testing for flexion, for example. If a fascial line is restricted, mobilizing these joints often results in only partial release.

- The patient's joints may have a tendency to be hypermobile, but they still present with decreased range of motion when active ROM is tested.

Vector analysis: load and listen test

This test derives from listening courses developed by Gail Wexler for the Barral Institute. These listening techniques differentiate active and passive listening. "Load and listen" encompasses both aspects of listening. I find it invaluable in helping to detect the primary myofascial vectors that may be impacting a joint.

When an accessory movement for a joint is assessed, not only is the resistance of this accessory movement noted, but, in this test, particular attention is paid to the release component of the accessory glide. In other words, when you let go of a correction, where does it pull you? This is what is termed vector analysis. Vector analysis in the Integrated Systems Model (ISM) approach has taken the "load and listen" concept of the Barral visceral approach and applied it to the musculoskeletal system, to help identify the underlying system impairment that is creating suboptimal alignment, biomechanics, and/or control of a body region.

- In a *healthy hip*, when the therapist glides the femoral head posteriorly, it floats back up to the surface, much like the type of "Soap on a Rope" that pops back up to the surface of the water after it has been pushed down (Diane Lee, personal communication).

- If the load and listen test points to an *articular restriction*, the therapist will feel that the accessory glide may be stiff with a relatively harder, capsular end feel. Upon the release of the accessory glide, a small amplitude movement occurs to allow the joint to re-establish a more neutral position.

- If the load and listen test points to a *myofascial restriction*, the therapist feels the resistance to the accessory movement but the end feel will not be as hard. More importantly, upon release of the glide, there will be a vector of pull towards the area that is "tugging" on the joint. This myofascial restriction may be a combination of neuromuscular vectors (increased tone in muscles due to increased neural drive), visceral vectors, muscular, and fascial vectors. (Keep in mind that fascia surrounds all of these systems.)

This test may be used as a "before" and "after" test, when using any type of release technique. It is particularly useful to use before and after a MMS technique. It guides the therapist as to which myofascial vector(s) have the most impact on a particular joint and encourages exploration of that myofascial vector. Release can be done both locally to the involved muscle and also along its myofascial line (based on *Anatomy Trains* myofascial meridians).

(Chapter 11 outlines the load and listen test for the hip joint.)

The same concepts for the load and listen test apply to other joints. For example, if the glenohumeral (GH) joint is positioned anteriorly in relation to the acromion, on the load and listen test we may find some limitation in the posterior glide of the GH joint (the loading aspect of the test): but upon the release of the anteroposterior (A/P) glide (the listening aspect of the test), we may feel a vector that pulls the humeral head caudally toward the biceps if the Superficial Front Arm Line is shortened. It is then appropriate to check the myofascial tissues of the Superficial Front Line. (Chapter 13 outlines the load and listen test for the GH joint.)

Dynamic stability tests

Dynamic instability may be defined as a patient exhibiting a failed load transfer when performing functional tasks such as the half squat or OLS (one leg stand) test. The failed load transfer (FLT) in these functional tests may present in one or several areas (Lee & Lee 2011):

- The pelvis: "unlocking" of the pelvis may occur. In this situation, the sacroiliac (SI) joint fails to maintain a position of sacral nutation in relation to the ilium (the position of optimal stability for the SI joint). The therapist may perceive this as the ilium moving into anterior rotation (relative counternutation of the sacrum) when doing a half squat or OLS test.

- The hip: ideally the femoral head should stay centered in relation to the pelvis throughout a OLS or a squat maneuver. A common clinical pattern of dysfunction is a femoral head that glides anteriorly and/or internally rotates instead of staying centralized.

- The foot: the foot should be able to maintain its neutral position, with the talus directly under the tibia, the forefoot in neutral position in relation to the hindfoot.

- The thorax: no lateral shift of the thoracic rings should occur with functional tests of OLS and squat (Lee & Lee 2011).

Patients with fascial dysfunction frequently exhibit signs of dynamic instability, especially in the area of fascial tightness. Recruiting muscles that help in motor control is often a frustrating experience for both the therapist and the client, as fascial tension is frequently a factor that inhibits these stabilizer muscles from "kicking in."

Assessment of the fascial system

Testing for fascial restriction with recurring joint dysfunction

If a joint restriction is recurrent despite good effects with previous treatment, good compliance with mobility and stability exercises, and awareness of posture, it may be that the fascial component to the restriction needs to be addressed. For example, if anteroposterior (A/P) mobilizations of the C4 and C5 levels are chronically stiff despite good release with treatment, we may consider whether this dysfunction is perhaps connected elsewhere along a fascial line, and whether this may possibly be a contributing factor toward its recurrence. If the therapist suspects that fascia may be a factor in movement restriction, he/she can then explore which line of tension is most problematic.

The MMS techniques described in this text have two components:

1. The therapist **stabilizes** an area of recurrent dysfunction with one hand – stabilizing either an accessory movement of a joint or a recurring myofascial trigger point.

2. The therapist's other hand becomes the hand that **explores and mobilizes** lines of fascia, always using the "star concept" (described below).

Continuing with the same example of the restricted A/P mobilization at C4, the C4 level can be stabilized with an A/P mobilization angled cranially and then the following considered:

- To explore the SFL the therapist may add:
  - an A/P mobilization to the ipsilateral or contralateral scapula
  - an A/P pressure directed caudally to the tissue anterior to the sternum
  - the rest of this line may then be explored with an A/P pressure directed caudally to the rectus abdominis area and/or the symphisis pubis (see Chapter 5 for details).

- To explore the DFL the therapist may add:
  - an A/P mobilization directed caudally to the tissue posterior to the sternum (pericardium)
  - an A/P mobilization directed caudally to the right and/or left diaphragm
  - active dorsiflexion/eversion of the ankles to pretense the DFL by putting a stretch on the tibialis posterior, which is at the tail end of this line (see Chapter 5 for details).

- To explore the Lateral Line the therapist may position the client in side-lying, stabilize the mid-cervical spine with an A/P mobilization and explore the intercostal fascia on the side of the trunk (see Chapter 5 for details).

How does the therapist know when a particular line of fascia is restricted?

The therapist will feel an almost immediate increase in tension of the stabilizing hand (in this case, the A/P mobilization of the C4) as he/she applies a gentle pressure on the anterior aspect of the sternum with the exploratory hand (for a SFL restriction). It is normal to feel a certain resistance between the two areas at the end of a caudal pressure on the sternum, but it is not normal to feel this resistance at the very start of the maneuver being performed by the exploratory hand. There should be (in Geoff Maitland's terms) a "toe region" where there is little resistance at the beginning of movement. (Please refer to the section on Maitland's grades of movement in Chapter 4.) When the fascial line is restricted, this toe region is absent or quite limited and early resistance between the two hands of the therapist will be felt. The patient may perceive this as the therapist pushing harder on the level being stabilized (in this case, C4) when in reality the therapist is simply preventing the fascial tissues at C4 from gliding caudally.

Using the star concept

The star concept implies that the therapist must not think along the lines of an articular glide but rather explore multiple directions, somewhat like the shape of a star. The aim is to discover where there is most tension between the stabilizing hand and the fascial tissues anterior to the sternum (for this example of a problem with the Superficial Front Line). The therapist "corrals" the myofascial tissue, "sniffing out" the vector where most tension between the two hands is felt. In the example above, the caudal pressure on the tissues anterior to the sternum may be done in a straight caudal direction, caudal to the right of the patient, caudal to the left of the patient, or perhaps in a medial/ lateral direction or even in a clockwise/counterclockwise direction. Restriction may be felt in several directions. Treatment begins by using the most restricted direction and, once released, exploring and releasing the other restricted directions in that fascial line.

The same "star concept" applies to any MMS technique, for any line of fascia.

Exploring lines of fascia

- Tom Myers's Anatomy Trains lines, although very pertinent to MMS, are not the only way a therapist can explore the fascia. The Anatomy Trains is simply a map of the "grain" in the myofascial fabric, and so, like most maps, only an indication of a good place to look (Myers 2014).

- The *nervous system* may also be used as a guideline (see the femoral nerve fascial technique in Chapter 9 as an example).

- The patient's *functional problems* may also give us a clue as to what to explore. Refer to Chapter 5 (Anterior cervical in relation to glenohumeral movements) for an example where the patient complains of arm pain with reaching forward as opposed to reaching sideways with abduction.

- "It hurts right here." The *location of the patient's main complaint of pain* may also be a good place to start, stabilizing that area and exploring fascial lines that may be "tethered" to that painful area. The area of pain is frequently a "victim" of another dysfunction nearby (e.g., the lower lumbar area may become symptomatic during standing or walking if it is compensating for an extension dysfunction in the upper lumbar area, and/or poor hip extension). However, the symptomatic area may also be tethered by a tight fascial line, and this may also play a role in its recurrence.

Reposition and test

Another way to help differentiate an accessory joint movement restricted by the joint capsule from one restricted by myofascial vectors, is to repeat an accessory movement with other regions of the body under tension. For example, an A/P mobilization of the C4 level in the mid-cervical region may be compared to the same mobilization (same grade of movement) with the ipsilateral arm in 70 degrees of abduction. If the A/P at C4 is stiffer (which may or may not reproduce pain), then it implies that fascia may be a factor in this recurrent restriction. The fascia may be related to the muscular system (e.g., scalenes), the clavicle, the neural system (e.g., median nerve), the visceral system (e.g., pericardium) or perhaps a combination of all four areas.

Another example is to explore the DFL of fascia in relation to the recurrent C4 dysfunction. This is done by stabilizing C4 as above and simply adding active (or passive) combined dorsiflexion/eversion of the ankles to see if this affects C4. (Keep in mind that tibialis posterior is at the tail end of Tom Myers's Deep Front Line, so adding dorsiflexion/eversion puts it under tension). If there is abnormal tension in the DFL of fascia, then adding dorsiflexion/eversion will cause an immediate increase in tension in the hand that is stabilizing C4 in an A/P glide (see Chapter 5 for MMS technique).

Testing for fascial restriction with a recurring muscle trigger point

Myofascial tension may have a tendency to recur if the following factors are not addressed:

- optimizing balance between muscle groups in the area (i.e., stretching tight muscles, strengthening weak ones)

- using dry needling or IMS techniques to de-facilitate muscles that are hypertonic secondary to increased neural drive

- considering other areas of the body that may be impacting the symptomatic area (ISM concept of drivers)

- last, but not least, considering that there may be a myofascial component to the restriction that needs to be addressed.

An example of this last concept using MMS is as follows:

Recurrent tension in the upper fibers of trapezius (UFT) may be due to tension of the Superficial Back Arm Line (SBAL), which needs to be addressed in order to get optimal results. In this example, the therapist "stabilizes" the recurrent myofascial trigger point in the UFT by pinching it in an A/P direction. If there is tension in the SBAL, the therapist will feel an immediate increase in tension of the "stabilizing" hand on the UFT as soon as he/she adds a component of passive wrist and finger flexion. Keep in mind that the wrist and finger extensors are at the tail end of the SBAL (see Chapter 2). Using oscillatory movements of wrist flexion while maintaining the pinch on the trigger point will help to release this line of tension (see Chapter 5 for MMS technique).

Testing for fascial restriction with a neural mobility test

In order to address problems of decreased mobility of a particular nerve, the usual approach in manual therapy is to mobilize the interfaces of the nerve in question. The median nerve, for example, may involve positioning the arm in some degree of shoulder abduction, external rotation, elbow extension, and wrist and finger extension (depending on irritability of the tissues and where first resistance is felt when doing the median nerve mobility test) and then adding A/P mobilizations or lateral shear movements at C5, C6, and C7. As well, the nerve mobility test itself may be used as a treatment technique, either as a sliding technique or a tensioning technique. If, however, tension of the nervous system persists despite this approach to treatment, it is suggested that the therapist explore a little more broadly than the usual interfaces of the nerves. For example, the therapist may use a mobilizing technique in the anterior cervical spine with the arm in abduction, external rotation, wrist and finger extension to pre-tense the median nerve and then explore the SFL of the trunk. Or the therapist may also explore other regions of the cervical spine, frequently as high as C1 or C2, that may have an impact on the mobility of the median nerve (see Chapter 5 for MMS techniques).

Indications/contraindications to MMS treatment

The contraindications to treatment with MMS are similar to the contraindications for manual therapy in general (Box 3.1). CNS, spinal cord or cauda equina disease and injury are an obvious contraindication to any manual therapy but there are also other conditions to consider such as vascular issues and metabolic and systemic contraindications (Canadian Physiotherapy Association).

BOX 3.1 Contraindications to manual therapy

Contraindications specific to the patient:

- lack of consent
- disturbed psychological or emotional state
- inability to communicate/unreliable historian
- inability to relax
- constant or continuous undiagnosed pain
- intoxication/highly medicated

Bone contraindications:

- relevant recent trauma (fractures, dislocations)
- past or present cancer that produces bone metastases (breast, bronchus, prostate, thyroid, kidney, intestine, lymphoma)
- active infection (osteomyelitis, tuberculosis, previous bone infection)
- significant foraminal or spinal canal reduction on radiography or other imaging examinations (for techniques done in extension)

Neurological contraindications:

CNS disease or injury

- extrasegmental pain increased by passive flexion of the neck
- bilateral or quadrilateral multisegmental paresthesia, augmented by passive flexion of the neck
- paresis or multisegmental paralysis
- hyperreflexia
- presence of Babinski/Oppenheim/Hoffmann/clonus
- ataxia
- neurological spasticity
- bladder or bowel dysfunction
- dysphagia/dysphasia
- Wallenberg syndrome (inferoposterior cerebellar artery)
- other signs/symptoms of cranial nerves
- nystagmus (if associated with dizziness/vertigo, requires more diagnostic differentiation)

Spinal cord injury or disease

- extrasegmental pain below the level of the lesion, which can increase with passive flexion of the neck
- bilateral or quadrilateral multisegmental paresthesia below the level of the lesion, which can increase with passive flexion of the neck
- bilateral or quadrilateral multisegmental weakness or spastic weakness below the level of the lesion
- hyperreflexia below the level of the lesion
- possible presence of hyporeflexia at the level of the lesion
- presence of Babinski or Oppenheim sign

- presence of Hoffmann's sign if the lesion is above C5–6
- clonus below the lesion level
- ataxia
- neurological spasticity below the level of the lesion
- reflex bladder (the bladder empties when it is distended)

Cauda equina compression

- hyporeflexia or areflexia (bilateral or multisegmental)
- paresthesia/bilateral or multisegmental pain
- initially overactive bladder (urgency and increased frequency) then paralysis of the bladder (overflow urination)
- fecal retention with overload and overflow of feces
- loss of genital sensation
- loss of erection reflex or ejaculation
- signs and symptoms of bilateral or multisegmental nerve root lesions

Vascular contraindications:

- vertebral artery insufficiency
- vascular disease (aneurysm)
- bleeding problems (e.g., hemophilia)

Contraindications related to collagen disease:

- Ehlers–Danlos syndrome
- Marfan syndrome
- osteogenesis imperfecta
- benign hypermobility syndrome (precaution) – laxity of the connective tissue
- acute post-traumatic phase (precautionary for 6–8 weeks)

Age-related contraindications:

- children (skeletal immaturity, consent issues)
- elderly (increased risk of osteoporosis, vascular disease, spinal stenosis)

Metabolic contraindications:

- bone disease (e.g., osteoporosis, Paget's disease)

Systemic contraindications:

- diabetes (precaution)
- asthma (pay attention to the side effects of corticosteroids)
- endocrine disorders (precaution) – hypothyroidism, hyperthyroidism, hyperparathyroidism
- endocrine disorders (contraindication if treated with drugs that affect collagen)
- pregnancy, contraindicated in the presence of:
  - any history of miscarriage
  - hypermobility/instability – recent postpartum (joint instability, risk of postpartum hemorrhage)

Medication:

- active inflammatory disease (e.g., rheumatoid arthritis, psoriatic arthritis, ankylosing spondylitis, Reiter's syndrome)
- inactive inflammatory disease (precaution)
- anticoagulants (Coumadin (warfarin), heparin) – pay attention to ASA (acetylsalicylic acid, aspirin)
- any medication that affects collagen – corticosteroids, tamoxifen
- any medication related to osteoporosis (see list below)
- antidepressants (precaution)
- harmful medications for bones

- glucocorticoids

  diseases treated with glucocorticoids

  rheumatoid arthritis, osteoarthritis, bursitis

  asthma, COPD, allergic rhinitis

  liver disease

  lupus, psoriasis, severe dermatitis

  cancers: leukemia, lymphoma

  ulcerative colitis, Crohn's disease

  multiple sclerosis

  post organ transplant

  inflammation and eye diseases (glaucoma)

- methotrexate

  diseases treated with methotrexate

  cancers

  immune disorders

  resistant arthritic conditions

- cyclosporin A

  diseases treated with immunosuppressive drugs

  post transplantation

  immune diseases

- other medicines

  heparin

  cholestyramine (control of blood cholesterol levels)

  thyroid hormones

  anticonvulsants

  antacids containing aluminum

MMS is particularly indicated for subacute or chronic conditions.

If the condition is acute, the therapist may work either proximally or distally (craniocaudally) to the symptomatic region, following Myers's fascial lines of tension. When first working with tissues that are in the subacute phase of healing, it is wise to use "listening techniques" rather than be too directive until such time that the body gives you a green light to go ahead (see Chapter 4 for principles of treatment with MMS).

Recent fractures must be given time to heal before using fascial techniques directly on the fracture site, but areas above and below the fracture may be explored and treated.

Summary

This chapter described the assessment of the fascial system and its relation to the overall physiotherapeutic assessment. Chapter 4 will focus on the principles of treatment with Mobilization of the Myofascial System (MMS).

Principles of treatment with Mobilization of the Myofascial System

The aim of this chapter is to introduce the reader to the concepts of using Mobilization of the Myofascial System (MMS) as a treatment for musculoskeletal problems.

MMS guidelines for treatment

Treat joints first

Generally speaking, if there is a true joint dysfunction, especially with a fibrotic or articular feel, it is best to treat these first, with graded mobilizations and/or manipulation. However, if several segments in the spine (as an example) are limited in flexion, there is commonly a myofascial component to this restriction on PIVM (passive intervertebral movement) testing. In this case, myofascial techniques should be used as a first approach to treatment, as it is then easier to focus on one or two levels that are truly restricted by the joint capsule.

Star concept

Treatment is directed by the fascial assessment (see Chapter 3 for assessment). One hand stabilizes the recurrent joint dysfunction or muscle trigger point. The therapist's other (exploratory) hand seeks the direction of most restriction between it and the anchoring hand, in relation to a particular fascial line, always using a "star" concept. For example, if the SFL of fascia has been found to be problematic in relation to recurrent A/P dysfunction of the C4 joint, the therapist will find early tension between the hand that is gently anchoring C4 with a cranial A/P glide and the exploratory hand that is performing a gentle A/P pressure on the tissues anterior to the sternum. This exploratory hand uses the star concept to determine the direction(s) of most tension between the therapist's two hands. The direction of the exploratory hand may be in a straight caudal direction, caudal to the right of the patient, caudal to the left of the patient, or perhaps in a medial/lateral direction or even in a clockwise/counterclockwise direction. Note that there may be several directions where restriction is felt

between the two hands of the therapist. Treatment begins by using the **most restricted** direction and, once released, exploring and releasing the other restricted directions in that fascial line. Once all directions have been released between the anchoring hand at C4 and the tissues anterior to the sternum, the therapist may then explore and treat the rest of the SFL, including the rectus abdominis in its entirety, all the way down to the symphysis pubis.

Depth of technique: understanding accessory movements and grades of movement

A review of Maitland's grades of passive movement is required here in order to explain the depth of technique needed for the MMS approach.

Manual physiotherapists have been taught that when assessing passive physiological or passive accessory movements of a joint, attention must be paid to the sensation throughout the whole movement and not simply the end feel of the movement.

Grades of passive movement

Grades of passive movement, as well as movement diagrams, were created as a means of communication between physiotherapists. They are not a science and should not be used in any scientific or rigid context. Movement diagrams are simply a means of allowing one person to express in pictorial form what they are feeling through their hands when they examine a passive movement (Maitland 2005). Grades of movement are used as an indication of where in the available range a treatment technique is being performed.

Historically, there have been two systems of grading passive movement. The system developed by Kaltenborn describes three stages of motion related to accessory glides (stages 1, 2, and 3).

R1 is defined as the start of the first resistance felt by the therapist when performing an accessory or passive physiological movement. R2 is defined as the second barrier or end range of the resistance to the movement performed. Stage 1, called the "toe region," is entirely before the start of resistance (R1). Stage 2, called "taking up the slack," stops between R1 and R2 so is well into the resistance. Stage 3, called "stretch," reaches R2 and attempts to move R2 further into range (Kaltenborn 2014).

In the system devised by Maitland, all joints have range of motion divided into two zones:

- A **neutral zone** (NZ) in which no resistance is felt. The NZ ends once the beginning of the first resistance to movement is perceived (R1).

- An **elastic zone** (EZ) in which the first resistance to movement (R1) gradually increases until firm resistance is felt (R2) at the end of range, the restriction due to tension in the ligaments and capsule of the joint.

Maitland's grades of mobilization are described as grade I through grade IV (Table 4.1). There are always four grades of mobilization, whether the range of motion is normal or limited. A Grade V is a grade that defines a manipulation technique, which is a high velocity short amplitude thrust at the end of the available range, at R2.

In this system, the grades I through IV are defined according to where they are in the range in relationship to R1 (first barrier of resistance) and R2 (second barrier or

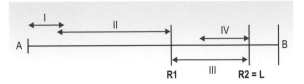

Figure 4.1
Maitland's grades of movement: R1 = first barrier of resistance; R2 = second barrier of resistance; L = limitation of range. The line A to B represents normal ROM. In this example, R2 is about 85 percent of full ROM

Table 4.2 The grades of movement into resistance can be defined as shown

Grade IV– or grade III–	Movement into the first third of resistance (often described as 25 percent of the distance between R1 and R2)
Grade IV or grade III	Movement in the middle of the resistance from a third to two-thirds of resistance (often described as 50 percent of the distance between R1 and R2)
Grade IV+ or grade III+	Movement into the last third of resistance (often described as greater than 75 percent of R and pushing into R2)

end range resistance) (Figure 4.1). *Grades I and II are found before R1* and are therefore found in the resistance-free range. *Grades III and IV are grades that penetrate the resistance* and can be found between R1 and R2.

Grades, therefore, are defined according to **resistance** and not to symptoms, although these will be taken into consideration for the appropriate choice of the grade in treatment.

To make the grades clinically more useful and a more accurate reflection of how we progress our treatment techniques, Maitland further defined the grades as plus (+) or minus (–) to indicate the amount of resistance into which the movement is performed (Table 4.2; Figure 4.2).

Table 4.1 Definition of Maitland's grades of mobilization

Grade I	Small amplitude movement near the beginning of the range
Grade II	Large amplitude movement within the resistance-free range; further than a grade I but before R1
Grade III	Large amplitude movement into resistance
Grade IV	Small amplitude movement into resistance

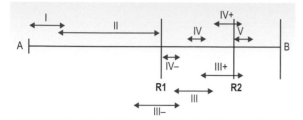

Figure 4.2
Maitland's grades of movement further broken down into plus (+) or minus (−) in relation to resistance. The line A to B represents normal ROM. In this example, R2 is about 80 percent of full ROM

For example, a grade IV− moves into less resistance than a grade IV, and a grade IV+ is into more resistance than a grade IV. Similarly, a grade III− moves into less resistance than a grade III, and a grade III+ is into more resistance than a grade III. Both grades IV+ and III+ push into R2. As grades III and IV reach the same point in range, the only difference between the two is their amplitude. A grade IV is therefore, not necessarily a progression of a grade III in treatment, in terms of where it is in the range. However, a grade III is a progression from a grade III− and a grade III+ is a progression from a grade III. Similarly, there is a progression from a grade IV− to a grade IV to a grade IV+.

The definitions given are subjective and can definitely vary from one therapist to the next. It has been difficult to use grades in research situations because our ability to determine the difference between 75 percent and 80 percent of the resistance is very poor to non-existent. We have to recognize that these definitions are more *guidelines* but may be of use during clinical reasoning as to the choice of treatment techniques (Maheu 2007).

When using MMS techniques, if we take the example above of a recurrent C4 restriction in relation to the SFL, it is normal to feel a certain resistance between C4 and the sternal tissues at the **end** of a caudal A/P pressure on the sternum. However, it is not normal to feel this at the very start of the maneuver being performed by the exploratory hand. Normally, if there is good mobility of a fascial line, there should be a "toe region" where there is little to no

resistance between the two hands of the therapist at the beginning of movement. The therapist should be able to perform a full (but gentle) A/P pressure on the sternal tissues without feeling a corresponding increase in tension in the anchoring hand until the very end of range.

The grades of movement most commonly used with MMS techniques are the large amplitude movements into the resistance of the tissues; that is, grades III−, III, and III+. The anchoring hand stabilizes the joint or muscle and the exploratory hand mobilizes the fascia, starting with a grade III− technique and then progressing to a grade III and finally a grade III+. The aim of the technique is to increase the NZ (neutral zone) between the two hands, working at the point where R1 is first perceived and gradually "pushing" R2 toward its normal limit (i.e., B on the movement diagram), where the therapist no longer feels an increase in tension at the anchor at C4. The release between the therapist's two hands is generally felt within 20–30 seconds (most probably a neurophysiological and/or hydration effect). Because of the quick response of the technique, during a single treatment session the therapist can easily assess and treat several directions of restriction in relation to one area of the body as well as several areas in a particular fascial line.

MMS treatment concepts

There are four treatment concepts to consider when using MMS techniques:

1. Choose a recurrent articular dysfunction or muscle trigger point and explore a fascial line in relation to it.

2. Convert a joint mobilization into a fascial technique.

3. Convert a nerve mobilization technique into a fascial technique.

4. Use the concept of "release with awareness."

Choose a recurrent articular dysfunction or muscle trigger point and explore a fascial line in relation to it

This is the most common technique used with the MMS approach. The idea is for the therapist to anchor him/herself to a recurrent articular dysfunction (or muscle trigger point) and explore fascial lines of tension in relation to the anchor, looking for early tension between the therapist's two hands.

There are a few ways to release this fascial tissue. The patient's response will always dictate the best approach to use with that particular patient.

- The therapist may work with *oscillations* (start with grade III–, progressing to grade III and then grade III+). The oscillations are continued until there is a sense of softening felt in the hands of the therapist. The patient often perceives this softening as "the therapist is not pushing so hard with the stabilizing hand" when, in reality, it is the neurophysiological and/or hydration reaction in the tissues that gives the therapist and the patient a sense of "release." The therapist will also feel an increase in the "toe region" between their two hands; that is, much less resistance.

When the therapist is able to perform a grade III+ mobilization with the exploratory hand and no longer feels an increase in tension in the stabilizing hand, then the rest of the fascial line may be assessed and treated in a similar way. For example, once the A/P mobilization at C4 has been released in relation to the sternal tissues of the SFL, the therapist may then explore and release the fascia over the rectus abdominis area and then the fascia over the symphysis pubis area. In this way the upper quadrant portion of the SFL may be explored and treated.

When working with oscillations, it is important to remember to come out of the range where initial resistance is felt (R1) as the oscillations are repeated.

From a teaching perspective there are two common errors that are noted when using this oscillatory technique. The first is that throughout this technique the stabilizing hand that is anchoring a joint or trigger point **should not move**. The oscillations are performed by the mobilizing hand that is exploring a fascial line in relation to the stable anchor.

The second common error that may occur is that the therapist continues the oscillations progressively into the range and does not come back to the point where R1 is felt. In other words, the therapist works progressively into R2, and ends up performing a "grade 10" maneuver. It is difficult to feel the sense of release if this point is not taken into consideration; that is, the therapist must come out of the range where R1 is felt before repeating the oscillatory movement they have chosen (grade III–, III, or III+).

- Work with *sustained pressure* – some bodies prefer a "listening" approach to treatment and do not necessarily respond well to oscillatory treatments. This is particularly true with patients whose tissues are in the subacute stage of healing or those with a sensitized nervous system. The concept behind using a listening approach is to load the fascial tissues between the anchoring hand and the exploratory hand (establish the first resistance in the line of tension), and then wait to see what the body wants to do with this tension. The therapist may feel the tension increase between the hands, with the body adding small micro-adjustments in multiple directions. The sensation is similar to that of twisted elastic that is attempting to unwind itself. The therapist follows this unwinding, preventing the tissues from going back to the direction from which they came. The tension tends to build up gradually and then suddenly release, with a fluid-like feel, often accompanied by a therapeutic pulse. Working in this way, it is rare for the patient to experience much treatment soreness as the therapist is not being directive and is following what the body will allow at that present time.

- Work with *"harmonics."* Dr Laurie Hartman, an osteopath from the UK, has demonstrated the harmonic technique in his courses on joint manipulation and describes it in his *Handbook of Osteopathic Techniques* (Hartman 1997). Harmonic technique is a technique where a passive oscillatory movement is performed to a joint or tissue. In this technique, the recoil of the tissues does the major part of the work and the therapist is only a catalyst to the maneuver. For example, the therapist may induce internal rotation of the thigh and allow external rotation to take place. The technique is done at a frequency of about one cycle per second, a frequency that facilitates the neurophysiological effects of treatment and promotes release. Certain fascial techniques lend themselves well to this approach (see Chapter 9, thoracolumbar fascia, for an example using harmonic technique).

Convert a joint mobilization into a fascial technique

Any joint mobilization technique that the therapist uses may be converted into a fascial technique simply by repeating the mobilization with a change in position of the body, so to increase tension in a particular fascial line. For example, an A/P mobilization of the talocrural joint, which is commonly performed to improve ankle dorsiflexion, may be converted into a fascial technique by repeating the same mobilization with the patient in a long sitting position, which will increase tension to the SBL of fascia (see Chapter 11). This approach is particularly useful if a plateau is reached with common physiotherapy joint mobilizations.

Convert a nerve mobilization technique into a fascial technique

The concept of neurodynamics and its importance as a contributor to pain mechanisms has been researched extensively (Butler 1991; Shacklock 2005). A positive neurodynamic test may result from a decrease in mobility of the actual nerve itself and/or may be due to problems with mobility of the myofascial tissues that interface with the nerve. Any nerve mobilization technique that the therapist uses may be converted into a fascial technique simply by adding a stabilizing maneuver in the area of the nerve mobilization and repeating the nerve mobilization technique (see Femoral nerve fascial technique in Chapter 9). The therapist may also like to explore a little more broadly than the usual interfaces of the nerves. For example, the therapist may use a mobilizing technique in the anterior cervical spine with the arm in abduction, external rotation, wrist and finger extension to pre-tense the median nerve and then explore the SFL of the trunk (see Chapter 5 for MMS technique).

Use the concept of "release with awareness"

Release with awareness (RWA) is a biofeedback technique developed by Diane Lee and L. J. Lee in which the patient is an active participant (Lee & Lee 2011). This technique is used to dampen down tone in the neural system and may also be progressed into full stretch, thereby affecting any adhesions in the fascial system. The patient is asked to bring their awareness to the muscle being palpated and to respond to various imagery cues to facilitate relaxation of the muscle. This involvement of the patient takes place as the therapist guides the release with feedback from their hands.

For an example of how this process of biofeedback works, we will consider the case where ankle dorsiflexion is decreased and there is a neuromuscular vector in the medial gastrocnemius muscle that is preventing the talus from rocking posteriorly to allow full dorsiflexion to occur (see Chapter 11). The therapist performs an accessory movement of an A/P rock to the talus with one hand, and maintains it at the point where initial resistance to the movement is felt. At the same time, the therapist palpates and monitors the area of the gastrocnemius muscle that has most connection with the restricted A/P rock of the talus; that is, an area where a gentle pressure and stretch of the medial gastrocnemius has an almost immediate impact on the accessory movement at the talus, giving the therapist the sensation that the talus is being pushed anteriorly. As the therapist provides manual input to the gastrocnemius, the patient is instructed to "soften the muscle, let it go, see if you can find a way to allow my fingers to sink into the muscle." At the same time, the therapist moves the joint or muscle to shorten origin and insertion, diminishing tension on the muscle spindle. The therapist then waits, allowing the patient and his/her system to cue into the release as the therapist gives manual and verbal cues to let go. Once maximum release is obtained, usually within 10–15 seconds, the muscle is gently taken through a full stretch, with the therapist listening to its response and avoiding recurrence of overactivity. A full A/P rocking movement is encouraged, using a sustained movement at the ankle. At the same time, the therapist may encourage a release of the muscle fascicle in a cranial direction, helping to release the "fuzz" of connective tissue that has lost its ability to elongate. Once released, the therapist may seek and explore other areas of the calf that may be limiting this accessory movement. I have found this technique to be very useful clinically. Involving the patient in the release seems to create a more long-lasting effect, and carry-over from one treatment to the next is excellent (Lee & Lee 2011).

Effects of manual therapy for the fascia (MMS)

What can we learn from research evidence pertaining to release techniques for the fascia? There are a number of hypotheses and theories as to why therapists feel a sense of "release" when using any type of fascial technique. Potential explanations include:

- freeing the fascial envelope which then helps to decrease muscle tension

- lengthening collagen fibers, breaking adhesions between the collagen fibers, elastin fibers and between the different layers of the fasciae, thereby changing fibrosis

- draining necrotic cell debris and toxins accumulated as a result of tissue degradation

- releasing trigger points

- causing a change in sol/gel chemistry of the ground substance

- improving hydration

- affecting neuromodulation via integrins/mechanotransduction

- affecting a shift in energy between the patient and the therapist.

The **mechanical model** suggests that the practitioner is altering the density, viscosity or arrangement of the collagen in the fascia through the application of manual pressure (Paoletti 2006).

Robert Schleip is a leader of the Fascia Research Group at the University of Ulm, Germany. In relation to the possibility of fascial techniques affecting the collagen in the fascia, he states:

In most systems of myofascial manipulation, the duration of an individual "stroke" or technique on a particular spot of tissue is between a few seconds and 1.5 minutes. Rarely is a practitioner seen – or is it taught – to apply uninterrupted manual pressure for more than 2 minutes. Studies on the subject of time and force dependency of connective tissue plasticity (in terms of creep and stress relaxation) have shown that either much longer amounts of time or significantly more force are required for permanent deformation of dense connective tissues (Currier & Nelson 1992). Additional models are needed to explain short-term plasticity. (Schleip 2003)

The **thixotrophic model** suggests that connective tissue can change from gel to fluid with heat or mechanical input. This model suggests that these changes take place primarily in the ground substance of the fascia (Myers 2014).

The **piezoelectric model** suggests that fascia is organized like a cross-hatched electrical grid that conducts pulses all over the body. Collagen in fascia is a semi-crystalline structure, which gives it electrical properties (crystals are piezoelectric, able to generate tiny electrical currents when an object is deformed by therapy and/or movement) (Keown 2014). This model suggests that manual therapies directed towards the fascia have a direct effect on function of cells by issuing electrical impulses. Manual pressure generates electrical current that stimulates fibroblasts and fibroclasts. This hypothesis may explain effects on the collagen in fascia (Myers 2014).

Hydration model: Jean-Claude's Guimberteau's seminal work on living fascia points to its chaotic fibrillar arrangement, with its varying polygonal shapes of a microvacuolar sliding system, filled with fluid and proteoglycans. His videos depicting living fascia in vitro clearly show how hydrated this tissue truly is and how it constantly changes shape as fibrils slide over one another with movement. This may also explain the fluid release felt in the hands of the therapist when using techniques that work the fascial system. We may be essentially opening up the microtubules and allowing the tissues to become more hydrated (Guimberteau 2015).

Neuromodulation model: slow adapting plasticity makes sense in order to adjust to patterns of long-term use, but we need another explanation for the rapid change we see in treatment. Perhaps the main effect of our treatments to the fascial system occurs via neuromodulation. We may effectively be changing sensory input into the nervous system to change motor output, bringing awareness to the patient about his/her tissues. Schleip's article on fascial plasticity describes the nervous system as a "wet tropical jungle" – much more than the traditional "switchboard system." He views the nervous system as primarily a liquid system in which fluid dynamics play a major role (Schleip 2003). This model suggests that only the patient can make a difference in their brain map, and the therapist is there to simply act as a coach.

Some might argue that, instead of identifying and treating biomechanical abnormalities with the intent of modulating pain, manual therapy should be used as a vehicle to engage the nervous system in order to modulate pain-related movement. Manual therapies such as mobilization, manipulation, massage, trigger point release, etc. could be conceived as a physical modality, similar to thermal and electrical modalities. Their role then is not to "fix" the underlying tissue dysfunction, but rather modulate pain to enable more successful participation in exercise and activities (Orthopaedic Division Review).

Because the fascia is highly innervated (see Chapter 1), it may be one of the most potent ways in which therapists can modulate the nervous system.

In the field of fascia research, there is one consensus emerging from several studies, namely the concept that the collagen in the fascia is actually NOT stretching. Robert Schleip sums it up nicely: "After years of research into the effects of manual therapies for the fascia,we must let go of concept that we are stretching collagen. What we experience as 'fascial plasticity' during our Rolfing strokes is in fact due to the plasticity of the neuromuscular system."

MMS in relation to the overall treatment approach

Patient responses to treatment

Generally speaking, when the MMS approach is used to release fascia, there is very little treatment soreness. This benefit contrasts with some mobilization or manipulation techniques, where treatment soreness occurs more frequently. Like any other soft tissue technique, the changes

to the tissues tend to rebound back a little from one treatment to the next, but much less than with traditional manual therapy. Techniques may need to be repeated for a few sessions in order to get optimal release, especially if the problem is long-standing and there are a few "layers of the onion" to work through. However, follow-up with exercises to maintain fascial mobility (see Chapter 14) and to re-educate motor control help to maintain effects of treatment.

Re-assessing functional tests for mobility and dynamic stability

Once a fascial line has been released, the therapist should re-evaluate the effect of this treatment on mobility tests and dynamic stability tests. This re-assessment of **mobility tests** could involve the following:

- active range of motion (e.g., re-assessing side-flexion of the lumbar spine following a release of the lateral line of fascia)

- joint mobility (using an accessory movement or a passive physiological movement (e.g., re-assessing passive wrist extension once the SFAL has been released)

- muscle flexibility (e.g., re-assessing flexibility of hip flexors once the DFL of fascia has been released).

Dynamic stability tests, such as a OLS (one leg stand) test or a half squat are also re-assessed. The test used should relate to a functional problem that the client is complaining of. For example, a half squat test can be used for those who complain of difficulty with sitting. A OLS test can be used for a problem with standing or walking. A common clinical finding is to find areas of fascial tightness in the region of the "instability," in particular dynamic instability, where non-optimal patterns of movement tend to occur. Dynamic stability is usually achieved with optimal motor control, but recruiting muscles that help motor control is often a frustrating experience for both the therapist and the client if there is some fascial tightness in the area. Fascial tension is a factor that inhibits stabilizer muscles from kicking in. When tight fascia is released, there is often improvement in dynamic stability tests – sometimes partially improved, sometimes completely. If the dynamic stability tests are completely improved (i.e., negative), it is not necessary to assess the stabilizer system. The patient can move directly towards functional and sport-specific training. If dynamic stability tests are still positive, then further tests are needed to see which strategies for motor control are best for the specific meaningful task required. This process may also include finding the drivers that are maintaining the non-optimal strategy for movement (Lee & Lee 2011).

Using IMS or dry needling to release any hypertonic muscles that may remain (see Chapter 1, section on trigger points as a fascia-related disorder, for the explanation about how these two approaches interact). Clinical experience has shown that myofascial trigger points and fascial dysfunction frequently coexist. Using MMS techniques first in order to release the fascia enables the therapist to treat fewer trigger points with IMS or dry needling.

Follow up with an active approach

The clinical reasoning framework for treatment prescription according to the Integrated Systems Model (Diane Lee and L. J. Lee) contains the acronym RACM (release, align, connect/control, move). Every treatment session has components of the following:

- **R: *release.*** This applies to cognitive, emotional, social, and physical barriers. A variety of techniques may be used to release overactive muscles and adhesions (myofascial, articular, neural and visceral impairments). The technique chosen depends on vector analysis. Release can be a joint mobilization or manipulation, a visceral technique or an MMS technique, depending on the findings of the vector analysis. It may also simply be a verbal cue ("let go of your hyoid," "lift your sternum," "create some space").

- **A: *align:*** cues/corrections to align the body both within and between regions. Teaching the patient to find their neutral spine is also included in this section.

- **C: *connect/control:*** cues for activation and co-ordination of the deep and superficial muscle systems. This phase involves extensive use of imagery to rewire brain pathways and maps.

- **M: *move.*** Use the principles of neuroplasticity to re-wire (re-set) brain maps and create more efficient strategies for function and performance in ways that have meaning to goals (Lee & Lee 2011).

The MMS approach to treatment is one of many techniques that may be used to remove barriers to achieving optimal alignment and movement strategies. (Other techniques may include joint mobilizations and/or manipulation, muscle energy, proprioceptive neuromuscular facilitation (PNF), etc.). Because fascia innervation is so widespread, the MMS approach has a powerful neurophysiological effect that allows the therapist an open window to re-pattern the brain map. Once the fascial tension related to the suboptimal strategy for movement has been released, it is much easier to align, connect, and move.

It is strongly recommended to follow up MMS approach to treatment with movement therapies that can optimally integrate the changes in the patient's body:

- exercise to maintain flexibility of fascial line

- ball release

- stretch with awareness

- yoga therapy

- using tools to enhance fascial mobility.

Chapter 14 has more information on this topic.

Summary

This chapter has described the guidelines and concepts used for treatment using MMS techniques. It has also defined how this approach may be used in the context of the overall treatment strategy that many physiotherapists use to manage musculoskeletal conditions. Finally, a brief summary, based on current research in the field of fascia, offers explanation of the possible ways in which fascial techniques may affect the body. The following Chapters, 5 through 13, are descriptions of MMS techniques that may be used in the various regions of the body.

Section 2
MMS techniques for fascia

The cervical spine

When treating patients with problems in the cervical spine, manual therapists are trained to assess and treat joints that are prone to limitations with a forward head posture. In particular, common findings in cases of joint restriction include a lack of flexion between the occiput and C1, a lack of extension in the C/Thx region and the mid-cervical area exhibiting limitations in both flexion and extension of the zygapophysial joints. Anterior palpation of the cervical spine (Maitland's A/P mobilizations) are also commonly used to mobilize periarticular tissue in the anterior aspect of the neck, which has been found to be useful in improving mobility of the cervical spine as well as treating interfaces for problems with decreased mobility of the nervous system.

In addition, the muscles of the upper quadrant are assessed and treated for imbalance between hypertonic, tight muscles and weak muscles. However, mobilizing joints and stretching and strengthening individual muscles can achieve only partial benefits if the fascial system is not taken into consideration.

This chapter will describe techniques to release the following fascial dysfunctions:

1. Craniovertebral area (occiput, C1, C2) in relation to the SBL and SFL.

2. Mid-cervical spine (C2–6) in relation to the SFL, the DFL, the glenohumeral (GH) joint, the scapula, the Lateral Line, the Spiral Line and the neural tissues of the upper extremity.

3. Cervicothoracic area (C7–T2) in relation to the Lateral Line and the DFL.

4. The upper fibers of trapezius (UFT) in relation to the SBAL and the SFL.

Indications for MMS for this chapter

1. Recurring neck pain despite the following treatment approaches:

- mobilization/manipulation of the cervical spine and thorax
- stabilization exercises for the cervical spine
- release of trigger points to the cervical muscles with manual or dry needling techniques.

2. Tension in the anterior cervical spine/throat area.

Postural analysis

Ideally, in the sagittal plane, a vertical line should pass through the external auditory meatus and the bodies of the cervical vertebrae. If a plumb line were to be dropped from the chin, it should contact the sternum. Postural analysis may be used as a guideline to explore particular fascial lines. For example, restriction of the Superficial (SFL) or Deep Front Line (DFL) of fascia may maintain a forward head posture. This tension can develop as a result of trauma, including surgical scars to the abdominal area. As well, certain activities of daily living, such as excessive time spent in a sitting position for work or leisure activities, can be a factor in creating these fascial lines of tension.

If there is restriction in the Lateral Line of fascia, this may create a lateral tilt or side shift of the thorax, the cervical spine, the lumbar spine or the pelvis, and contribute to recurring issues with these areas.

If there is restriction of the Spiral Line of fascia, it may also contribute to a lateral tilt or side shift of the thorax or the cervical spine, as well as unilateral tension in the abdominal oblique muscles. It may also impact the position of the scapula and therefore, the function of the shoulder complex. Postural analysis should be re-assessed after using MMS techniques in order to evaluate their impact on global posture.

Positional tests

The therapist takes note of the position of the cervical spine in relation to the patient's meaningful task (sitting or standing). The occiput should sit squarely on top of C1, with no side-flexion or rotation – the position of the ears may be used to determine the relative alignment. There should be no global deviation in relation to the thorax or shoulder girdle. Intersegmental palpation of the cervical spine should not reveal any lateral shifts (usually associated with contralateral rotation in the mid-cervical spine). Any shifts and deviations may be due to restriction of a particular segment (either articular or myofascial) or due to a lack of dynamic control of that region. Positional tests should be assessed before and after using MMS techniques.

Active range of motion tests

Cervical movement testing should be performed before and after MMS techniques, in order to evaluate the impact of the techniques on ROM. These movements include cervical flexion, extension, rotation and side-bending as well as craniovertebral flexion, extension and cervicothoracic flexion and extension. The therapist evaluates the quality and quantity of movement as well as reproduction of any symptoms. The emphasis should be on movements that most correspond to the patient's functional problem(s).

Functional tests

Sitting arm lift (SAL). This test is a variation of the prone arm lift test, developed by Linda-Joy Lee as a test for evaluating dynamic stability of the thorax and cervical spine (Lee 2003). It evolved from the active straight leg raise test (ASLR) (Mens et al. 1999, 2001). The sitting patient is asked to flex their arm from a neutral position to approximately 90 degrees of flexion and to note any difference in effort required to lift the right or left arm. (Does one arm seem heavier or harder to lift?) The strategy used to stabilize the cervical spine during this task is observed. The cervical spine should not laterally shift or rotate during this task. It is important to observe what happens to the cervical spine during the moment that the arm begins to lift and not simply at the end of the required shoulder flexion. If there is movement in the cervical spine during this task, the therapist corrects the cervical segment passively towards the midline (e.g., if a segment laterally shifts to the right, the therapist corrects the segment by gently shifting it towards the midline (left) and de-rotates the segment towards neutral). The SAL is repeated and any change in effort and/or pain is noted. This test may also be used to

assess the strategy to stabilize the thoracic spine and the scapula (Lee 2003). This test should be assessed before and after using MMS techniques, as fascial restrictions may inhibit the dynamic neck stabilizers from working optimally. If the test is still positive after releasing tight fascia in relation to the cervical spine, then the therapist should assess and treat the stabilizer function of the cervical muscles.

Concepts of treatment using MMS

For this chapter, we will be using primarily the first concept of treatment when using MMS techniques; that is, choose a recurrent articular dysfunction or myofascial trigger point and explore a fascial line in relation to it. The therapist anchors him/herself to a recurrent articular dysfunction or myofascial trigger point and assesses the fascial lines of tension in relation to the anchor, looking for early tension between their two hands.

The following approaches may be used, depending on how the tissues respond:

- work with oscillations (grades III−, III, III+)
- work with sustained pressure
- work with "harmonics" (Laurie Hartman).

Please refer to Chapter 4 for further detail on concepts of treatment using MMS.

The following techniques are suggested for addressing fascial restrictions in the cervical spine.

MMS techniques: craniovertebral region in relation to the Superficial Back Line of fascia (SBL)

Tom Myers's description of the Superficial Back Line of fascia involves the scalp fascia, the occipital ridge, the erector spinae muscles, the lumbosacral fascia, the posterior aspect of the sacrum, the sacrotuberous ligament, hamstring muscles, gastrocnemius/Achilles tendon, plantar fascia and short toe flexors. (Refer to Chapter 2 for a full description and illustration of this line of fascia.) These fascial connections become very apparent when working with the MMS techniques described in this chapter.

Techniques for the SBL are described below:

MMS central occiput with the cervicothoracic region (SBL) (Figure 5.1)

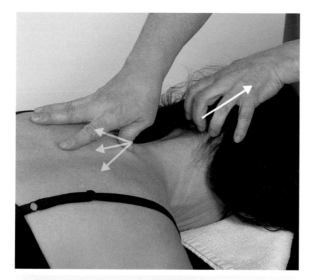

Figure 5.1
MMS central occipitalis with the C/Thx region

Stabilizing hand The patient is in a prone position. The therapist anchors onto the central suboccipital region with the one hand (third finger of the hand at the most central point) and pulls it gently in a cranial direction, maintaining the tension on this region.

Mobilizing hand The therapist then explores the area of the C/Thx spinous processes or facet joints, first by slowly sinking into the tissues of the C/Thx region in a postero-anterior direction and then gently pushing in a caudal direction, all the while maintaining the depth of the fascial line. The therapist looks for the angle where he/she perceives immediate tension in the hand palpating the occiput. The tension between the two hands of the therapist may be felt most with the mobilizing hand performing A/P pressures in a simple caudal direction, or caudal to the right of the patient or caudal to the left. This technique can be explored anywhere from C7 to the T4 level (spinous pro-

cesses or facet joint area). If no tension is perceived, then the SBL of fascia in relation to this region is not tight. If this fascial line is tight, the therapist will feel an increase in tension in the anchoring hand, as if the suboccipital tissues were being pulled caudally. The patient perceives this as the therapist increasing his/her pressure on the occipital region. If tension is perceived (quick resistance is felt between the two hands of the therapist), then it can be mobilized as per the approaches outlined in Chapter 4.

MMS right occiput with the cervicothoracic region (SBL) (Figure 5.2)

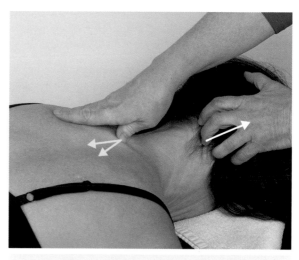

Figure 5.2
MMS right occipitalis with the C/Thx region

Stabilizing hand The therapist anchors onto the right suboccipital region with the one hand and pulls it gently in a cranial direction.

Mobilizing hand As per the technique above. Both the left and the right occipital region may be explored in a similar fashion.

Note that the craniovertebral region can also be explored down the spine and into the sacrum. This area is also part of the SBL and, depending on the depth of the technique, may also be a way to mobilize the posterior dura (see Chapter 7).

MMS techniques: craniovertebral region in relation to the Superficial Front Line (SFL) of fascia

The occipital region is frequently tight in relation to the SFL as well. This line involves the scalp fascia, sternocleidomastoid (SCM), sternochondral fascia, rectus abdominis to the symphysis pubis. It then begins again at the origin of the rectus femoris and includes the quadriceps muscles, the patellar tendon, the short and long toe extensors, tibialis anterior, and the anterior crural compartment. Although we may think of the occipital region as a posterior structure and part of the SBL of fascia, Tom Myers describes a fascial connection between both SCM muscles that extends towards the back of the occiput like a sling (refer to Chapter 2 for illustrations and a full description of this line of fascia). This sling of fascia is what connects the occipital region to the SFL of fascia.

The techniques for this line are described below. Although the techniques described here are for the right side of the craniovertebral region, they may also be performed on the left side.

MMS right occipitalis with A/P pressures of the contralateral Cx (Figure 5.3)

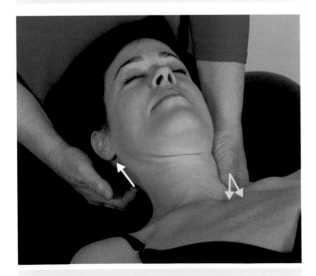

Figure 5.3
MMS right occipitalis with A/P pressures of the contralateral Cx

Stabilizing hand The patient lies in a supine position. The therapist anchors onto the right suboccipital region and/or the occipitalis muscle (an area about 3 cm square) with the right hand and pulls it gently in a cranial direction, maintaining the tension on this region.

Mobilizing hand The therapist uses their left hand to explore the tissues of the contralateral mid-cervical spine, using A/P pressures (Maitland technique) from C1 to C6 on the left side. The therapist looks for the angle where he/she perceives immediate tension in the hand that is stabilizing the occiput. The tension between the two hands of the therapist may be felt most with the mobilizing hand performing A/P pressures in a simple caudal direction, or caudal to the right of the client or caudal to the left. If this fascial line is tight, the therapist will feel an increase in tension in the anchoring hand, as if the tissues of the right occipitalis were being pulled caudally. The patient perceives this as the therapist increasing his/her pressure on the occipitalis. If tension is perceived (quick resistance is felt between the two hands of the therapist) then it can be mobilized as per the approaches outlined in Chapter 4.

MMS right occipitalis with A/P pressures of the ipsilateral cervical spine (Figure 5.4)

Stabilizing hand As per the technique above except that the therapist uses their left hand to anchor the right occipitalis.

Mobilizing hand As per the technique above except that the therapist uses their right hand to explore the tissues of the ipsilateral mid-Cx spine with A/P pressures.

The SFL also includes the pectoral region, which contributes to the "turtle" position in forward head posture, where the shoulder girdle area is held anteriorly. Mobilizing the fascia of the occipital region in relation to the shoulder girdle is often helpful to re-establishing a more optimal posture. It can be mobilized as follows:

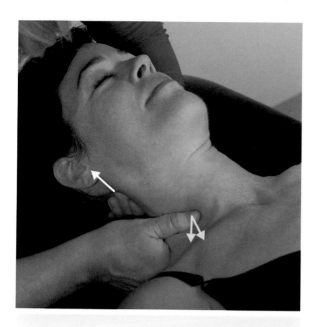

Figure 5.4
MMS right occipitalis with A/P pressures of the ipsilateral Cx

MMS right occipitalis with anteroposterior caudal glides of the shoulder region – ipsilateral or contralateral (SFL) (Figures 5.5, 5.6)

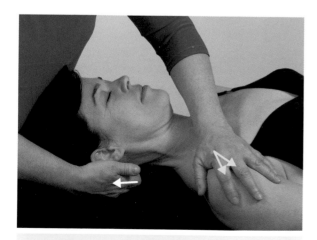

Figure 5.5
MMS occipitalis with anteroposterior-caudal "glides" of the shoulder region – ipsilateral

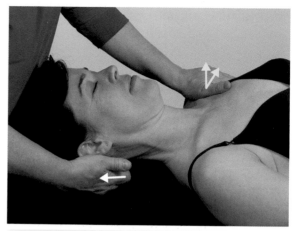

Figure 5.6
MMS occipitalis with anteroposterior-caudal "glides" of the shoulder region – contralateral

Stabilizing hand For this technique, the therapist's right hand uses the same anchor on the right occipitalis region, as described above.

Mobilizing hand The therapist's left hand explores the shoulder and shoulder girdle area with an "anteroposterior caudal glide" of the tissues in the area of the lateral clavicle and/or the GH joint, using the "star concept" to find the direction of most tension between their two hands. Sometimes tension is felt most with a posterior tilt or lateral "glide" of the scapula. Both the ipsilateral and contralateral shoulder girdle may be explored in this fashion. If this fascial line is tight, the therapist will feel an increase in tension in the anchoring hand, as if the occipitalis moves caudally. The patient perceives this as the therapist increasing his/her pressure on the occiput. If no tension is perceived, then the SFL of fascia in relation to this region is not tight. If tension is perceived (quick resistance is felt between the two hands of the therapist) then it can be mobilized as per the approaches outlined in Chapter 4. The therapist maintains the anchor on the occiput to prevent it from moving as he / she performs repeated A/P mobilizations of the ipsilateral or the contralateral shoulder area.)

NB This technique may be progressed by exploring the occipitalis in relation to the rest of the SFL of fascia; that is, the sternal region, the rectus abdominis and the symphysis pubis (described below in relation to the mid-cervical spine).

Chapter 5

MMS techniques: mid-cervical region in relation to the Superficial Front Line (SFL)

Techniques for this line are described below. Although described for the right side of the mid-cervical spine, they may also be performed on the left side:

> **MMS A/P pressures of the right mid-Cx in relation to the sternum (SFL) (Figure 5.7)**

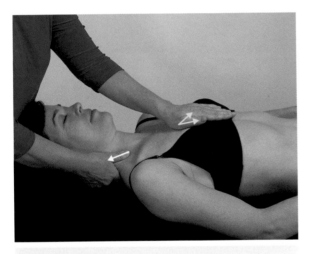

Figure 5.7
MMS A/P pressures of the mid-Cx with the sternum (SFL)

Stabilizing hand The patient is in a supine position. The therapist's right hand anchors to an area of the anterior mid-cervical spine that is chronically stiff (often C4), using an A/P mobilization in a cranial direction (grade IV–).

Mobilizing hand The therapist's left hand explores the manubrial and sternal area with an anteroposterior caudal glide of the tissues, making sure that the touch is light and stays in the plane of the SFL. The therapist looks for the angle where he/she perceives immediate tension in the hand anchoring the anterior cervical spine. That tension may be felt most when the mobilizing hand moves the fascia in a simple caudal direction, or caudal to the right of the client, or caudal to the left. Sometimes the tension is most felt when moving the sternal tissues mediolaterally or in a clockwise/counterclockwise direction, always maintaining the depth of

the tissue. If this fascial line is tight, the therapist will feel an immediate increase in tension in the anchoring hand, as if the mid-Cx region translates anteriorly and caudally. The patient perceives this as the therapist increasing his/her pressure on the anterior Cx spine. If no tension is perceived, then the SBL of fascia in relation to this region is not tight. If tension is perceived (quick resistance is felt between the two hands of the therapist) then it can be mobilized as per the approaches outlined in Chapter 4. (The therapist maintains the A/P pressure to prevent the segment from moving as he/she performs repeated A/P mobilizations of the manubrial/sternal area in the direction(s) of most restriction.)

> **MMS A/P pressures of the right mid-Cx in relation to the rectus abdominis (SFL) (Figure 5.8)**

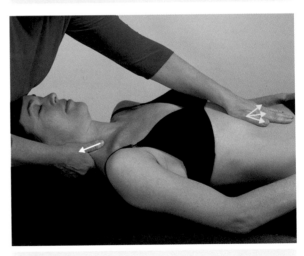

Figure 5.8
MMS A/P pressures of the mid-Cx with the rectus abdominis (SFL)

Stabilizing hand As per the technique above.

Mobilizing hand As per the technique above except that the therapist explores the rectus abdominis (ipsilateral and contralateral) caudally towards its insertion at the symphysis pubis. If tension is perceived (quick resistance is felt between the two hands of the therapist) then it can be mobilized as per the approaches outlined in Chapter 4.

MMS A/P pressures of the right mid-Cx in relation to the symphysis pubis (SFL) (Figure 5.9)

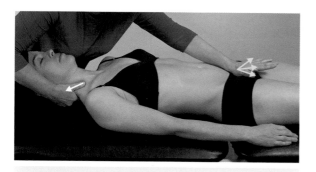

Figure 5.9
MMS A/P pressures of the mid-Cx with the symphysis pubis (SFL)

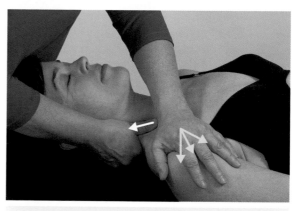

Figure 5.10
MMS A/P pressures of the mid-Cx with anteroposterior-caudal "glides" of the shoulder region – ipsilateral (SFL)

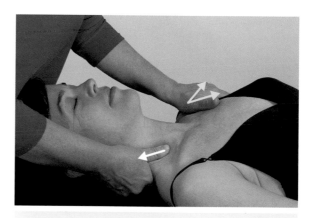

Figure 5.11
MMS A/P pressures of the mid-Cx with anteroposterior-caudal "glides" of the shoulder region – contralateral (SFL)

Stabilizing hand As per the technique above.

Mobilizing hand As per the technique above except that the therapist explores the area of the symphysis pubis (right, left, and center).

MMS A/P pressures of the right mid-Cx with anteroposterior caudal glides of the shoulder region – ipsilateral or contralateral (SFL) (Figures 5.10, 5.11)

This is a similar technique to that described in relation to the occipital region except that the anchor is at the mid-cervical spine.

Stabilizing hand As per the technique above.

Mobilizing hand The therapist's left hand explores the shoulder and shoulder girdle area with an anteroposterior caudal glide of the tissues in the area of the lateral clavicle and/or the GH joint, always looking for the immediate line of tension between the therapist's two hands as a gentle pressure of the caudal hand is performed. Sometimes tension is felt most with a posterior tilt of the scapula. If this fascial line is tight, the therapist will feel an immediate increase in tension in the anchoring hand, as if the mid-Cx region translates anteriorly and caudally. The patient perceives this as the therapist increasing his/her pressure on the anterior cervical spine. Similar concepts for mobilizing this line of fascia apply as per previous techniques.

MMS techniques: Cx in relation to the Deep Front Line of fascia (DFL)

Tom Myers's description of the Deep Front Line of fascia involves the temporomandibular joint (TMJ) muscles, the longus colli and capitis, infrahyoid and suprahyoid muscles, the cranium and facial bones, as well as the pericardium, anterior diaphragm, posterior diaphragm, central tendon of the diaphragm, psoas, iliacus, pelvic floor fascia, anterior sacral fascia, adductor magnus, adductor brevis, adductor longus, popliteus, and finally the tibialis posterior and the long toe flexors. A number of the fascial techniques to evaluate and treat tension of the DFL make particular use of combined dorsiflexion/eversion of the ankle, thereby increasing tension of the distal aspect of the DFL. Deep inspiration may also be used, which involves the diaphragm. These fascial connections become very apparent when working with the MMS techniques described below. (Refer to Chapter 2 for illustrations and a full description of this line of fascia.)

Techniques for this line are described below. Although the techniques described here are for the right mid-cervical spine, they may also be performed on the left side.

MMS A/P pressures of the right mid-Cx in relation to the pericardium (DFL) (Figure 5.12)

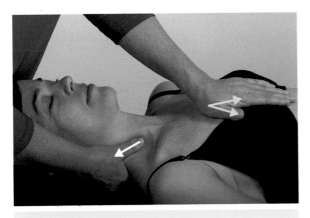

Figure 5.12
MMS A/P pressures of the mid-Cx with the pericardium (DFL)

Stabilizing hand As per the techniques for the Cx in relation to the SFL, using a grade IV– A/P mobilization in a cranial direction.

Mobilizing hand Using the left hand, the therapist explores the area of the pericardium, first by slowly sinking into the tissues **posterior** to the sternum and then, gently moving in a caudal direction, all the while maintaining the depth of the fascial line posterior to the sternum. The therapist looks for the angle where he/she perceives immediate tension in the hand anchoring the mid-cervical spine with an A/P pressure. That tension may be felt most in the pericardial area in a simple caudal direction, or caudal to the right of the client or caudal to the left. Sometimes the tension is most felt when moving the pericardial tissues mediolaterally or in a clockwise/counterclockwise direction, always maintaining the depth of the tissue. If no tension is perceived, then the DFL of fascia in relation to the anterior cervical spine is not tight. If this fascial line is tight, the therapist will feel an increase in tension in the anchoring hand, as if the mid-Cx region translates anteriorly and caudally. The patient perceives this as the therapist increasing his/her pressure on the anterior cervical spine. Similar concepts for mobilizing this line of fascia apply as per previous techniques.

MMS A/P pressures of the right mid-Cx in relation to the diaphragm (ipsilateral/contralateral) (DFL) (Figures 5.13, 5.14)

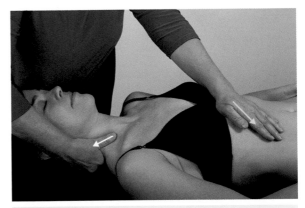

Figure 5.13
MMS A/P pressures of the mid-Cx with the ipsilateral diaphragm (DFL)

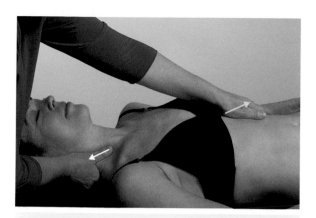

Figure 5.14
MMS A/P pressures of the mid-Cx with the contralateral diaphragm (DFL)

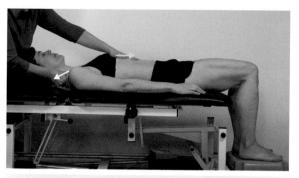

Figure 5.15
MMS A/P pressures of the mid-Cx with knee flexion (both SFL and DFL)

MMS A/P pressures of the right mid-Cx with knee flexion + shoulder flexion (both SFL and DFL) (Figure 5.16)

Stabilizing hand As per the technique above.

Mobilizing hand The therapist's left hand explores the anterior diaphragm area with a caudal/lateral glide of the tissues, always looking for the immediate line of tension between the two hands. Appropriate depth of tissues is required. The fascia around the rectus abdominis and oblique abdominal muscles may be accessed with this technique if the technique is done superficially (this would be a technique for the SFL). However, in order to access the diaphragm which is part of the DFL, the therapist must first slowly sink into the tissues posterior to the lower ribs and then gently move in a caudal/lateral direction. This technique may be done with either the ipsilateral or the contralateral diaphragm.

MMS A/P pressures of the right mid-Cx with hips extended, knees flexed (both SFL and DFL) (Figure 5.15)

All techniques in the section above may be further progressed by positioning the patient in supine, with the hips extended and knees flexed, and the table adjusted in height to ensure a comfortable position for the client's low back. This position puts additional tension on both the SFL and the DFL of fascia.

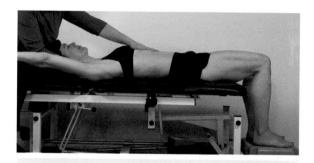

Figure 5.16
MMS A/P pressures of the right mid-Cx with knee flexion + shoulder flexion (both SFL and DFL)

The techniques above may be further progressed by adding bilateral shoulder flexion.

MMS A/P pressures of the right mid-Cx with ankle dorsiflexion/eversion (DFL) (Figure 5.17)

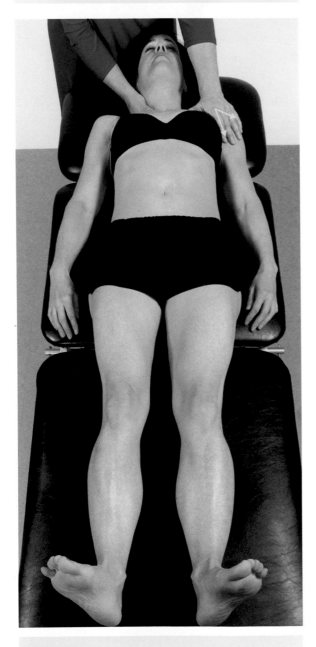

Figure 5.17
MMS A/P pressures of the mid-Cx with ankle DF/eversion (DFL)

Another way to progress the techniques is to add a combined movement of ankle dorsiflexion/eversion, thereby stretching the tibialis posterior muscle, the tail end of the DFL of fascia. The patient is asked to actively dorsiflex and evert both ankles, which increases the tension of the DFL from below. If the line is very tight, simply adding active dorsiflexion/eversion will immediately increase the tension in the mid-cervical area where the therapist is anchoring with an A/P pressure, directed cranially. If this fascial line is tight, the therapist will feel an increase in tension in his/her hands, as if the tissues of the anterior cervical spine were being dragged in an anterior and caudal direction. The therapist maintains the anchor of the mid Cx in a postero/cranial direction and waits until a softening of the system is perceived. The patient then releases the feet; the therapist may feel that the A/P pressure "gives" a little more in a postero/cranial direction. The slack of the tissues is taken up by the therapist as the patient continues to actively dorsiflex/evert the ankles. This continues until there is no further change perceived in the therapist's hands, and generally requires approximately five or six cycles. This technique can be progressed further by including the diaphragm, and asking the patient to take deep breaths in and out. Finally, the techniques may be progressed by asking the patient to maintain dorsiflexion/eversion as the therapist explores the pericardium, diaphragm, etc. This approach applies to all the techniques outlined in the above section.

Case report 5.1 Caroline's story*

This 52-year-old patient consulted for complaints of chronic, persistent right cervical pain, felt both anteriorly and posteriorly. There was history of mild whiplash two years prior to treatment, as well as a history of adhesive capsulitis in her right shoulder four years ago, which was treated with distension arthrography and physiotherapy with 85 percent return of ROM. She wore orthotics in her shoes and had previously been treated by a manual therapist for the articular dysfunctions in both her feet. She presently had no complaints of foot pain. X-rays and magnetic resonance imaging (MRI) showed some mild degenerative changes in the mid-cervical spine.

Her neck was sensitive to her husband's "abrupt driving habits" and this made the patient very nervous about her neck if she was a passenger in her husband's car. She had had previous treatment for her neck by another physiotherapist, who had used cervical mobilizations, ROM exercises, and dry needling techniques, with only partial relief of symptoms. On examination, it was noted that there were some pain-sensitizing issues and yellow flags, as she discussed her husband's contribution to her symptoms. Keeping this in mind, we proceeded with the assessment of her condition and found slight articular restrictions, with a lack of flexion at C4–5 and C5–6 as well as stiffness reproducing local pain with A/P pressures at C4, C5, and C6 on the right side. The craniocervical flexion test (CCFT) was done to assess the action and endurance of her deep neck stabilizers. Her score was low, being able to maintain only 22 mgHg pressure for 5 seconds. In addition there was a deficit in the cervical proprioceptive function. Evaluation of the fascial system revealed tension in the Superficial and Deep Front Lines of fascia, with restrictions noted particularly between the A/P pressures of C4–6 on the right with the sternum, symphysis pubis and right anteroposterior caudal glides of the shoulder region (SFL techniques) as well as the pericardium and right anterior diaphragm (DFL techniques). All of these issues were treated with the appropriate techniques and her pain decreased by 60 percent from the initial treatment. After eight treatments she had hit a plateau. By then, her CCFT testing was normal and the deep extensors of the cervical spine also tested as within normal limits. Cervical proprioception tests had much improved and there was no longer any tension with the fascial techniques above. Taking into consideration her previous history of foot problems, I then explored and treated the anterior cervical spine fascial techniques with movement of her feet (dorsiflexion/eversion), which pre-tenses the DFL. It was only after we released this fascial line all the way down to her feet that her chronic cervical symptoms resolved. We could then surmise that her previous foot dysfunctions may have contributed to tension in the DFL of fascia, affecting the cervical spine. Perhaps her "back-seat driver" habits of putting pressure on imaginary brakes increased tension in the cervical spine via the DFL!

* Please note that the patient's name has been changed to protect her privacy

MMS techniques: mid-cervical region in relation to the glenohumeral joint

Fascial restrictions between the mid-Cx spine and the GH joint is a factor that must be considered in cases of persistent "shoulder" restriction, cervical tension, and a loss of mobility of the neural system. Described below are a few common patterns of fascial restriction. Any movement of the GH joint may be used with these techniques. Shoulder abduction, external rotation and flexion are demonstrated below.

MMS A/P pressures of the right mid-Cx with passive GH abduction (Figure 5.18)

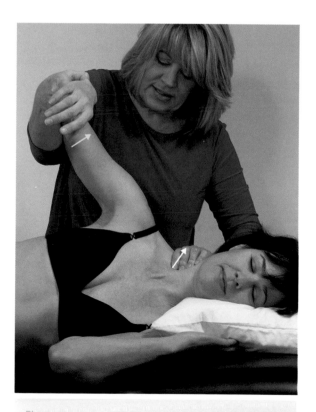

Figure 5.18
MMS A/P pressures of the mid-Cx with GH passive abduction

Stabilizing hand The patient is in left side-lying position. The therapist's left hand anchors to an area of the anterior mid-Cx spine that is chronically stiff (often C4) using an A/P mobilization.

Mobilizing hand The therapist's right hand supports the uppermost upper extremity and performs a passive physiological movement of the GH joint into abduction, stopping as soon as an increase in tension is perceived in the hand palpating the mid-cervical spine in an A/P direction (to the first resistance or R1 of Maitland's movement diagram). If there is tension in this line of fascia, it will seem like the mid-Cx region translates anteriorly before full GH abduction can be achieved (usually around 90–100 degrees of abduction). The therapist maintains the A/P pressure and simply prevents the segment from moving anteriorly. The patient perceives this as the therapist increasing his/her pressure on the cervical spine. The therapist performs repeated passive physiological abduction of the shoulder while maintaining a steady pressure on the cervical spine, always to when R1 is perceived (a grade III– passive physiological movement in Maitland terms). This movement is repeated until a release is felt between the therapist's two hands, progressing from a grade III– to a grade III and finally a grade III+. It generally requires approximately five to eight cycles.

> MMS A/P pressures of the right mid-Cx with passive glenohumeral external rotation (Figure 5.19)

Stabilizing hand As per the technique above.

Mobilizing hand As per the technique above except that the therapist performs a passive physiological GH external rotation movement.

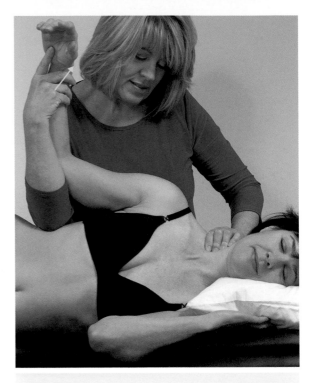

Figure 5.19
MMS A/P pressures of the mid-Cx with GH passive ER

> MMS A/P pressures of the right mid-Cx with passive glenohumeral flexion (Figure 5.20)

Stabilizing hand As per the technique above except that the therapist uses their right hand to stabilize the mid-Cx.

Mobilizing hand As per the technique above except that the therapist uses their left hand to perform a passive physiological GH flexion movement.

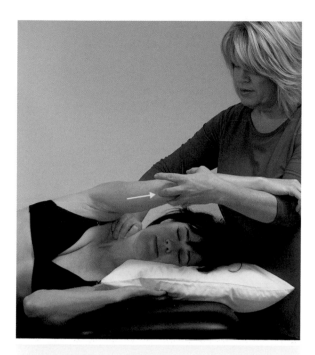

Figure 5.20
MMS A/P pressures of the mid-Cx with GH passive flexion

Case report 5.2 Beverly's story

This 45-year-old patient had initially come for treatment with complaints of tension in her right arm whenever she performed reaching movements requiring abduction. Evaluation revealed positive neurodynamic tension tests for the median and radial nerve on the right, with mobility issues at the interfaces of the mid-cervical spine, especially with lateral shears to the left and A/P mobilizations from C2 to C7. Treatment was directed to improving the mobility of the median nerve (positioning the arm in abduction, external rotation, elbow extension and wrist and finger extension) and then adding A/P mobilizations and lateral shear movements from C2 to C7. (Keep in mind that fascia around the nerve extends beyond the usual levels of C5 to C7.) As well, the nerve mobility test itself was used as a treatment technique, both as a sliding technique and a tensioning technique. A similar approach was used for the radial nerve, the only difference being that the arm was positioned in internal rotation and the wrist and fingers were flexed. Three treatments later, she reported that abduction movements were no longer problematic but that when she reached forward into flexion to get something from a cupboard, she could still feel her arm symptoms. Previously positive tests and techniques were negative, so I then proceeded to test the mobility of the anterior cervical fascia in left side-lying with passive physiological shoulder flexion (technique above). Although she had very little tension in the mid-Cx with passive shoulder abduction and external rotation, 45 degrees of shoulder flexion increased tension in the anterior mid-Cx, as if the myofascial tissues in this direction were tethering the cervical spine anteriorly. We used this MMS technique until she was able to obtain full shoulder flexion without subsequent pull on the mid-Cx and successfully treated her remaining symptoms. Prior to this case, I had not explored the anterior cervical fascia with shoulder flexion. This was a perfect case of "listen to the patient. He/she will tell you what the problem is and how to treat it" (Maitland 1992; Vail IFOMPT Conference, Vail, Colorado, 1992).

MMS techniques: mid-cervical region in relation to the scapula

Fascial restrictions are also common between the mid-cervical spine and the scapula. A similar approach is used but this time, the mid-Cx is assessed in relation to the scapular movements rather than shoulder movements. Ideally, the therapist should not feel the mid-Cx translate anteriorly before the scapula attains full movement in any direction (particularly scapular elevation, depression, retraction, and upward rotation). This technique can be useful for cases of persistent scapular dysfunctions despite exercise programs or in cases of chronic cervical tension.

MMS A/P pressures of the right mid-Cx with scapular depression (Figure 5.21)

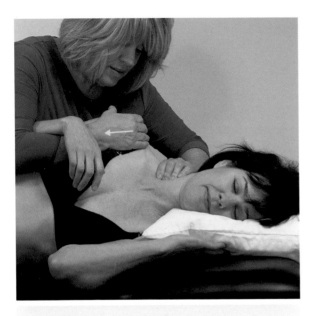

Figure 5.21
MMS A/P pressures of the mid-Cx with scapular depression

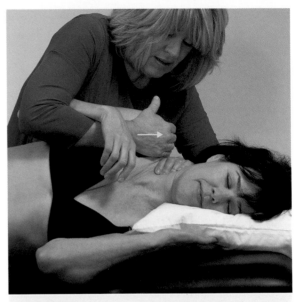

Figure 5.22
MMS A/P pressures of the mid-Cx with scapular elevation

Stabilizing hand As per the technique above, in left side-lying.

Mobilizing hand As per the technique above except that the therapist performs a passive physiological depression of the scapula.

MMS A/P pressures of the right mid-Cx with scapular elevation (Figure 5.22)

Stabilizing hand As per the technique above.

Mobilizing hand As per technique above except that the therapist performs a passive physiological elevation of the scapula.

MMS A/P pressures of the right mid-Cx with scapular retraction (Figure 5.23)

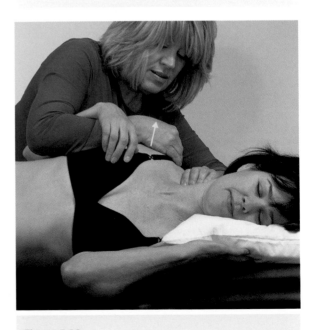

Figure 5.23
MMS A/P pressures of the mid-Cx with scapular retraction

Stabilizing hand As per the technique above.

Mobilizing hand As per the technique above except that the therapist performs a passive physiological retraction of the scapula.

MMS techniques: mid-cervical region in relation to the Lateral Line

Tom Myers's description of the Lateral Line of fascia involves the splenius capitis, the SCM, external and internal intercostals, ribs, lateral abdominal obliques, iliac crest, anterior and posterior superior iliac spines (ASIS and PSIS), gluteus maximus, tensor fasciae latae, iliotibial band (ITB), fibular head, peroneal muscles, and the lateral crural compartment. (Refer to Chapter 2 for illustrations and a full description of this line of fascia.) The technique below may be considered in cases of persistent tension/pain in the cervical or thoracic area.

MMS right lateral mid-Cx with lateral ribcage (Figure 5.24)

Stabilizing hand The patient is in a left side-lying position. Using the left hand, the therapist stabilizes the lateral aspect of the cervical spine with a lateral to medial pressure of the tissues (i.e., toward the plinth). This hand-hold involves both the articular components as well as the lateral cervical musculature, including the scalene muscles and levator scapulae. In addition, the patient's shoulder may be flexed to increase tension on the latissimus dorsi and its fasciae.

Mobilizing hand The therapist's right forearm explores the lateral ribcage/intercostal area, using the star concept. The therapist may explore moving the lateral ribcage in a number of possible directions:

- in a caudal direction (toward the patient's feet)

- in a caudal-anterior direction (the therapist must adjust their forearm to begin the maneuver slightly posterior to the lateral ribcage), and/or

- in a caudal posterior direction (the therapist must adjust their forearm to begin the maneuver slightly anterior to the lateral ribcage).

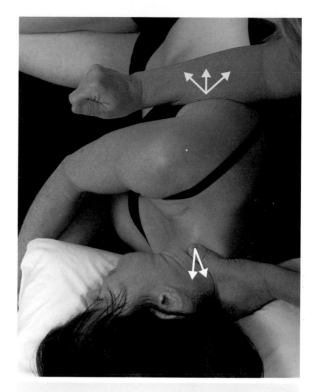

Figure 5.24
MMS: lateral mid-cervical spine with lateral ribcage

Note that the directions of the mobilizing forearm follow the diamond shape of the intercostal muscles. The ribcage may be explored in this manner both in the lower thoracic region and in the middle thoracic region. This is a general technique and not specific to a thoracic ring, although correcting a specific thoracic ring may also be done with this technique. The therapist looks for the angle and the area(s) on the ribcage where he/she perceives immediate tension in the hand palpating the mid-cervical spine (to the first resistance or R1 of Maitland's movement diagram). If there is tension in this line of fascia, it will seem like the mid-cervical region translates laterally before full caudal glide of the thoracic ribcage can be achieved. The therapist maintains the medial pressure of the cervical spine and simply prevents the segment from moving laterally. The patient perceives this as the therapist increasing his/her pressure on the cervical spine. Similar concepts for mobilizing this line of fascia apply as per previous techniques.

MMS techniques: mid-cervical region in relation to the Spiral Line

Besides restrictions in the SBL of fascia, persistent tension or pain in the craniovertebral (Cr/V) area (occiput and C2) may also be due to restrictions with the Spiral Line of fascia. Exploring these two areas in relation to the opposite thorax is frequently beneficial if the spiral line is a problem. (Refer to Chapter 2 for a full description and illustration of this line of fascia.)

> ### MMS unilateral P/A of C2 on the right in relation to the right Spiral Line (Figure 5.25)

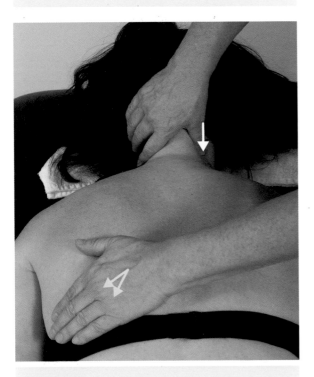

Figure 5.25
MMS unilateral P/A of C2 in relation to the right Spiral Line

Stabilizing hand The patient is in a prone position. The therapist uses his/her right thumb to perform a unilateral P/A pressure on the lamina of C2 on the right side (grade IV–).

Mobilizing hand The therapist's left hand explores the thoracic ribcage on the left side with a caudal/lateral glide of the tissues, always looking for the immediate line of tension between the two hands. Appropriate depth of tissues is required: sometimes tension is found with a more superficial glide of the ribcage; sometimes with a deeper/more anterior component to the caudal/lateral glide. If no tension is perceived, then the spiral of fascia in relation to C2 is not tight. If this fascial line is tight, the therapist will feel an immediate increase in tension in the anchoring hand, as if C2 pulls into right rotation, relative to C3. The patient perceives this as the therapist increasing his/her pressure on C2. If tension is perceived (quick resistance is felt between the two hands of the therapist), the therapist performs repeated caudal/lateral movement of the ribcage on the left while maintaining a steady pressure on C2 on the right, always to when R1 is perceived. This is repeated until a release is felt between the therapist's two hands; this generally requires approximately five to eight cycles.

> ### MMS right occiput in relation to the right Spiral Line (Figure 5.26)

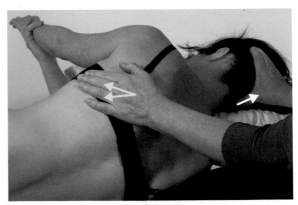

Figure 5.26
MMS right occiput in relation to the right Spiral Line

Stabilizing hand The patient is in a right side-lying position. The therapist uses his/her right thumb to perform a flexion (cranial glide) of the occiput on the right side. The arms of the patient may be offset (uppermost arm more anterior) in order to further protract the scapula and add more tension to this line.

Mobilizing hand As per the technique above.

MMS techniques for the cervicothoracic region

The fascia of the cervicothoracic (C/Thx) region may be explored in relation to the lateral line as well as the deeper fascia of the DFL. The following techniques are suggested:

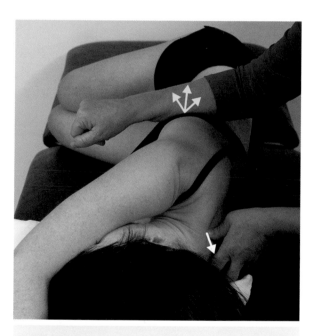

Figure 5.27
MMS C/Thx spine with lateral ribcage

MMS right C/Thx spine with lateral ribcage (Figure 5.27)

Stabilizing hand The patient is in a left side-lying position. The therapist stabilizes the lateral aspect of the spinous processes of the C/Thx spine (C7–T2) with a lateral to medial pressure of the tissues (i.e., towards the plinth).

Mobilizing hand As per the technique for MMS right lateral mid-Cx with lateral ribcage.

MMS C/Thx spine with right anterior cervical area

This particular technique does not address either Tom Myers's SFL or his SBL. It addresses the fascial tension that can occur between the anterior and posterior structures of the cervical region (DFL?) and thus contribute towards a forward head posture.

MMS C/Thx spine with right anterior cervical region (ipsilateral) (Figure 5.28)

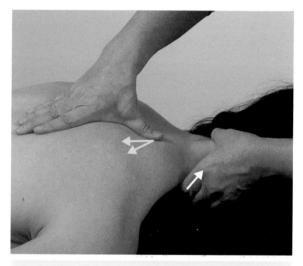

Figure 5.28
MMS C/Thx spine with right anterior cervical region (ipsilateral)

Stabilizing hand The patient is in a prone position. The therapist stabilizes the anterior cervical spine on the right side with an anteroposterior pressure directed cranially – this technique can be performed at several levels of the mid-cervical spine, notably C4, C5, and C6 levels.

Mobilizing hand The therapist then uses their left hand to explore the area of the right C/Thx spinous processes or facet joints, first by slowly sinking into the tissues of the C/Thx region and then gently pushing in a caudal direction, while maintaining the depth of the fascial line. The therapist looks for the angle where he/she perceives immediate tension in the hand palpating the anterior cervical region.

Tension may be felt most when the C/Thx spine is mobilized in a simple caudal direction, or caudal to the right of the client or caudal to the left. This technique can be explored anywhere from C7 to around T4 (spinous processes or facet joint area). The therapist may also explore the upper ribs, especially ribs 1 and 2, using a caudal glide of the costotransverse joint of the rib as a handle to explore this fascia. If no tension is perceived, then the fascia in between the anterior cervical spine and the C/Thx region is not tight. If this fascia is tight, the therapist will feel an immediate increase in tension in the anchoring hand, as if the mid-Cx region translates anteriorly and caudally. The patient perceives this as the therapist increasing his/her pressure on the anterior Cx spine. Similar concepts for mobilizing this line of fascia apply as per previous techniques.

MMS C/Thx spine with right anterior cervical region (contralateral) (Figure 5.29)

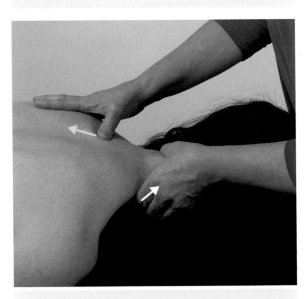

Figure 5.29
MMS C/Thx spine with right anterior cervical region (contralateral)

Stabilizing hand As per previous technique.

Mobilizing hand The therapist explores the tissues of the left C/Thx region, including the upper ribs. The technique is similar to the previous one.

MMS upper fibers of trapezius

The upper fibers of trapezius (UFT) are frequently hypertonic and facilitated. Dry needling may help restore a more normal tone to this muscle; however, tight fascia around the muscle may contribute to its tendency to be recalcitrant. The UFT are part of Tom Myers's Superficial Back Arm Line, and as such, may be put under tension with the addition of wrist and finger flexion. (Refer to Chapter 2 for a full description and illustration of this line of fascia.)

MMS UFT with wrist and finger flexion (SBAL) (Figure 5.30)

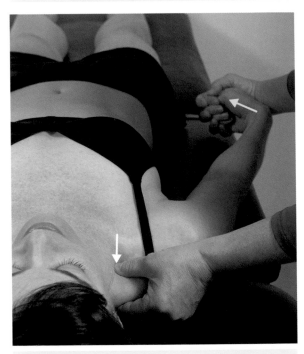

Figure 5.30
MMS UFT with wrist and finger flexion

Stabilizing hand The therapist "pinches" the UFT between the thumb and fingers and may explore the muscle along its length for tension.

Mobilizing hand The therapist flexes the patient's wrist and fingers, stopping as soon as an increase in tension is perceived in the hand palpating the UFT. If there is tension in this line of fascia, it will seem like the tension in the UFT increases before full wrist and finger flexion can be achieved. The therapist maintains the pinch of the UFT and simply prevents the tissues from gliding caudally. The patient perceives this as the therapist increasing his/her pressure on the muscle. The therapist performs repeated caudal movement of the wrist while maintaining a steady pressure on the UFT, always to when R1 is perceived. This action is repeated until a release is felt between the therapist's two hands; this generally requires approximately five to eight cycles.

Although not technically part of Tom Myers's SFL, the UFT muscle is often fascially tight in relation to this line. It may be mobilized as follows:

MMS UFT with the SFL

Stabilizing hand As per the previous technique.

Mobilizing hand The caudal hand explores the manubrial and sternal area with an anteroposterior caudal glide of the tissues, making sure that the touch is light and stays in the plane of the SFL similar to the technique for the anterior cervical spine in relation to the SFL. The therapist looks for the angle where he/she perceives immediate tension in the hand anchoring the UFT. That tension may be felt most when the moving hand mobilizes the fascia in a simple caudal direction, or caudal to the right of the client or caudal to the left. Sometimes the tension is most felt when moving the sternal tissues mediolaterally or in a clockwise/counterclockwise direction, always maintaining the depth of the tissue. If no tension is perceived, then the SFL of fascia in relation to this region is not tight. If tension is perceived (quick resistance is felt between the two hands of the therapist) then it can be mobilized as per the approaches outlined in Chapter 4.

This technique can also be used to explore the SFL all the way down to the rectus abdominis and symphysis pubis, as well as the shoulder/lateral clavicle area as per the MMS technique mid-Cx with anteroposterior caudal glides of the shoulder region   ipsilateral or contralateral. (Technique not pictured.)

For the following techniques, we will be using primarily the third concept of treatment when using MMS tech-

niques; that is, convert a nerve mobilization technique into a fascial technique. (Refer to Chapter 4 for further detail on concepts of treatment using MMS.)

MMS techniques: mid-cervical region in relation to neural tissues of the upper extremity

Indications

- Persistent tension/pain in the cervical spine and/or upper extremity.

- To mobilize the neural interfaces in relation to the upper extremity.

MMS A/P pressures of the right mid-Cx with scapular retraction, arm in upper ULNT2a position for the median nerve (Figure 5.31)

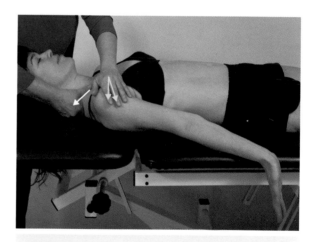

Figure 5.31
MMS A/P pressures of the mid-Cx with scapular retraction, arm in ULNT2a position for median nerve

Stabilizing hand The patient's arm is placed in about 30 degrees of abduction, with the wrist and fingers extended to pre-tense the median nerve; the therapist's right hand anchors to an area of the anterior mid-cervical spine that is chronically stiff (often C4) using an A/P mobilization in a cranial direction.

Mobilizing hand The therapist's left hand explores the ipsilateral shoulder and shoulder girdle area with an anteroposterior caudal glide of the tissues in the area of the lateral clavicle and/or the GH joint, always looking for the immediate line of tension with gentle pressure of the caudal hand. Sometimes tension is felt most with a posterior tilt or a lateral glide of the scapula. This technique can be explored anywhere from C1 to C7. Similar concepts for mobilizing this line of fascia apply as per previous techniques.

MMS A/P pressures of the right mid-Cx with scapular retraction, arm in ULNT2b position for the radial nerve (Figure 5.32)

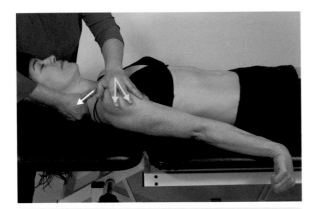

Figure 5.32
MMS A/P pressures of the Cx with scapular retraction, arm in ULNT2b position for radial nerve

Stabilizing hand As per the technique above, with the patient's arm placed in about 30 degrees of abduction, the wrist and fingers and thumb flexed to pre-tense the radial nerve.

Mobilizing hand As per the technique above.

MMS A/P pressures of the right mid-Cx with scapular retraction, arm in ULNT3 position for the ulnar nerve (Figure 5.33)

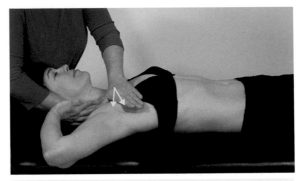

Figure 5.33
MMS A/P pressures of the mid-Cx with scapular retraction, arm in ULNT3 position for ulnar nerve

Stabilizing hand As per the technique above, with the patient's arm placed in about 80 degrees of abduction, with the elbow flexed, forearm pronated, wrist and fingers extended, to pre-tense the ulnar nerve.

Mobilizing hand As per the technique above.

MMS: Mid-Cx in relation to the shoulder girdle/clavicle

The mid-Cx may also be explored in relation to the shoulder girdle and clavicle (see Chapter 12).

MMS: C/Thx, mid-Cx and Cr/V area in relation to mobility of the dura

The mid-Cx may also be explored in relation to the dura (see Chapter 7).

Summary

This chapter has described MMS techniques that may be used for each region of the cervical spine: the craniovertebral area, the mid-cervical region and the cervicothoracic area. These techniques have been described in relation to Tom Myers's fascial lines, in particular the Superficial Back Line, the Superficial Front Line, the Deep Front Line, the Lateral Line, and the Spiral Line. MMS techniques for the cervical spine have also been described in relation to the glenohumeral joint and the scapula, along with an MMS technique for trigger points in relation to the upper fibers of trapezius. This concept may apply to any recurrent trigger point associated with dysfunction of the cervical spine. The next chapter will focus on techniques for the craniofacial region and the temporomandibular joint (TMJ).

The craniofacial region (cranium, temporomandibular joint)

When treating headaches, manual therapists are trained to assess and treat the joints of the cervical spine (especially the upper cervical spine), the temporomandibular joints (TMJ), and the muscles of the upper quadrant (looking for imbalance between hypertonic, tight muscles and weak muscles of the cervical spine and scapula). However, mobilizing joints and stretching individual muscles can achieve only partial benefits if the fascial system is not addressed.

This chapter will describe the clinical findings of restriction in the fascial lines in relation to the following areas:

- the muscles of the temporomandibular joint (TMJ) in relation to the SFL and the DFL
- the fascia of the scalp (epicranial fascia) in relation to the SFL and the Spiral Line
- the tongue in relation to the SFL and the DFL.

Although the techniques for the dura and fascia within the cranium are relevant to this chapter (because these tissues are frequently problematic in clients with head and facial pain), they are described separately in Chapter 7.

Indications for MMS for this chapter

1. Recurring craniofacial pain despite the following treatment approaches:
   - mobilization/manipulation of the cervical spine and thorax
   - stabilization exercises for the cervical spine and thorax
   - mobilization of the TMJ
   - release of trigger points to the cervical, thoracic and/or TMJ muscles with manual or dry needling techniques
   - treatment of cranial dysfunctions.
2. Tension in the anterior cervical spine/throat area.

Postural analysis

If there is restriction of the DFL of fascia, this may have an impact on posture, in particular the forward head posture that is so common. This tension can develop as a result of trauma, including surgical scars to the abdominal area. (One may think of the impact of caesarean section scars, old appendectomy scars, hernia repairs, etc.) As per the cervical spine, excessive time spent in the sitting position can also be a factor in creating these fascial lines of tension.

If there is restriction in the Lateral Line of fascia, this may create a lateral tilt or side shift of the thorax, the cervical spine, the lumbar spine, or the pelvis. It may also become a contributing factor for dysfunctions of the Lateral Line, more notably recurring issues with TMJ dysfunctions and headaches.

Concepts of treatment using MMS

For this chapter, we will be using primarily the first concept of treatment when using MMS techniques; that is, choose a recurrent articular dysfunction or myofascial trigger point and explore a fascial line in relation to it. The therapist anchors him/herself to a recurrent articular dysfunction or myofascial trigger point and assesses the fascial lines of tension in relation to the anchor, looking for early tension between their two hands.

The following approaches may be used, depending on how the tissues respond:

- work with oscillations (grades III−, III, III+)
- work with sustained pressure
- work with "harmonics" (Dr Laurie Hartman).

Please refer to Chapter 4 for further detail on concepts of treatment using MMS.

TMJ muscles: anatomical overview and palpation

The muscles around the TMJ are common sites of recurrent tension and frequently involved in dysfunction of the fascial lines (Figures 6.1, 6.2). They include temporalis, superficial masseter, medial pterygoid, mylohyoid, buccinator, and the supra- and infrahyoid muscles.

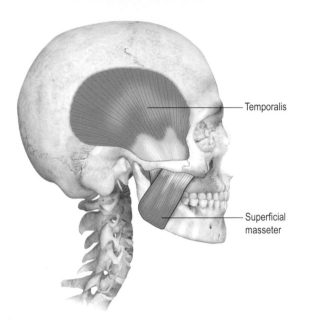

Figure 6.1
Temporalis and superficial masseter muscles

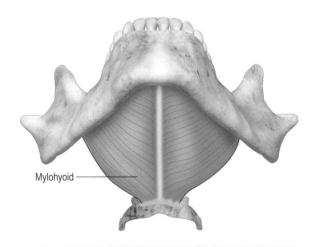

Figure 6.2
Mylohyoid muscle

Anchoring onto the TMJ muscles

Anchoring onto the temporalis muscle (Figure 6.3)

The temporalis muscle may be palpated along its entire breadth, including the anterior, middle, and posterior portions of the muscle belly itself as well as the tenoperiosteal junction of the muscle in the area of the greater wing of the sphenoid bone. The therapist looks for recurrent tension in the various parts of the muscle, which is frequently accompanied by pain on palpation. The therapist "hooks onto" the area of the muscle where there is most tension and pulls with both hands in a cranial direction.

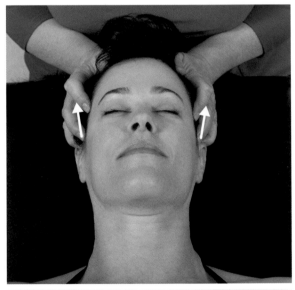

Figure 6.3
Anchoring onto temporalis

Anchoring onto the superficial masseter (Figure 6.4)

The superficial masseter muscle may be palpated along its entire breadth, including the zygomatic attachment, the mandibular attachment and the mid-portion of the muscle. The muscle may also be explored from its anterior portion, posteriorly towards the ear. The therapist looks for recurrent tension in the various parts of the muscle, which is

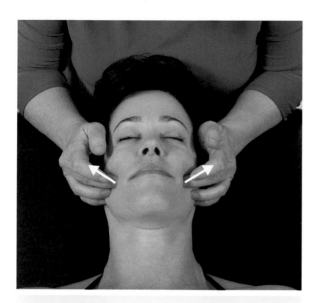

Figure 6.4
Anchoring onto superficial masseter

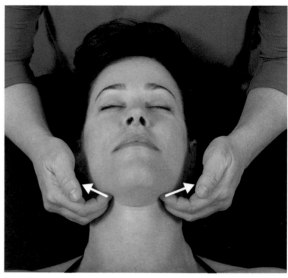

Figure 6.5
Anchoring onto medial pterygoid

frequently accompanied by pain on palpation. The therapist gently hooks onto the area of the muscle where there is most tension (often the anterior aspect of the mid-portion of the muscle) and pulls with both hands in a combined lateral/cranial direction.

Anchoring onto the medial pterygoid (Figure 6.5)

The medial pterygoid muscle is best palpated along its attachment under the mandible of the jaw. The muscle may also be explored from its anterior portion, posteriorly towards the ear. The therapist looks for recurrent tension in the various parts of the muscle, which is frequently accompanied by pain on palpation. The therapist gently hooks onto the area of the muscle where there is most tension and pulls with both hands in a combined lateral/cranial direction.

Anchoring onto the mylohyoid (Figure 6.6)

The mylohyoid muscle is best palpated along its attachment under the mandible, close to the center. The muscle may also be explored from its anterior portion and posteriorly towards the ear, about 2 cm on either side. The therapist looks for recurrent tension in the various parts of the muscle,

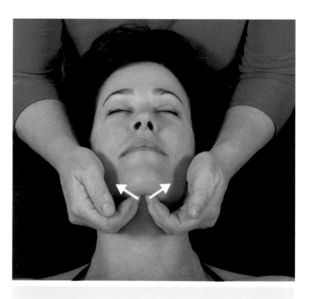

Figure 6.6
Anchoring onto mylohyoid

which is frequently accompanied by pain on palpation. The therapist gently hooks onto the area of the muscle where there is most tension and pulls with both hands in a combined lateral/cranial direction.

MMS techniques: temporomandibular joint muscles in relation to the SFL of fascia

Tom Myers's description of the SFL of fascia involves the scalp fascia, SCM, sternochondral fascia, pectoral muscles, rectus abdominis to the symphysis pubis. It then begins again at the origin of the rectus femoris and includes the quadriceps muscles, the patellar tendon, short and long toe extensors, tibialis anterior, and the anterior crural compartment. (Refer to Chapter 2 for a full description and illustration of this line of fascia.) These fascial connections become very apparent when working with the MMS techniques described in this chapter. The following techniques are demonstrated in relation to the superficial masseter muscle; however, any of the TMJ muscles may be explored in a similar fashion.

> MMS right superficial masseter with antero-posterior caudal glides of the shoulder region (SFL) (Figures 6.7, 6.8)

Stabilizing hand For this technique the therapist's right hand uses the anchor onto the right superficial masseter muscle (described above).

Mobilizing hand The therapist's left hand explores the shoulder and shoulder girdle area with an antero-posterior caudal glide of the tissues in the area of the lateral clavicle and/or the glenohumeral (GH) joint, using the "star concept" to find the direction of most tension between their two hands. Sometimes tension is felt most with a posterior tilt or lateral glide of the scapula. If this fascial line is tight, the therapist will feel an increase in tension in the anchoring hand, as if the superficial masseter muscle moves medially and caudally. The patient perceives this as the therapist increasing his/her pressure on the superficial masseter. If no tension is perceived, then the SFL of fascia in relation to this region is not tight. If tension is perceived (quick resistance is felt between the two hands of the therapist) then it can be mobilized as per the approaches outlined in Chapter 4. (The therapist maintains the anchor on the superficial masseter to prevent it from moving as he/she performs repeated A/P mobilizations of the ipsilateral or the contralateral shoulder area.)

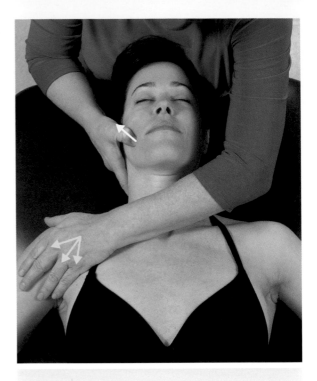

Figure 6.7
MMS right superficial masseter with anteroposterior-caudal "glides" of the shoulder region (SFL) – ipsilateral shoulder

NB This technique may be progressed by exploring the superficial masseter in relation to the rectus abdominis and the symphysis pubis, thereby exploring the upper quadrant aspect of the SFL. (See Chapter 5 for similar techniques in relation to the anterior mid-cervical area.)

Although demonstrated on the superficial masseter, this technique may be used with any of the TMJ muscles.

MMS techniques: TMJ muscles in relation to the DFL of fascia

Tom Myers's description of the Deep Front Line (DFL) of fascia involves the TMJ muscles, the longus colli and capitis, infrahyoid and suprahyoid muscles, the cranium and facial bones as well as the pericardium, anterior diaphragm, posterior diaphragm, central tendon of the diaphragm, psoas,

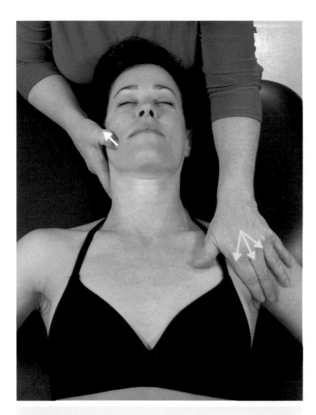

Figure 6.8
MMS right superficial masseter with anteroposterior-caudal "glides" of the shoulder region (SFL) – contralateral shoulder

MMS right superficial masseter in relation to the pericardium (DFL) (Figure 6.9)

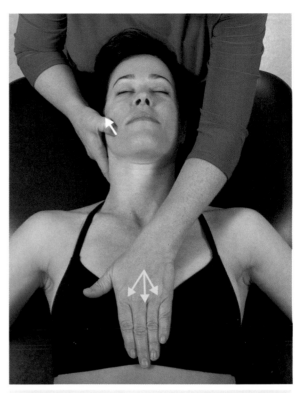

Figure 6.9
MMS right superficial masseter in relation to the pericardium (DFL)

iliacus, pelvic floor fascia, anterior sacral fascia, adductor magnus, adductor brevis, adductor longus, popliteus, and finally the tibialis posterior and the long toe flexors. A number of the fascial techniques to evaluate and treat tension of the DFL makes particular use combined dorsiflexion/eversion of the ankle, thereby increasing tension of the distal aspect of the DFL. Deep inspiration may also be used, which involves the diaphragm. These fascial connections become very apparent when working with the MMS techniques described below. (Refer to Chapter 2 for illustrations and a full description of this line of fascia.)

Note that the photos for the techniques below are demonstrated using the superficial masseter; however, all the TMJ muscles noted above may be used with these techniques.

Stabilizing hand Using the right hand, the therapist anchors onto the superficial masseter and pulls it gently in a craniolateral direction, maintaining the tension on this muscle.

Mobilizing hand The therapist then uses the left hand to explore the area of the pericardium, first by slowly sinking into the tissues **posterior** to the sternum and then gently pushing them in a caudal direction, all the while maintaining the depth of the fascial line posterior to the sternum. The therapist looks for the angle where he/she perceives immediate tension in the hand palpating the superficial masseter. Using the star concept to find the direction of most tension is useful here. That tension may be felt most in a simple caudal direction, or caudal to the right of the client or caudal to the left. Sometimes the tension is most felt when moving the pericardial tissues mediolaterally or in a clockwise/counterclockwise direction, always maintaining the depth of the tissue. If no tension is perceived, then the DFL of fascia in relation to this muscle is not tight. If this fascial line is tight, the therapist will feel an increase in tension in the anchoring hand, as if the superficial masseter muscle pulls medially and caudally. The patient perceives this as the therapist increasing his/her pressure on the superficial masseter. Similar concepts for mobilizing this line of fascia apply as per previous techniques.

MMS right superficial masseter in relation to the diaphragm (DFL) (Figures 6.10, 6.11)

Stabilizing hand As per technique above.

Mobilizing hand The therapist's left hand explores the anterior diaphragm area with a caudal/lateral glide of the tissues, always looking for the immediate line of tension between the two hands. Appropriate depth of tissues is required. The fascia around the rectus abdominis and oblique abdominal muscles may be accessed with this technique if the technique is done superficially. (This would be a technique for the SFL.) However, in order to access the diaphragm which is part of the DFL, the therapist must first slowly sink into the tissues posterior to the lower ribs and then gently push in a caudal/lateral direction. This technique can be done with either the ipsilateral or the contralateral diaphragm.

MMS superficial masseter with dorsiflexion/eversion of the ankle (pre-tensing the DFL via the tibialis posterior) (Figure 6.12)

Stabilizing hands For this technique the therapist's hands use the same anchor on both superficial masseter muscles

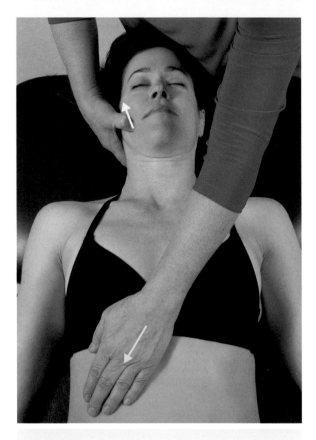

Figure 6.10
MMS right superficial masseter in relation to the ipsilateral diaphragm (DFL)

at the same time and the therapist pulls both hands gently in a cranial-lateral direction.

Movement The patient is asked to actively dorsiflex and evert both ankles and take a deep breath in, thereby increasing the tension of the DFL from below. If this fascial line is tight, the therapist will feel an increase in tension in their hands, as if the tissues were being pulled in a caudal-medial direction. The therapist maintains the hold towards a cranial-medial direction with both hands until a softening of

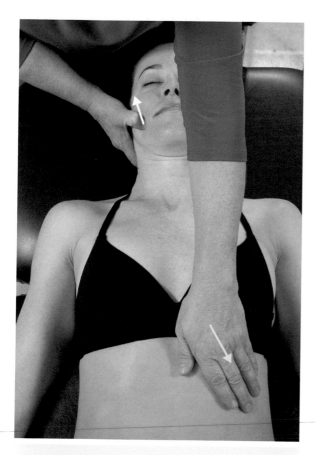

Figure 6.11
MMS right superficial masseter in relation to the contralateral diaphragm (DFL)

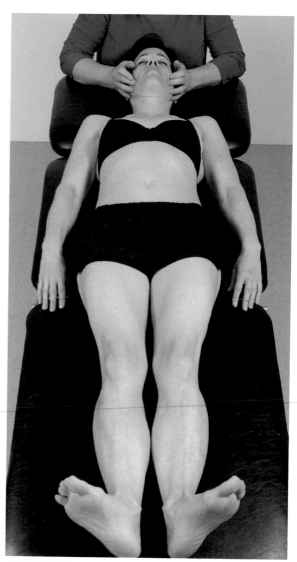

Figure 6.12
MMS superficial masseter with ankle DF/eversion (DFL)

the system is perceived. The client then releases the feet and breathes normally: the therapist may feel that both hands can glide a little more cranially. The slack of the tissues is taken up by the therapist as the patient continues to actively dorsiflex/evert the ankles and take deep breaths. This sequence continues until there is no further change perceived in the therapist's hands and generally requires approximately five or six cycles.

Finally, the techniques may be progressed by asking the patient to maintain dorsiflexion/eversion as the therapist explores the pericardium, diaphragm, etc.

This applies to all the techniques outlined in the above section.

NB This technique may be used with any of the TMJ muscles.

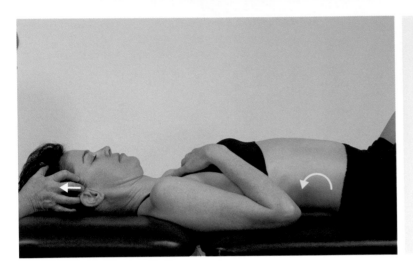

Figure 6.13
MMS temporalis with anterior pelvic tilt

MMS temporalis with anterior pelvic tilt (Figure 6.13)

Stabilizing hands As per technique above except that the therapist anchors onto both temporalis muscles (see anchoring technique at the start of the chapter).

Movement The patient is asked to perform an anterior pelvic tilt, thereby increasing the tension of the DFL from below. If this fascial line is tight, the therapist will feel an increase in tension in their hands as if the tissues were being pulled in a caudal direction. The therapist maintains the hold with both hands towards a cranial direction until a softening of the system is perceived. The patient then releases the pelvis back to a more neutral position – the therapist may feel that both hands can glide a little more cranially. The slack of the tissues is taken up by the therapist as the patient continues to actively do an anterior pelvic tilt. This continues until there is no further change perceived in the therapist's hands and generally requires approximately five or six cycles.

NB This technique may be used with any of the TMJ muscles.

MMS techniques: temporomandibular joint muscles in relation to the Lateral Line of fascia

Tom Myers's description of the Lateral Line of fascia involves the splenius capitis, SCM, external and internal intercostals, ribs, lateral abdominal obliques, iliac crest, anterior and posterior superior iliac spines (ASIS and PSIS), gluteus maximus, tensor fasciae latae, iliotibial band (ITB), fibular head, peroneal muscles, and lateral crural compartment. Although technically not part of the Lateral Line, the TMJ muscles have clinical connections with this line. (Refer to Chapter 2 for illustrations and a full description of this line of fascia.)

MMS right superficial masseter with the lateral ribcage (Figures 6.14–6.16)

Stabilizing hand The patient is in a left side-lying position. The therapist's left hand anchors onto the superficial masseter, using a craniolateral "hook."

Mobilizing hand The therapist's right forearm explores the lateral ribcage/intercostal area, using the star concept. The therapist may explore moving the lateral ribcage in a number of possible directions:

- in a caudal direction (toward the patient's feet)
- in a caudal-anterior direction (the therapist must adjust their forearm to begin the maneuver slightly posterior to the lateral ribcage), and/or
- in a caudal-posterior direction (the therapist must adjust their forearm to begin the maneuver slightly anterior to the lateral ribcage).

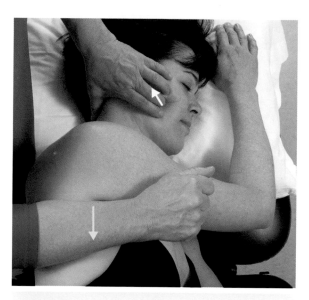

Figure 6.14
MMS right superficial masseter with the lateral ribcage (caudal direction)

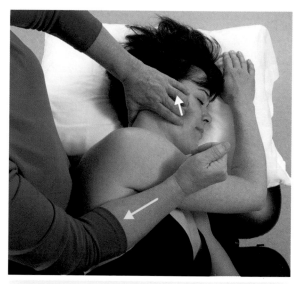

Figure 6.16
MMS right superficial masseter with the lateral ribcage (caudal-posterior direction)

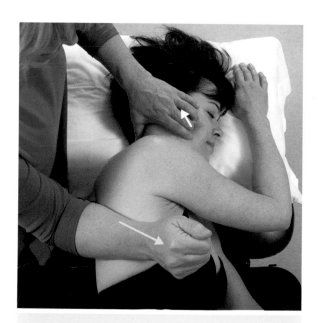

Figure 6.15
MMS right superficial masseter with the lateral ribcage (caudal anterior direction)

Note that the directions of the mobilizing forearm follow the diamond shape of the intercostal muscles. The ribcage may be explored in this manner both in the lower thoracic region and the middle thoracic region. This is a general technique, but it may also be used in relation to a specific thoracic ring. The therapist looks for the angle and the area(s) on the ribcage where he/ she perceives immediate tension in the hand anchoring the right superficial masseter. If this fascial line is tight, the therapist will feel an increase in tension in their anchoring hand, as if the tissues were being pulled in a caudal direction. If tension is perceived (quick resistance is felt between the two hands of the therapist), then it can be mobilized as per the approaches outlined in Chapter 4.

MMS temporalis with lateral ribcage (Figure 6.17)

This technique is performed as above except that the therapist anchors onto the temporalis muscle (anterior, middle and/or posterior aspect) and also explores the muscle in its entirety.

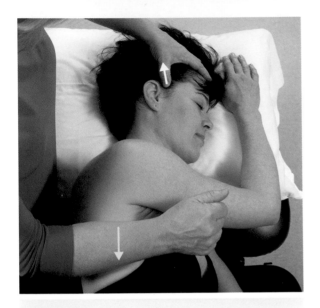

Figure 6.17
MMS right temporalis with lateral ribcage

MMS techniques: TMJ muscles in relation to the Spiral Line

As with the Lateral Line, the TMJ muscles have clinical anecdotal evidence of their involvement with the Spiral Line. (Refer to Chapter 2 for illustrations and a full description of this line of fascia.)

MMS temporalis with lumbar rotation (Figure 6.18)

Stabilizing hands For this technique the therapist's hands use the same anchor on both superficial masseter muscles or both temporalis muscles at the same time. The therapist pulls both hands gently in a cranial direction.

Movement The patient is in a crook-lying position. He/she is asked to let their knees slowly drop to the right, thereby inducing lumbar rotation to the left. If the Spiral Line is tight, the therapist will feel an increase in tension in their hands as if the tissues were being pulled in a caudal direction. The patient perceives this as the therapist increasing

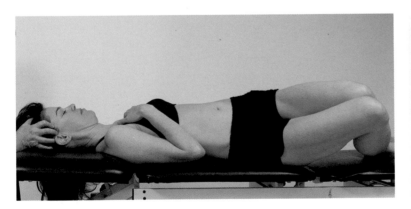

Figure 6.18
MMS temporalis with lumbar rotation

his/her pressure on the superficial masseter muscles or the temporalis muscles. The therapist maintains the hold with both hands in a cranial direction until a softening of the system is perceived. The patient then brings the knees back to a more neutral position – the therapist may feel that both hands can glide a little more cranially. The slack of the tissues is taken up by the therapist as the patient continues to actively rotate to the right or the left. This continues until there is no further change perceived in the therapist's hands and generally requires approximately five or six cycles.

NB This technique may be used with any of the TMJ muscles.

Case report 6.1 Lois's story*

Lois was a 40-year-old university English professor with complaints of chronic pain in the area of the temporal and occipital regions bilaterally, as well as tooth pain in the left lower mandibular area (tooth 37). She also had a history of cervical and scapular pain that had resolved a couple of months earlier. This head and tooth pain interfered with her sleep and was particularly bad in the morning. At its worst, she was unable to concentrate, experienced nausea, and was unable to tolerate the upright position. The pain began after a neck injury in a car accident two years prior, followed shortly thereafter by a dental laser procedure that exacerbated her cervical, scapular, head, and tooth pain. The dental injury affected her bite so that her upper and lower teeth no longer touched on the right side. A dental specialist had recommended shaving down the teeth in order to normalize the patient's bite, but the patient did not go through this procedure. She had had a number of treatments to address her issues: Botox, acupuncture, dry needling, dental appliances, cranial and general osteopathy, lidocaine injections (administered by doctors in a pain clinic). These approaches helped her cervical and scapular pain but not her tooth pain and provided only

temporary relief of her head pain. Chronic pain is usually multifactorial and this case was no exception. The initial physiotherapy evaluation revealed problems with articular mobility in the cervical and craniovertebral joints, muscle imbalance issues in the upper quadrant, including weakness of the cervical and scapular stabilizers, decreased dural mobility, and hypertonic TMJ muscles. All of these issues were addressed with the appropriate techniques. However, it was not until the fascial techniques in relation to the TMJ were introduced that the patient began to show subjective improvement in her head pain symptoms. As well, her dentist testified that her bite had returned to a fully normal position. Treatment of the fascia of the TMJ muscles (temporalis, deep masseter, medial and lateral pterygoid muscles, buccinator complex) in relation to the DFL, Spiral Line and Lateral Line techniques were used as well as MMS techniques to the occipitalis (see Chapter 5) and the anterior sacral fascia (see Chapter 10). In addition, the fascia of the problematic tooth was found to be tight and was released, both in relation to its mandibular attachment and also in relation to the DFL of fascia. This approach to treatment solved her tooth pain and decreased her head pain to the point where she was able to concentrate, sleep better, and resume her writing. A combination of MMS along with movement therapies (Qi gong, Pilates, aerobic exercise) is the program that allows this patient to now be more functional.

* Please note that the patient's name has been changed to protect her privacy.

Buccinator/pharyngeal constrictor complex and its fascia (Figure 6.19)

Clinical implications

This muscle complex comprises the buccinator muscle, which runs from the orbicularis oris muscle surrounding the mouth,

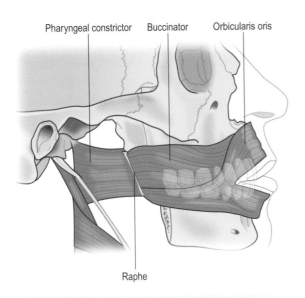

Pharyngeal constrictor   Buccinator   Orbicularis oris

Raphe

Figure 6.19
Buccinator/pharyngeal constrictor complex

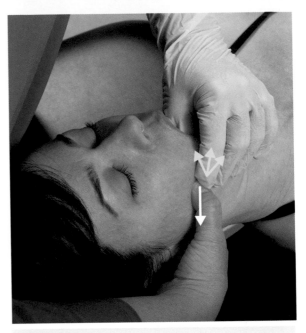

Figure 6.20
MMS right buccinator with raphe

and then connects to a fascial raphe that is easily palpable just anterior to the superficial masseter muscle. It then continues posteriorly to connect with the pharyngeal constrictor muscle, which attaches to the occiput and to the anterior aspect of the body of C2. The pterygoid plates of the sphenoid bone also have a fascial connection to this complex. It is frequently problematic with cases of recurrent TMJ dysfunction, as tension here may retract the mandible, leading to TMJ disc dysfunction and myofascial TMJ pain. Releasing this complex often helps to release other frequently tight TMJ muscles, such as the masseter and pterygoid muscles.

MMS right buccinator with raphe (Figure 6.20)

Stabilizing hand To release the right buccinator/pharyngeal constrictor complex and its fascia, the therapist uses the thumb of the right hand to palpate the raphe on the outside of the patient's right cheek and anchor it with a gentle pull towards the occiput – the rest of his/her hand encompasses the head and occiput.

Mobilizing hand The therapist's left hand "pinches" the right cheek, as close to the raphe as possible, with the left thumb inside the mouth and the index on the outside of the cheek. Using the left hand, the therapist pulls gently towards the patient's mouth, using the star concept to seek a direction where there is the most tension between the therapist's two hands (there may be a cranial or caudal component to the medial pull). The therapist maintains the hold with both hands until a softening of the system is perceived. The patient's respiration may be used to facilitate release.

MMS right buccinator with sphenoid (Figure 6.21)

Stabilizing hand The therapist's left hand maintains the same position in the mouth but now becomes the stabilizer, as the therapist pulls the tissues gently in a caudal direction.

Mobilizing hand The therapist changes the position of their right hand to encompass the greater wings of the patient's sphenoid bone, just lateral to the eyes (anchoring both the left and right side of the sphenoid). The therapist gently pulls the sphenoid bone in a cranial direction,

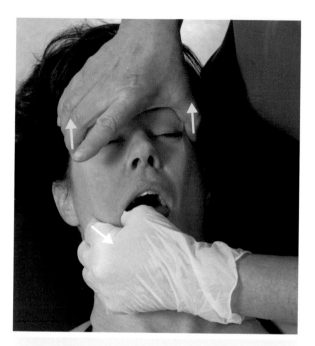

Figure 6.21
MMS right buccinator with sphenoid

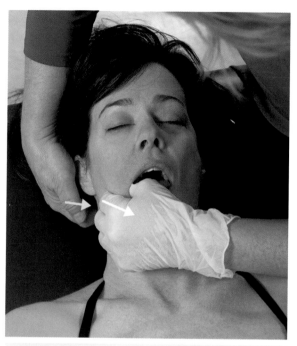

Figure 6.22
MMS right buccinator with occiput

looking for early tension between the two hands. If there is tension in this fascial line, the therapist will feel an increase in tension of their anchoring hand. The patient perceives this as the therapist increasing his/her pressure on the raphe of the buccinator. The therapist maintains the hold with both hands until a softening of the system is perceived. The patient's respiration may be used to facilitate release.

MMS right buccinator with occiput (Figure 6.22)

Stabilizing hand As per the previous technique.

Mobilizing hand The therapist changes the position of his/her right hand to encompass the occiput, with the index and middle fingers focused on the right occipital condyle, and pulls this occipital area in a medial direction, looking for early tension between the two hands. The patient's respiration may be used to facilitate release.

Adding the fascial component

These three techniques to release the buccinator/pharyngeal constrictor muscle complex can be progressed by adding a gentle active chin-nod movement to the fascial technique. It may also be assessed and treated in relation to the DFL by simply adding bilateral ankle dorsiflexion/eversion or anterior pelvic tilt and repeating the process.

Anterior cervical fascia: supra- and infrahyoid region

This area is important to explore, especially with those patients complaining of tension in the throat, or those with persistent cervical or TMJ pain.

MMS right suprahyoid fascia (Figure 6.23)

Stabilizing hand The therapist's left hand hooks onto the right side of the hyoid bone, pulling it gently towards the left and slightly caudally.

Mobilizing hand The therapist's right hand explores the muscles and fascia of the caudal edge of the mandible on the right side, pulling them gently in a cranial and lateral direction. If this fascial line is tight, the therapist will

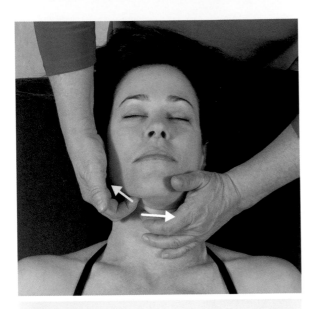

Figure 6.23
MMS right suprahyoid fascia

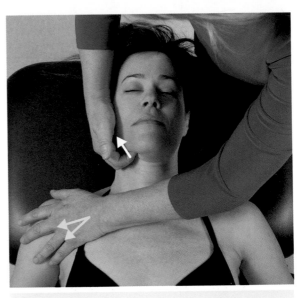

Figure 6.24
MMS right suprahyoid fascia with clavicle – ipsilateral

feel an immediate increase in tension in their stabilizing hand. The therapist maintains the hold with both hands until a softening of the system is perceived. The patient's respiration may be used to facilitate release. The fascia can also be assessed and worked in relation to the DFL by simply adding bilateral ankle dorsiflexion/eversion or anterior pelvic tilt. The slack of the tissues is taken up by the therapist, as the patient continues to actively do an anterior pelvic tilt and/or dorsiflex/evert the feet. This continues until there is no further change perceived in the therapist's hands; this generally requires approximately five or six cycles.

MMS right suprahyoid fascia with clavicle (SFL)
(Figures 6.24, 6.25)

Stabilizing hand The therapist's right hand explores the muscles and fascia of the caudal edge of the mandible on the right side, pulling it gently in a cranial and lateral direction.

Mobilizing hand The therapist's left hand explores the shoulder and shoulder girdle area with an antero-posterior caudal glide of the tissues in the area of the whole clavicle and/or the GH joint, using the star

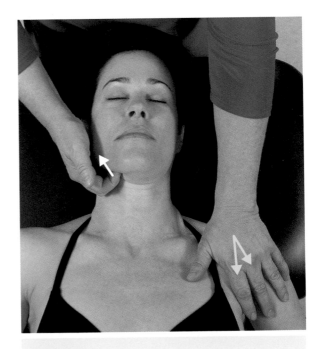

Figure 6.25
MMS right suprahyoid fascia with clavicle – contralateral

concept to seek the direction where an immediate line of tension is felt between the therapist's hands as gentle pressure is applied with the caudal hand. This can be done using either the ipsilateral or the contralateral clavicular/shoulder area, as the therapist explores the SFL of fascia. If this fascial line is tight, the therapist will feel an immediate increase in tension in the hand anchoring the suprahyoid region. The therapist maintains the hold with both hands until a softening of the system is perceived. The patient perceives this as the therapist increasing his/her pressure on the mandible. If no tension is perceived, then the SFL of fascia in relation to this region is not tight. If tension is perceived (quick resistance is felt between the two hands of the therapist) then it can be mobilized as per the approaches outlined in Chapter 4. (The therapist maintains the anchor on the suprahyoid region to prevent it from moving as he/she performs repeated A/P mobilizations of the ipsilateral or the contralateral shoulder area.)

MMS right suprahyoid fascia with pericardium (DFL)

The area of the manubrium, sternum, and pericardium may also be explored in this fashion (for the DFL of fascia). The fascia can also be assessed and worked in relation to the DFL by simply adding bilateral ankle dorsiflexion/eversion or anterior pelvic tilt. The slack of the tissues is taken up by the therapist as the patient continues to actively do an anterior pelvic tilt and/or dorsiflex/evert the feet. This continues until there is no further change perceived in the therapist's hands; this generally requires approximately five or six cycles. (Technique not shown.)

MMS right infrahyoid fascia with pericardium (Figure 6.26)

Stabilizing hand To release the right infrahyoid fascia in relation to the SFL or DFL, the therapist's left hand hooks onto the right side of the hyoid bone, pulling it gently toward the left and slightly cranially.

Mobilizing hand As per the above two techniques for the suprahyoid fascia. Figure 6.26 depicts the technique performed in relation to the pericardial fascia (for the DFL of fascia).

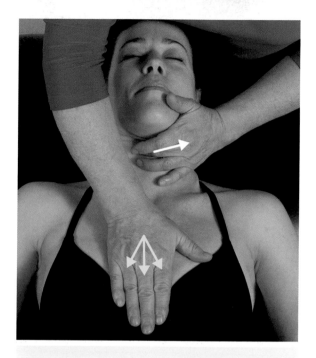

Figure 6.26
MMS right infrahyoid fascia with pericardium

MMS techniques: scalp fascia

Tension in the fascia of the epicranium is a common problem with those patients who suffer from tension headaches. The epicranium is also connected to the intracranial fascia and, if tight, can maintain cranial dysfunction (Paoletti 2006). Patients with this problem report decreased head pain if they or someone else pulls on their hair (large sections of hair, not individual hairs!). The hair (if present) can be a useful lever to move and tension the epicranial fascia below it.

MMS scalp fascia (epicranium): "hair-pull technique" (Figure 6.27)

For this technique, the therapist grasps the patient's hair (global hold) and pulls gently in a cranial direction. Various parts of the scalp and epicranial fascia can be accessed this way. If the client has little to no hair, the scalp fascia can be accessed by using a lumbrical grip of

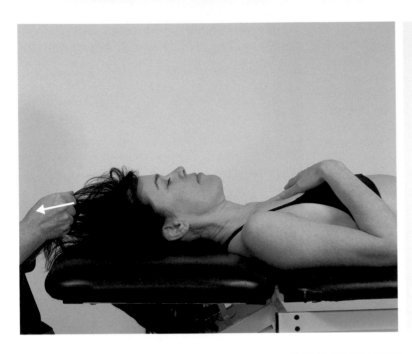

Figure 6.27
MMS scalp fascia (epicranium) – "hair-pull technique"

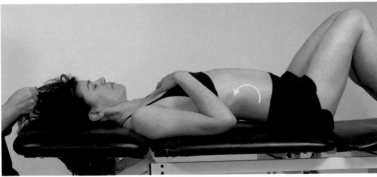

Figure 6.28
Adding anterior pelvic tilt to "hair-pull"

the therapist's fingertips to gently pull the scalp tissue in a cranial direction.

A number of movements from below may be added to this hair-pull technique to explore the SFL and/or the DFL of fascia. For example:

Add anterior pelvic tilt to "hair-pull" (Figure 6.28)

While the therapist maintains the "hair-pull" the patient is asked to perform an anterior pelvic tilt, thereby increasing the tension of the SFL or DFL from below. If these fascial lines are tight, the therapist will feel an increase in tension in their hands. The patient perceives this as the therapist pulling harder on the hair or scalp. The therapist maintains the hold with both hands toward a cranial direction until a softening of the system is perceived (usually within a few seconds). The patient then releases the pelvis back to a more neutral position; the therapist may feel that both hands can glide a little more cranially. The slack of the tissues is taken up by the therapist as the patient continues to actively perform an anterior pelvic tilt. This action

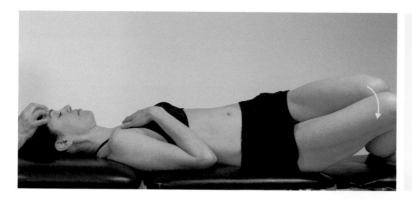

Figure 6.29
MMS scalp fascia in relation to the Spiral Line – shown using frontalis

continues until there is no further change perceived in the therapist's hands and generally requires approximately five or six cycles.

MMS scalp fascia in relation to the Spiral Line (Figure 6.29)

(shown using frontalis muscle)

The therapist maintains the "hair-pull" or tension on the frontalis, as shown. The patient is asked to let flexed knees slowly move to the right, thereby inducing lumbar rotation to the left. If the spiral line is tight, the therapist will feel an increase in tension in one or both hands. The therapist maintains the hold with both hands towards a cranial direction until a softening of the system is perceived, usually within a few seconds. The patient then brings the knees back to a more neutral position; the therapist may feel that one or both hands can glide a little more cranially. The slack of the tissues is taken up by the therapist as the patient continues to actively rotate to the right or the left. This sequence continues until there is no further change perceived in the therapist's hands; this generally requires approximately five or six cycles.

MMS techniques: the tongue and its fascia (DFL)

Tom Myers's dissections of the Deep Front Line have shown that the tongue is one of the most prominent cranial components of this line (Figure 6.30). Working with the patient's tongue has been found to be clinically useful

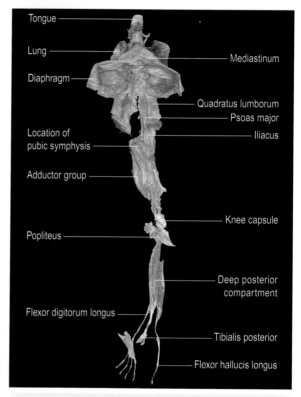

Figure 6.30
Dissection of DFL including tongue. Reproduced from *Anatomy Trains: Myofascial Meridians for Manual and Movement Therapists*, 3rd edition. With kind permission from Elsevier

with those clients complaining of tension in the area of the throat and mandibular area.

MMS tongue with pericardium (DFL) (Figure 6.31)

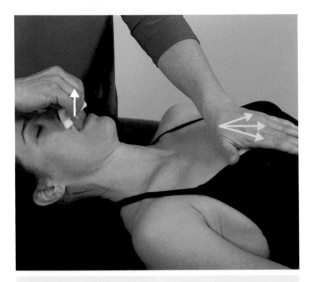

Figure 6.31
MMS tongue with pericardium (DFL)

MMS tongue with shoulder: ipsilateral or contralateral (SFL) (Figure 6.32)

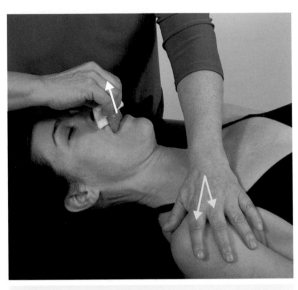

Figure 6.32
MMS tongue with shoulder – ipsilateral or contralateral (SFL)

Stabilizing hand The therapist holds onto the patient's tongue (using a paper towel) and gently pulls it anteriorly and in a cranial direction. Other directions may be explored as a progression, such as (gently) pulling the tongue in a cranial direction to the right or in a cranial direction to the left.

Mobilizing hand The therapist then explores the area of the pericardium in a posterior and caudal direction, looking for the angle where the therapist perceives immediate tension in the hand holding the tongue. If no tension is perceived, then the DFL of fascia in relation to the tongue is not tight. If there is tension in this line it will feel to the therapist as though the tongue wants to pull back posteriorly toward the throat area. The patient perceives this as the therapist pulling harder on the tongue when in reality the therapist is simply stopping the tongue from moving. If tension is perceived (quick resistance is felt between the two hands of the therapist), then it can be mobilized as per the approaches outlined in Chapter 4.

Stabilizing hand As per the technique above.

Mobilizing hand Using the caudal hand, the therapist explores the shoulder and shoulder girdle area with an anteroposterior caudal glide of the tissues in the area of the lateral clavicle and/or the GH joint, always looking for the immediate line of tension with gentle pressure of the caudal hand. This technique can be performed using either the ipsilateral or the contralateral shoulder area. If the ipsilateral shoulder is explored, the tension of the tongue fascia may be felt more easily by adding contralateral movement of the tongue in addition to an anterior and cranial pull (i.e., pulling the tongue to the right if using the left shoulder area and vice versa).

This technique may be used to explore the Superficial Front Line of fascia all the way down to the symphysis pubis, as well as the fascia of the DFL. The following case report illustrates this point.

Case report 6.2 Rita's Popsicle story

This 47-year-old patient had come for therapy with complaints of pain in the area of the right TMJ, noting difficulty chewing French bread. There was no history of trauma to the TMJ and her medical history noted a long-standing problem with irritable bowel syndrome, presently controlled with medication. Initial assessment and treatment of her condition involved the cervical spine and the TMJ, noting articular and myofascial restrictions in both areas. She responded well to manual therapy and exercises to address muscle imbalances in both areas. After three treatments, her initial problem was no longer a factor, but she noted that licking a Popsicle reproduced pain in her TMJ. The previously noted problems were re-assessed but the biomechanical exam was negative. Considering that the tongue was involved in this latest subjective complaint, it too was evaluated for mobility and strength. That test too, revealed no problems. However, using the techniques above, it was noted that there was considerable tension in the DFL of fascia, with tension noted between the tongue and pericardium, followed by the tongue and abdominal area. These techniques reproduced her craniofacial pain. One treatment to release this DFL solved her Popsicle problem. We may hypothesize from this case report that the patient's many bouts of inflammation secondary to her IBS created some fascial tension in the abdominal area, thus increasing tension into the tongue via the DFL of fascia.

Summary

The techniques in this chapter have focused on the myofascial connections in relation to the TMJ muscles, the epicranium, and the tongue. These tissues are frequently problematic in cases of persistent head, face, and TMJ pain and should be explored using MMS techniques. The next chapter will focus on MMS techniques for the dura and fascia within the cranium.

Dural mobility

When treating headaches or spinal pain, manual therapists are trained to assess and treat the mobility of the dura via techniques such as the straight leg raise (SLR) and/or slump technique. However, using this single approach to treatment may be insufficient, as the interfaces for neural structures must also be taken into account. We must consider that the dura does not end at the craniovertebral region, but extends to the cranium.

The cranium has a number of connections to the pelvic floor:

- articular connections: coccyx, sacrum, pelvis, lumbar spine, thorax, cervical spine, cranium

- myofascial connections: Deep Front Line of fascia (including the diaphragm), dura, falx cerebri, tentorium cerebellum

- neural connections: phrenic nerve, vagus nerve, dura, falx cerebri, tentorium cerebellum.

This chapter will focus on the myofascial connections between the cranium and the pelvic floor, as these tissues are frequently problematic in cases of persistent head pain, spinal pain, coccyx pain, and pelvic floor pain.

Of note is that the dura, falx cerebri, and tentorium cerebellum are all considered to be myofascial tissues as well as neural tissues (Diane Lee, personal communication). Within the cranium, the falx cerebri of the dura attaches to the crista galli of the ethmoid bone, which can be palpated indirectly via the glabella of the frontal bone (this feels like a small indentation on the forehead). This area will be used as a hook to anchor the falx cerebri.

The tentorium cerebelli is a horizontal fascia on either side of the falx cerebri that envelops the cerebellum and attaches to the falx cerebri within the cranium, at a junction called Sutherland's fulcrum (Figure 7.1). Pulling on the ears in a posterolateral inferior direction provides for the practitioner a lovely lever by which the tentorium cerebellum can be tensioned.

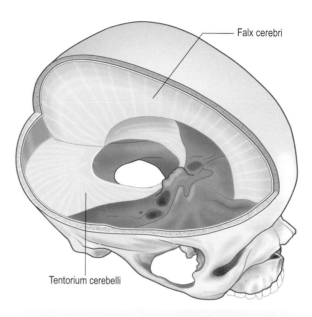

Falx cerebri

Tentorium cerebelli

Figure 7.1
Falx cerebri (a vertical structure that runs from front to back and separates the brain into right and left halves) and tentorium cerebelli (a horizontal fascia that connects to the falx cerebri and to both temporal bones)

The falx cerebri and the tentorium cerebellum are continuous with the dura that surrounds the brain. The dura then extends caudally to surround the spinal cord and ultimately ends at its attachment to the coccyx. The dura must have some inherent flexibility in order to accommodate movement of the spine. The spinal canal elongates as much as 9 cm during flexion of the whole spine (Louis 1981), but the sliding of the neural structures in the spine is complex and not fully understood. Neck flexion produces cephalad sliding of neural contents in the lumbar region (Breig & Troup 1979). However, the SLR produces caudal sliding of nerve roots in the lumbosacral intervertebral foramina (Goddard & Reid 1965; Breig & Troup 1979). Movement of the spine around neural structures is a complex series of lending and borrowing of neural tissue, producing convergence toward C5–6 and L4–5, the most mobile of spinal segments (Shacklock 2005; Louis 1981; Adams & Logue 1971).

The dura has a number of areas where mobility is naturally more tethered. These are at the junction of occiput/C1, C2/3, the cervicothoracic junction, the midthorax (T4–6), the thoracolumbar junction, the lumbosacral junction, S2/3 and the coccyx. Recurrent pain in these areas is not uncommon. It is also interesting to note that a number of horizontal fascial structures attach to the dura at many of these levels (the diaphragm at the Th/L levels, the thoracic inlet at the C/Thx levels, and the pelvic diaphragm).

The posterior dura is closer to the spinous processes than the anterior dura and is generally stretched in slump position (Figure 7.2). The anterior dura is closer to the anterior longitudinal ligament and is tensioned along with the DFL of fascia. As such, lumbar extension, knee and hip extension are maneuvers that will tension the anterior dura.

Signs and symptoms of dural mobility dysfunction include the following:

- headache and retro-orbital pain via the nerve supply of the dural membranes (trigeminal and vagus nerves, 1st, 2nd, and 3rd cervical nerves)

- face pain and abnormal tone of the temporomandibular joint (TMJ) muscles via the trigeminal nerve and the trigeminal ganglion, which is covered with dura and vulnerable to dural stress (Liem 2005)

- limitation in mobility of the cranial bones, the sacrum, and the coccygeal bone (Liem 2005)

- neurodynamic mobility issues, such as a positive slump test or upper limb neural techniques (ULNTs)

- in the ISM approach, if no corrections make the patient feel significantly better, the problem is frequently not in the skeleton but in the dura/nervous system.

The dura may also be impacted by dysfunctions in the craniosacral system, as these dysfunctions affect tension in the cerebral falx and/or tentorium cerebellum. In addition, the dura may be impacted by dysfunctions in the neck,

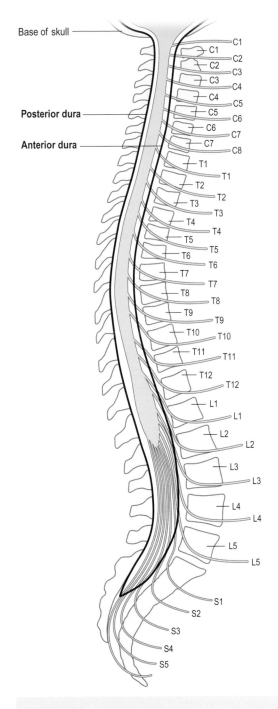

Figure 7.2
Posterior and anterior dura

clavicle, thorax, and/or sacrum, so the whole body should be considered (ISM model).

This chapter will describe the MMS techniques that are used to restore mobility of the following:

- the posterior dura
- the anterior dura
- the coccyx
- the anterior sacral fascia.

As well, the following MMS balancing techniques will be described:

- balancing the falx cerebri and the tentorium cerebellum
- balancing the occiput with the sacrum.

Indications for these techniques include the following:

- trauma to the head (post concussion)
- trauma or surgical techniques involving the dura (for example, post epidural)
- fall on the buttocks or the coccyx
- recurrent tension in the slump and/or ULNT position despite using slider or tensioner techniques.

Please note that treatment of the craniosacral system, an osteopathic approach, may also be necessary for full resolution of the patient's head pain. Despite my initial skepticism, I have found this approach invaluable for treatment of head pain. The scope of this book does not cover this method, although the balancing techniques described below are based on some of the craniosacral techniques.

Concepts of treatment using MMS

For this chapter, we will be using primarily the first concept of treatment for using MMS techniques. However, instead of choosing a recurrent articular dysfunction or myofascial trigger point, the therapist will anchor onto the areas of the dura that have a tendency to bind down when its mobility is impaired. If early tension is found between the hands of the therapist, the following approaches may be used, depending on how the tissues respond:

- work with oscillations (grades III– , III, III+)
- work with sustained pressure.

Please refer to Chapter 4 for further detail on concepts of treatment using MMS.

MMS techniques: posterior dura

The following techniques may be used to assess and treat the mobility of the posterior dura. The astute reader may remark that these techniques may also be considered a way to release tension in the Superficial Back Line of fascia (SBL) that encompasses the erector spinae muscles. The difference is in the depth of the technique and the intention of the therapist – the posterior dura is deeper than that of the fascia of the SBL of the back.

MMS posterior dura: thoracolumbar junction in relation to S2/3 (Figures 7.3, 7.4)

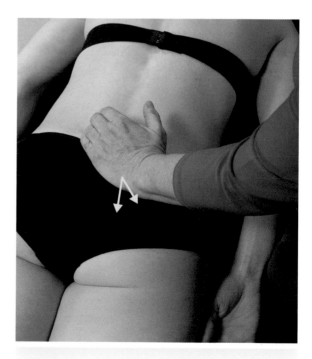

Figure 7.3
Posterior dura – hand position P/A S2/3 ®

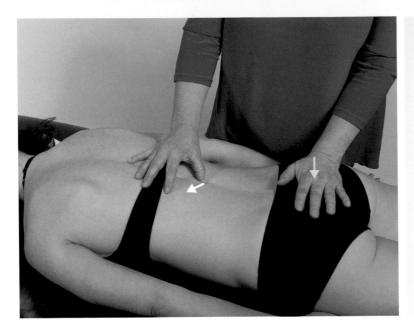

Figure 7.4
Posterior dura – P/A S2/3 ® + Th/L

Stabilizing hand The patient is in prone position. The therapist anchors onto the Th/L junction (T11–L1) via a cranially directed P/A on the right side of the spinous process. The inferior aspect of the spinous process provides a perfect "hook" that the therapist can use to stabilize this level.

Mobilizing hand The therapist then applies a P/A pressure to the right S2/3 region of the sacrum.

If the posterior dura is tethered at this level, the therapist will perceive an immediate increase in pressure on the thumb that is stabilizing the right side of the spinous process of T11 (and/or T12, L1), at the same time that a gentle P/A pressure of S2/3 is performed (Figure 7.4). The patient perceives this as the therapist pushing harder on T11, when, in reality, the therapist is simply preventing T11 from moving caudally. The therapist may use oscillations at S2/3 (grade IV– to grade IV to grade IV+) until no further increase in tension is perceived at T11. This may be repeated for levels T12 and L1 if tension is found at these levels.

MMS posterior dura: mid-thoracic spine in relation to S2/3 (Figure 7.5)

Stabilizing hand The therapist anchors onto the mid-Thx region (T4–6) via a cranially directed P/A on the right side of the spinous process. The inferior aspect of the spinous process provides a "hook" that the therapist can use to stabilize this level.

Mobilizing hand The therapist then applies a P/A pressure to the right S2/3 region of the sacrum, as per the previous technique. If the posterior dura is tethered at this level, the therapist will perceive this as an immediate increase in pressure on the thumb stabilizing the right side of the spinous process of T4 (and /or T5, T6), at the same time that a gentle P/A pressure of S2/3 is performed. Similar concepts for mobilizing this line of fascia apply as per the previous technique.

This technique may be repeated for levels T5 and T6 if tension is found at these levels.

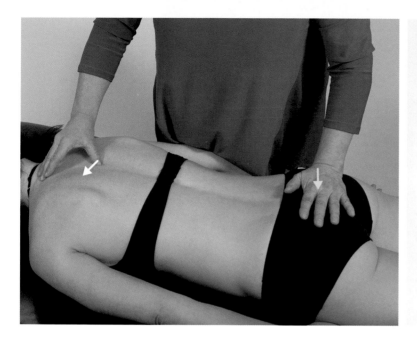

Figure 7.5
Posterior dura – P/A S2/3 ® + mid-Thx

MMS posterior dura: C2 in relation to S2/3 (Figure 7.6)

Stabilizing hand The therapist anchors onto C2 via a unilateral P/A pressure on the right side of the lamina of C2.

Mobilizing hand The therapist then applies a P/A pressure to the right S2/3 region of the sacrum, as per the technique above. If the posterior dura is tethered at this level, the therapist will perceive an immediate pressure on the thumb stabilizing the right lamina of C2, at the same time that a gentle P/A pressure of S2/3 is performed. The patient perceives this as the therapist pushing harder on C2, when, in reality, the therapist is simply preventing C2 from moving into right rotation relative to C3. Similar concepts for mobilizing this line of fascia apply as per the previous technique.

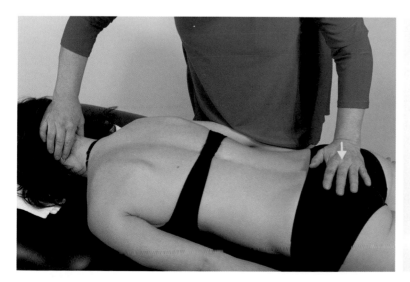

Figure 7.6
Posterior dura – P/A S2/3 ® + C2

MMS posterior dura: occipital flexion in relation to S2/3 (Figure 7.7)

MMS posterior dura: thoracolumbar junction in relation to L5/S1 (Figure 7.8)

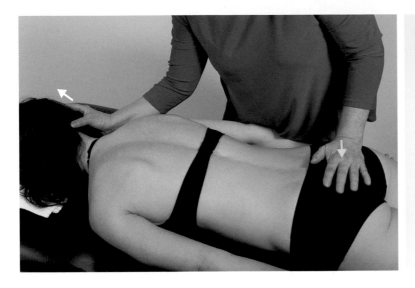

Figure 7.7
Posterior dura – P/A S2/3 ® + Occ flex

Stabilizing hand The therapist anchors onto the ipsilateral occiput via a cranially directed P/A pressure on the right side of the occiput. An area about 2 cm square may be explored at the occiput using this technique.

Mobilizing hand The therapist then applies a P/A pressure to the right S2/3 region of the sacrum, as per the previous technique. If the posterior dura is tethered at this level, the therapist will perceive this as an immediate increase in pressure on the thumb stabilizing the occiput, at same time that a gentle P/A pressure of S2/3 is performed. The patient perceives this as the therapist "pushing harder" on the occiput, when, in reality, the therapist is simply preventing the occiput from moving caudally. Similar concepts for mobilizing this line of fascia apply as per the previous technique.

The above techniques may also be explored in relation to the lumbosacral junction, an area that is frequently involved in tethering of the posterior dura. The example below shows how the above technique may be altered to work this particular interface. It can be used for the mid-thoracic region, as well as for C2 and the occiput.

Stabilizing hand The therapist anchors onto the Th/L junction (T11–L1) as per the technique for the posterior dura in relation to S2/3.

Mobilizing hand The therapist then applies a caudally directed P/A pressure to the center of the sacrum using their forearm, looking for the immediate line of tension between their two hands. If the posterior dura is tethered at this level, the therapist will perceive an increase in pressure on the thumb that is stabilizing the right side of the spinous process of T11 (and /or T12, L1), at the same time that a gentle caudal P/A pressure of L5/S1 is performed. The patient perceives this as the therapist pushing harder on T11, when, in reality, the therapist is simply preventing T11 from moving caudally. The therapist may use oscillations at L5/S1 (grade IV– to grade IV to grade IV+) until no further increase in tension is perceived at T11. This may be repeated for levels T12 and L1 if tension is found at these levels.

MMS techniques: anterior dura

The following techniques may be used to assess and treat the mobility of the anterior dura. The anterior dura is

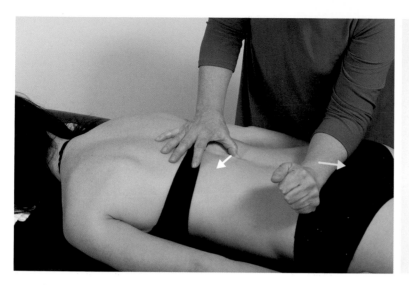

Figure 7.8
Posterior dura – P/A caud sacrum +
Th/L

considered part of the Deep Front Line of fascia (DFL),
which may be tensioned via knee flexion in prone, as well
as by adding dorsiflexion/eversion of the ankle (which tensions the tibialis posterior muscle, the tail end of the DFL).

MMS anterior dura: thoracolumbar junction in
relation to ipsilateral knee flexion +/– dorsiflexion/
eversion ankle (Figure 7.9)

Stabilizing hand The therapist anchors onto the Th/L
junction (T11–L1) via a cranially directed P/A on the right
side of the spinous process. The inferior aspect of the
spinous process provides a "hook" that the therapist can
use to stabilize this level.

Mobilizing hand The therapist then performs a passive physiological movement of right (ipsilateral) knee
flexion, looking for the immediate increase in tension
of the stabilizing hand. If the anterior dura is tethered
at this level, the therapist will perceive this as an immediate increase in pressure on the thumb stabilizing the
right side of the spinous process of T11 (and /or T12, L1),
before 90 degrees of knee flexion has been achieved. The
patient perceives this as the therapist pushing harder on
T11, when, in reality, the therapist is simply preventing
T11 from moving caudally. The therapist may use repeated passive physiological movements of knee flexion in an
oscillatory manner (grade IV– to grade IV to grade IV+)

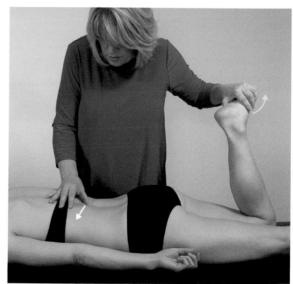

Figure 7.9
Anterior dura – DF/EV + knee flex + Th/L

until no further increase in tension is perceived at T11.
This may be repeated for levels T12 and L1 if tension is
found at these levels.

Progression Once 90 degrees of knee flexion has been
attained without a corresponding increase in tension at the
Th/L levels, the therapist may then progress the technique

by adding passive physiological dorsiflexion/eversion of the ipsilateral ankle at 90 degrees of knee flexion. As per the above technique, the similar concept of perceiving an increase in tension at the stabilizing hand exists, and is treated in a similar manner.

MMS anterior dura: mid-thoracic spine region in relation to ipsilateral knee flexion +/− dorsiflexion/eversion ankle (Figure 7.10)

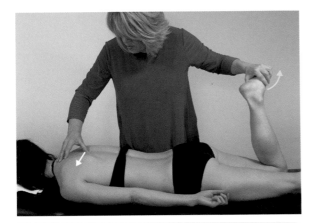

Figure 7.10
Anterior dura – DF/EV + knee flex + mid Thx

Stabilizing hand The therapist anchors onto the mid-thoracic spine region (T4–6) via a cranially directed P/A on the right side of the spinous process, as per the technique for the posterior dura in relation to S2/3.

Mobilizing hand The therapist then performs a passive physiological movement of right (ipsilateral) knee flexion, as per the technique above. Similar concepts for mobilizing this line of fascia apply. This may be repeated for levels T5 and T6 if tension is found at these levels.

Progression As per the above technique, the therapist may then progress the technique by adding passive physiological dorsiflexion/eversion of the ipsilateral ankle at 90 degrees of knee flexion. It is treated in a similar manner.

MMS anterior dura: C2 in relation to ipsilateral knee flexion +/− dorsiflexion/eversion ankle (Figure 7.11)

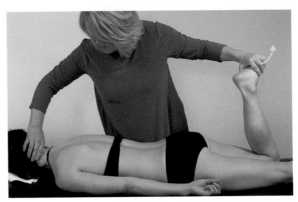

Figure 7.11
Anterior dura – DF/EV + knee flex + C2

Stabilizing hand The therapist anchors onto C2 via a unilateral P/A pressure on the right side of the lamina of C2, as per the technique for the posterior dura in relation to S2/3.

Mobilizing hand The therapist then performs a passive physiological movement of right (ipsilateral) knee flexion, looking for the immediate increase in tension of the stabilizing hand. If the anterior dura is tethered at this level, the therapist will perceive an immediate increase in pressure on the thumb stabilizing the right side of the lamina of C2 before 90 degrees of knee flexion has been achieved. The patient perceives this as the therapist pushing harder on C2, when, instead, the therapist is simply preventing C2 from moving into right rotation relative to C3. The therapist may use repeated passive physiological movements of knee flexion in an oscillatory manner (grade IV− to grade IV to grade IV+) until no further increase in tension is perceived at C2.

Progression As per the above technique, the therapist may then progress the technique by adding passive physiological dorsiflexion/eversion of the ipsilateral ankle at 90 degrees of knee flexion. It is treated in a similar manner.

MMS anterior dura: occiput in relation to ipsilateral knee flexion +/– dorsiflexion/eversion ankle (Figure 7.12)

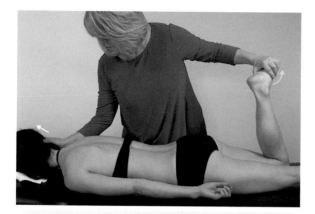

Figure 7.12
Anterior dura – DF/EV + knee flex + Occ

Stabilizing hand The therapist anchors onto the ipsilateral occiput via a cranially directed P/A pressure on the right side of the occiput. An area about 2 cm square may be explored at the occiput using this technique.

Mobilizing hand The therapist then performs a passive physiological movement of right (ipsilateral) knee flexion, looking for the immediate increase in tension of the stabilizing hand. If the anterior dura is tethered at this level, the therapist will perceive an immediate increase in pressure on the thumb stabilizing the right occiput before 90 degrees of knee flexion has been achieved. The patient perceives this as the therapist pushing harder on the occiput, when, in reality, the therapist is simply preventing the occiput from moving caudally. Similar concepts for mobilizing this line of fascia apply.

Progression As per the above technique, the therapist may then progress the technique by adding passive physiological dorsiflexion/eversion of the ipsilateral ankle at 90 degrees of knee flexion. It is treated in a similar manner.

MMS techniques: coccyx

The following techniques may be helpful in cases of coccydynia as well as in problems with dural mobility.

MMS A/P coccyx on the right + P/A base of sacrum on the right (Figures 7.13, 7.14)

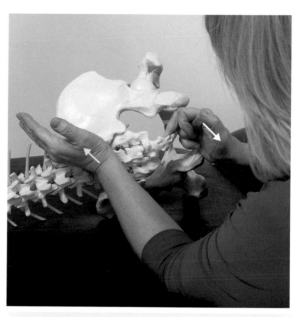

Figure 7.13
MMS A/P coccyx on the right + P/A base of sacrum on the right – skeleton

Stabilizing hand The patient is in a left side-lying position. The therapist **gently** anchors onto the anterior aspect of the right side of the coccyx using their third digit and performs a unilateral A/P pressure on the right side of the coccyx.

Mobilizing hand The therapist then applies a P/A pressure to nutate the right side of the sacrum (right S1 segment) using the pisiform area of the cranial hand, and looks for the immediate line of tension between the two hands. If the dura is tethered at this level the therapist will

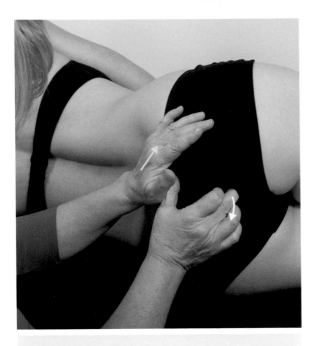

Figure 7.14
MMS A/P coccyx on the right + P/A base of sacrum on the right

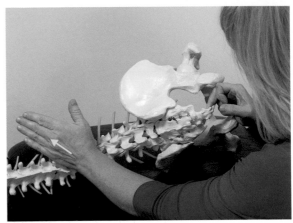

Figure 7.15
MMS A/P coccyx + P/A Th/L – skeleton

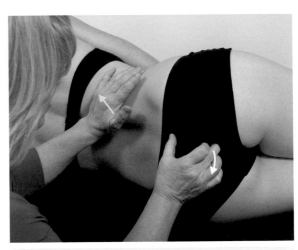

Figure 7.16
MMS A/P coccyx + P/A Th/L junction

perceive this as immediate pressure on their third digit performing the A/P on the coccyx, at the same time that a gentle P/A pressure of the right S1 is performed. The patient perceives this as the therapist pulling harder on coccyx, when, in reality, the therapist is simply preventing the coccyx from moving anteriorly. The therapist may use oscillations at the right sacral base (grade IV– to grade IV to grade IV+) until no further increase in tension is perceived at the coccyx. For sensitive patients, a non-oscillatory or "listening" technique may be more appropriate for this region.

Progression The stabilizing hand remains the same. The mobilizing hand may explore other areas where the dura may bind down, such as the Th/L area (Figures 7.15, 7.16), the mid-Thx area, C2 and the occiput (not shown).

The technique above may also be performed on the left side of the coccyx with the patient in a right side-lying position. In addition, the coccyx A/P maneuver may be performed centrally, with the patient lying on either side.

Balancing the falx cerebri and the tentorium cerebellum

The following techniques are useful to help balance the dura within the cranium. They are a way to integrate the entire dura, from the cranium to the feet. These techniques are also very useful at the end of an MMS treatment for any part of the body, and, in particular, for those patients who are prone to headaches and/or have highly reactive nervous systems.

Balancing the falx cerebri

There are two basic positions of the therapist's hands that may be used to connect to the dura and falx cerebri within the cranium. The hand-holds are the stabilizing aspect of these techniques. Either or both may be used.

- **Hold 1: occiput/ethmoid (Figure 7.17)**

The middle finger of the therapist's cranial hand is on the glabella, an indentation felt on the frontal bone, the index and ring ringers on either side of the frontal bone in line with the glabella. The therapist's caudal hand cups the occiput. Both hands pull gently in a cranial direction.

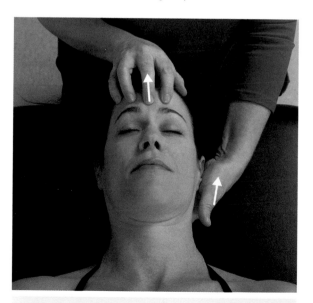

Figure 7.17
Balancing the falx cerebri – hold 1: occiput/ethmoid

- **Hold 2: occiput/frontal-nasal (alternate hold) (Figure 7.18)**

The therapist's second and third digits are on either side of the frontal bone next to the nasium (fronto-nasal sutures). The therapist's caudal hand cups the occiput. Both hands pull gently in a cranial direction.

As the therapist maintains their position on the patient's cranium, movement from below is added:

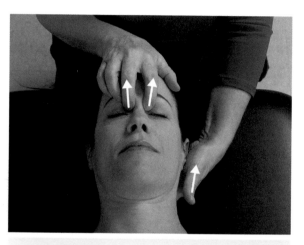

Figure 7.18
Balancing the falx cerebri – hold 2: occiput/frontal-nasal

A. Add ankle dorsiflexion and plantarflexion (Figures 7.19, 7.20)

The therapist maintains a cranial glide of both hands as the patient performs active ankle dorsiflexion (DF) and plantarflexion (PF). If the falx cerebri is tight, the therapist will feel that the tissues under their hands will want to move in a caudal direction with ankle PF. The therapist maintains the hold with both hands towards a cranial direction until a softening of the system is perceived. The client then returns to DF, and the therapist may feel that both hands can glide a little more cranially. The slack of the tissues in a cranial direction is taken up by the therapist as the patient

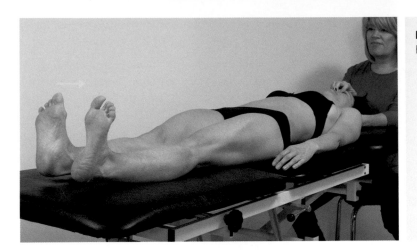

Figure 7.19
Falx cerebri + ankle DF

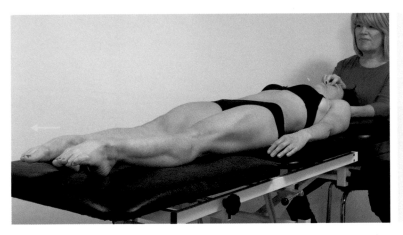

Figure 7.20
Falx cerebri + ankle PF

continues to actively DF and PF the ankles; this is repeated until no further change is perceived in the therapist's hands. It generally requires approximately five or six cycles of ankle DF/PF.

B. Add eye movement

The muscles of the eyes have strong fascial connections to both the falx cerebri and the tentorium cerebellum. As such this can be used to mobilize these fasciae inside the cranium, in particular when the patient complains of pain related to movement of the eyes and with reading.

The same hold on the head is maintained as per technique A; however, the patient is asked to actively move his/her eyes in a variety of directions. For the falx cerebri the most common restriction is noted with movement of the eyes in a cranial or caudal direction.

Falx cerebri with eye movement up (Figure 7.21)

While the therapist maintains the cranial hold above, the patient moves his/her eyes up towards the top of the head. Usually this movement increases the slack on the falx, allowing the therapist to further glide these tissues in a cranial direction.

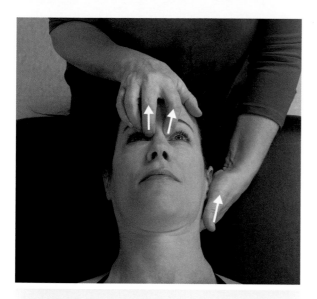

Figure 7.21
Falx cerebri with eye movement up

Falx cerebri with eye movement down (Figure 7.22)

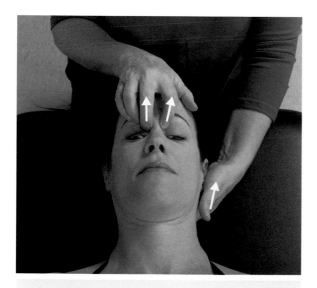

Figure 7.22
Falx cerebri with eye movement down

While the therapist maintains the cranial hold above, the patient moves his/her eyes down toward their feet. This movement usually increases the tension on the falx. The therapist perceives this tension as a tendency for both of their hands on the cranium wanting to move in a caudal direction. The patient perceives this tension as the therapist pulling harder in a cranial direction. The therapist simply maintains the original tension of the falx in a cranial direction until a softening of the system is perceived. Movement of the eyes up and down is repeated until the therapist perceives no further increase in tension with eye movement.

Falx cerebri with both ankle and eye movement together (feet and eyes up/feet and eyes down)

This technique is a progression of the technique described above. If both ankle dorsiflexion and plantarflexion and eye movement up and down no longer increase the tension on the cranium, the therapist may proceed with the combined technique below.

While the therapist maintains the cranial hold above, the patient moves his/her eyes up toward the top of the head at the same time as active dorsiflexion of the ankles is performed. Usually this movement increases the slack on the falx, allowing the therapist to further glide these tissues in a cranial direction. The patient is then asked to move the eyes down toward their feet at the same time as active plantarflexion of the ankles is performed. Usually this movement increases the tension on the falx. The therapist perceives this tension as a tendency for both of their hands on the cranium wanting to move in a caudal direction. At the same time, the patient perceives this tension as the therapist pulling harder in a cranial direction. The therapist simply maintains the original tension in a cranial direction until a softening of the system is felt. Movement of the eyes up with ankle dorsiflexion and eyes down with ankle plantarflexion is repeated until the therapist senses no further increase in tension with this combination of movement. (This technique is not pictured.)

The falx cerebri can also be mobilized in relation to the DFL of fascia by adding dorsiflexion/eversion of the ankle and inspiration to move the diaphragm.

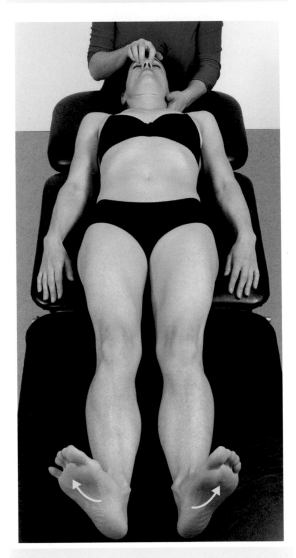

Falx cerebri with tension of the DFL: DF/eversion + deep inspiration (Figure 7.23)

Figure 7.23
Falx cerebri with tension of the DFL – DF/eversion + deep inspiration

While the therapist maintains the cranial hold, the patient moves both ankles into a combined movement of dorsiflexion/eversion, which increases tension on the DFL of

fascia. If the DFL is tight, this movement will increase the tension on the falx. The therapist perceives this tension as a tendency for both of their hands on the cranium wanting to move in a caudal direction. The patient perceives this tension as the therapist pulling harder in a cranial direction. The therapist simply maintains the original tension in a cranial direction until a softening of the system is perceived. Movement of both ankles in and out of combined dorsiflexion/eversion is repeated until the therapist perceives no further increase in tension with eye movement.

Progression This technique may be progressed by asking the patient to take a deep breath in at the same time as he/she performs active dorsiflexion/eversion of the ankles. The deep breath activates the diaphragm, which is also an important part of the DFL.

Balancing the tentorium cerebellum within the cranium

"Ear-pull" technique for the tentorium cerebellum (Figure 7.24)

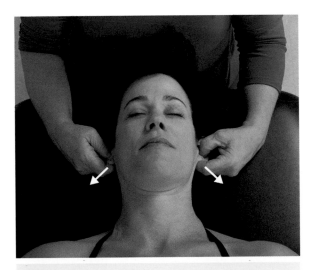

Figure 7.24
"Ear-pull" technique for the tentorium cerebellum

The ear-pull technique is commonly taught in the craniosacral approach to treatment. It is a way to improve mobility of the temporal bones as well as the tentorium cerebellum, a horizontal fascia on either side of the falx cerebri that encompasses the cerebellum and attaches to the falx cerebri within the cranium (Magoun 1976). The falx cerebri is continuous with the dura and may be affected by tension in the tentorium cerebellum.

The technique is performed as follows: the patient is lying in a supine position. The therapist's thumbs are inside the ear canal, and care is taken not to block the canal. The therapist's fingers gently grasp the posterior aspect of the ears, as close to the cranium as possible. The therapist then gently pulls simultaneously in three directions (posterior, inferior, lateral) at a 45 degree angle until the slack of the tissues between the two hands is taken up. If there are no articular restrictions of the sutures around the temporal bone, the therapist should have a membranous end-feel between their two hands. This membranous feel is considered optimal.

Fascia around the eye muscles and the optic nerve is intimately related to the intracranial fascia; therefore, restrictions in mobility of the fasciae in this area may contribute to dysfunctions of eye movement. This may translate clinically as difficulty with reading and headache. Adding eye movement to the ear-pull technique is a way to mobilize this intracranial interface.

Add eye movement (Figure 7.25–7.27)

The therapist maintains the pull on the ears as the patient actively moves the eyes to the right. Ideally, the therapist should feel no increase in tension of the tentorium cerebellum with eye movement. If there is tension in the tentorium, it will be perceived by the therapist as an increase in tension of the hand holding the left ear – as if the tissues on the left ear will want to "pull in" to the cranium at the same time as the patient moves the eyes to the right. The therapist simply maintains the ear-pull, but the patient perceives it as the therapist pulling harder on the left ear. The position is maintained until a softening in the system is perceived. The patient then brings the eyes back to the center. This action generally needs to be repeated only two to three times, until

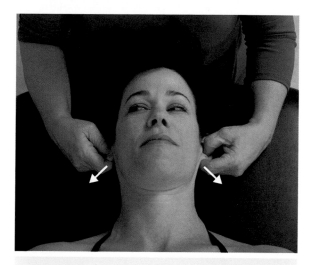

Figure 7.25
Eyes to the right while maintaining "ear-pull"

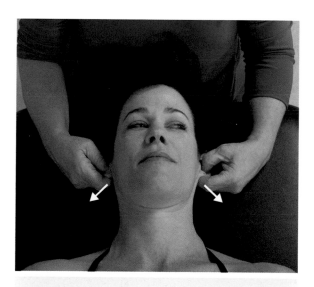

Figure 7.26
Eyes to the left while maintaining "ear-pull"

no further change is felt between the therapist's hands as the patient moves the eyes to the right.

Other directions may also be added, such as moving the eyes to the left. If the right tentorium cerebellum is tight, the therapist will feel an increase in tension of the right

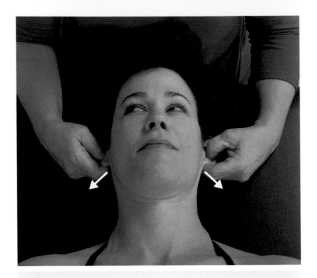

Figure 7.27
Eyes to the right and up in a diagonal while maintaining "ear-pull"

ear. Generally speaking, moving the eyes up or down has little effect on the tentorium cerebellum. However, moving the eyes in a diagonal direction often increases the pull and is worked in a similar way to that described above. The diagonal directions to be explored are as follows:

- up to the right corner
- down to the right corner
- up to the left corner
- down to the left corner.

Ear-pull with tension of the DFL: dorsiflexion/eversion + deep inspiration (Figure 7.28)

The tentorium cerebellum may also be affected by movements of the DFL of fascia (dorsiflexion/eversion + deep inspiration). While the therapist maintains the ear-pull, the patient moves both ankles into a combined movement of dorsiflexion/eversion, which tensions the DFL of fascia. If the DFL within the cranium is tight, this movement will increase the tension on the tentorium cerebellum. The therapist perceives this tension as a tendency for one or both of the hands on the temporal bones wanting to move towards the center of the head. The patient perceives this

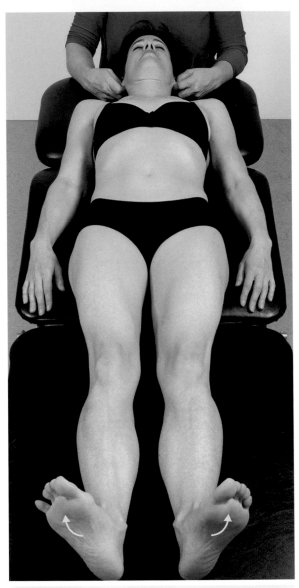

Figure 7.28
With tension of the DFL – DF/eversion + deep inspiration while maintaining "ear-pull"

tension as the therapist pulling harder on the ears. The therapist simply maintains the original tension in a postero-inferior-lateral (PIL) direction until a softening of the system is perceived. Movement of both ankles in and out of combined dorsiflexion/eversion is repeated until the therapist perceives no further increase in tension.

Balancing the occiput with the sacrum

The craniosacral mechanism is hypothesized to work based on a reciprocal tension membrane system. During the phase of physiological cranial flexion, the sacrum should move into counternutation; that is, the base of the sacrum should tilt posteriorly as the apex of the sacrum moves anteriorly. The opposite occurs during the cranial extension phase – the sacrum moves into nutation (Figure 7.29).

This rhythmical movement occurs at a frequency of between 8 and 14 cycles per minute, according to the craniosacral approach, and can be readily palpated by trained therapists. A common dysfunction is one in which the occiput is felt to move into physiological cranial flexion and extension but the sacrum is stagnant; that is, it does not exhibit the gentle physiological rocking motion of nutation and counternutation that occurs with cranial flexion and extension. This stagnation may occur after a fall on the buttocks or a blow on the head. Another dysfunction is one in which the occiput and the sacrum do not move synchronously; that is, as the occiput moves into cranial flexion, the sacrum nutates and vice versa. The following technique can resolve both of these issues.

Occiput-sacral balancing (Figure 7.30)

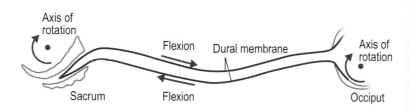

Figure 7.29
Craniosacral mechanism: during the flexion phase of the craniosacral movement, the sacrum should move into counternutation as the occiput moves into cranial flexion (similar to the biomechanics of craniovertebral extension movement but with a different axis of motion)

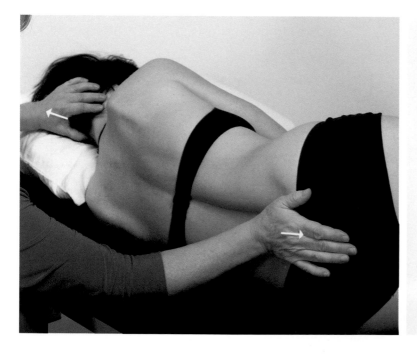

Figure 7.30
Occiput-sacral balancing

The therapist faces the back of the patient, who is in a side-lying position. This is a central technique so either side-lying position may be used.

One hand cups the occiput, with the palm of the hand or the therapist's fingers as close as possible to the base of the occiput. The therapist's other hand cups the sacrum, with the palm of the hand as close as possible to the sacral base (S1). The therapist sinks into the tissues, feeling the myofascial tissue release as they do so. The therapist then applies a gentle but firm distraction between their two hands until they feel the connection between their two hands. This technique is best done using sustained pressure. The idea behind a listening approach is to load the fascial tissues; that is, establish the first resistance in the line of tension, and then wait to see what the body wants to do with this tension. The therapist may feel the tension increase between the hands, with the body adding small micro-adjustments in multiple directions. The sensation is similar to that of twisted elastic that is attempting to unwind itself. The therapist follows this unwinding, preventing the tissues at the sacrum and/or the occiput from going back into the direction from which they came. The tension tends to build up gradually and then suddenly releases, often within a minute. This release is accompanied by a fluid-like feel and often, a therapeutic pulse.

MMS anterior sacral fascia

This technique is demonstrated in Chapter 10 on MMS techniques for the pelvic floor.

Summary

The techniques in this chapter have focused on the myofascial connections between the cranium and the pelvic floor, primarily the posterior and anterior dura and the tentorium cerebellum. These tissues are frequently problematic in cases of persistent head pain, spinal pain, and pelvic floor pain. These techniques are also valuable as a way to "calm down" the nervous system post treatment. They are particularly beneficial for those patients who tend to experience treatment soreness or post-treatment headaches. The next chapter will focus on techniques for the thorax.

The thorax

When treating the thorax, manual physiotherapists are trained to assess and treat the thoracic zygapophysial joints, the costotransverse and costovertebral joints, as well as the anterior sternochondral and costochondral joints. The scapular and trunk muscles are assessed for muscle imbalance issues, and a variety of techniques may be used to decrease tone in hypertonic muscles, as well as train/strengthen weak muscles. However, there has been less emphasis on myofascial tissues that have a strong impact on the biomechanics of the thoracic rings, and therefore play a role in the optimal functioning of the thorax. These myofascial tissues include the following:

- the diaphragm

- the intercostal muscles

- the muscles that connect the thorax to the scapula (serratus anterior, serratus posterior)

- the muscles that connect the thorax to the pelvis (quadratus lumborum, abdominal muscles, erector spinae muscles).

These muscles form part of every line described in Tom Myers's book, *Anatomy Trains*. If tension persists in these muscles despite using techniques to decrease tone and promote muscle balance, then we must consider the myofascial lines related to the affected muscle.

Indications for MMS for this chapter

1. Recurring thoracic pain despite the following treatment approaches:

   – mobilization/manipulation of the thoracic spine
   – stabilization exercises for the thorax
   – release of trigger points to the thoracic muscles with manual or dry needling techniques.
2. Tension in the anterior thorax area (sternum, diaphragm, abdominals).

The diaphragm

The diaphragm, apart from its primary role in respiration, has many other functions that affect the health of the body. It is important for spinal stability and plays a role in the optimal functioning of the pelvic floor and the floor of the mouth. It is also essential for proper organ function and for the function of the vascular and lymphatic systems, as the aorta, the inferior vena cava, and the esophagus all pass through the diaphragm (Clifton-Smith & Rowley 2011). When the diaphragm functions properly, and allows even distribution of breath into the lungs, it creates a balance between the front and back body (Holly Herman, personal communication).

An issue that has become common in modern times is lack of tone in the diaphragm, and as a result, poor function. As children we are constantly running, jumping, yelling, and singing: activities that keep the diaphragm fit and functioning at top form. As we age and move toward a more sedentary lifestyle, the diaphragm experiences less demand and loses its tone. Following this pattern, a diaphragm that ought to comfortably move 5–6 inches vertically might only move 1–3 inches.

Improper breathing patterns can create a variety of physiological problems (reduced availability to oxygen, respiratory alkalosis, "anxiety breathing," headaches, general fatigue, etc.). These poor respiratory patterns can also have biomechanical implications as well, including restricted thoracic spine movement, increased forward head posture, altered shoulder function and scapular mechanics, increased tone of the erector spinae muscles and accessory breathing muscles (sternocleidomastoid (SCM), scalenes, upper trapezius) and decreased pelvic floor strength, leading to potential instability of the lumbar spine (Clifton-Smith & Rowley 2011).

Despite its complexities, at the end of the day, the diaphragm is simply a muscle. Like any other muscle in the body, it needs to be maintained in order to function at its best. The importance of breath in yoga practice encourages proper tone in the diaphragm, which can increase lung capacity, and, in turn, longevity.

Lack of mobility of the diaphragm may impact not only the vascular and digestive systems, but also the thoracic spine joints. Persistent thoracic pain may be due to adhesions in the DFL of fascia, where there is insufficient play in the tissues between the thorax posteriorly and the diaphragm anteriorly. Similar issues can occur with the thorax in relation to the pericardial tissues, as the pericardium attaches to anterior aspect of T4, T2, C6, and the thoracic rings. Any type of cardiac or abdominal surgery tends to exacerbate the tension in these tissues.

This chapter will focus on the myofascial connections between the thorax and the pelvis and explore fascial lines that may be affected. These include the following:

- antero-posterior fascia of the thorax in relation to the pericardium and the diaphragm (DFL)

- antero-posterior fascia of the cervicothoracic region in relation to the pericardium and the diaphragm (DFL)

- antero-posterior fascia of the thoracolumbar region in relation to the pericardium and the diaphragm (DFL)

- iliacus fascia in relation to both the SFL and the DFL

- quadratus lumborum fascia in relation to the Lateral Line

- serratus anterior fascia

- serratus posterior inferior fascia.

Additional techniques that explore the thorax in relation to other areas of the body are discussed in other chapters:

- The techniques that explore the thorax in relation to the cervical spine are described in Chapter 5.

- Those that explore the thorax in relation to the cranium and temporomandibular joint (TMJ) are described in Chapter 6.

- Those that are in relation to the mobility of the dura are described in Chapter 7.

- Those techniques that are in relation to the mobility of the lumbar spine are found in Chapter 9 and those in relation to the pelvic floor are found in Chapter 10.

- The techniques that explore the thorax in relation to the shoulder girdle and upper extremity are described in Chapters 12 and 13.

These divisions are, of course, artificial, as the thoracic myofascia, like all myofascial tissue, is a continuum, all the way from the top of the head down to the toes. The techniques introduced in this book have been sorted into various regions simply to facilitate learning.

Postural analysis

A forward head posture is a frequent finding in the general population and in particular with those suffering from chronic spinal pain. As manual therapists, we are trained to mobilize joints of the thoracic spine that are prone to limitations with a forward head posture. The common findings in the thorax are an increase in kyphosis, often accompanied by articular restriction of the zygapophysial and costotransverse joints of the thorax. However, the mid-thoracic region may also exhibit flatness, demonstrated by a lack of flexion in this part of the thorax. In both cases, the restriction may be articular (decreased antero-superior glide of the facet joints and/or decreased antero-superior glide at the costotransverse joints for a flexion dysfunction; decreased postero-inferior glide of the facet joints and/or decreased postero-inferior glide at the costotransverse joints for a extension dysfunction). Restrictions of the thorax may also be due to non-optimal mechanics of the thoracic rings. The ISM approach looks for areas of lateral "ring shifts" in the thorax, indicating a ring that is rotated in relation to the one above and/or below it.

Regardless of the approach used (traditional manual physiotherapy or the ISM approach), the therapist must also consider that restrictions in the thorax may also be myofascial in origin. Joint or muscle dysfunction cannot fully explain all sources of restriction for the thorax. For example, restriction of the SFL or DFL of fascia may maintain a forward head posture. This tension can develop as a result of trauma, including surgical scars to the abdominal area. In addition, certain activities of daily living such as excessive time spent in the sitting position for work or leisure activities, can be a factor in creating these fascial lines of tension.

If there is restriction in the Lateral Line of fascia, this may create a lateral tilt or side shift of the thorax. If there is restriction of the Spiral Line of fascia, it may also contribute to a lateral tilt or side shift of the thorax, as well as unilateral tension in the abdominal oblique muscles. It may also impact the position of the scapula and therefore function of the shoulder complex. Both of these lines may also contribute to scoliosis.

Concepts of treatment using MMS

For this chapter, we will be using primarily the first concept of treatment when using MMS techniques; that is, choose a recurrent articular dysfunction or myofascial trigger point and explore a fascial line in relation to it. The therapist anchors him/herself to a recurrent articular dysfunction or myofascial trigger point and assesses the fascial lines of tension in relation to the anchor, looking for early tension between their two hands.

The following approaches may be used, depending on how the tissues respond:

- work with oscillations (grades III−, III, III+)
- work with sustained pressure
- work with "harmonics" (Dr Laurie Hartman).

Techniques applied in relation to serratus anterior respond particularly well to the release with awareness (RWA) approach. This is the fourth treatment concept for MMS that is outlined in Chapter 4. Please refer to this chapter for further detail on concepts of treatment using MMS.

Figure 8.1 depicts several layers of fascia found between the sternum and the cervicothoracic and mid-thoracic spine:

- the superficial (investing) cervical fascia (which connects the hyoid bone to the sternum)
- the deep cervical fascia, including:
  - the pre-trachial fascia (which surrounds the trachea, esophagus, and thyroid and is continuous to the mediastinum and pericardial fascia)
  - the pre-vertebral fascia (which surrounds the vertebral column and muscles in the posterior cervical spine).

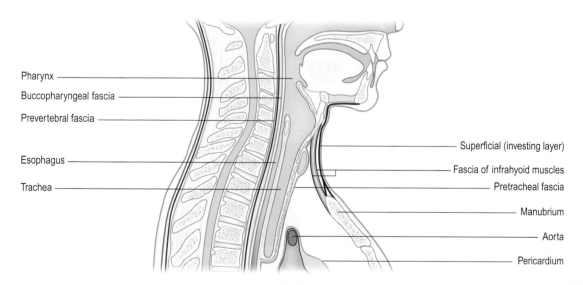

Pharynx
Buccopharyngeal fascia
Prevertebral fascia
Esophagus
Trachea

Superficial (investing layer)
Fascia of infrahyoid muscles
Pretracheal fascia
Manubrium
Aorta
Pericardium

Figure 8.1
Fascial layers of the cervical spine

Figure 8.1 helps the therapist understand the following techniques that were developed to help restore the mobility of the fascia "in between" the anterior and the posterior aspects of the body. Restoring mobility of these tissues helps to decrease symptoms in the posterior thorax as well as the front of the chest and abdomen. It may also facilitate the correction of an excessive thoracic kyphosis.

MMS techniques: anterior/posterior thorax

A/P thorax on the right in relation to the pericardium (DFL) (Figures 8.2–8.4)

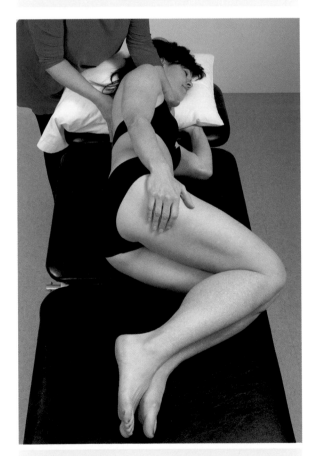

Figure 8.2
MMS A/P thorax with lumbar spine neutral

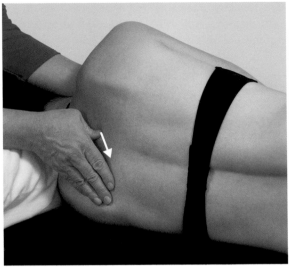

Figure 8.3
MMS techniques ant/post thorax – stabilizing hold on the thorax

Stabilizing hand The patient is in the left side-lying position with the thorax and lumbar spine in a neutral position, hips and knees bent.

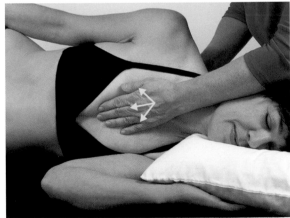

Figure 8.4
MMS A/P thorax in relation to the pericardium

The therapist anchors onto the mid-thoracic region (T3–10) via a caudally directed P/A on the right side of the spinous process. Note that this example is for the right side of the thorax – the left side of the thorax is treated similarly, but with the patient in right side-lying position and the therapist stabilizing the left side of the spinous processes of the mid-thorax region.

Mobilizing hand The therapist explores the area of the pericardium, first by slowly sinking into the tissues posterior to the sternum and then gently pushing in a caudal direction, all the while maintaining the depth of the fascial line posterior to the sternum. The therapist looks for the angle where he/she perceives immediate tension in the hand anchoring the mid-thoracic spine with a caudal P/A pressure. The star concept is a useful approach to determine which vectors pull the most on the stabilizing hand. The tension may be felt most when the pericardial tissues are pushed in a simple caudal direction, or caudal to the right of the client or caudal to the left. Sometimes the tension is most apparent when moving the pericardial tissues mediolaterally or in a clockwise/counterclockwise direction, always maintaining the depth of the tissue. The patient perceives this tension as the therapist pushing harder on the thoracic vertebra when, in reality, the therapist is simply preventing the thoracic spinous process from moving. If no tension is perceived, then this part of the DFL of fascia in relation to the thorax is not tight. If tension is perceived (quick resistance is felt between the two hands of the therapist), then it can be mobilized as per the approaches outlined in Chapter 4. (The therapist maintains the pressure on the spinous process of the thorax to prevent it from moving as he/she performs repeated A/P mobilizations of the pericardial fascia in the direction(s) of most restriction.) This may be repeated for all thoracic levels if tension is found at these levels.

A/P thorax in relation to the diaphragm (DFL) (Figure 8.5)

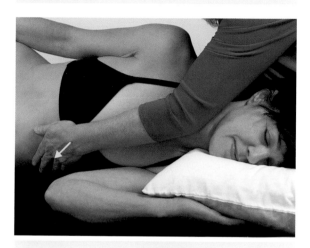

Figure 8.5
MMS A/P Thx in relation to the diaphragm

The three previous techniques can be explored equally in relation to the diaphragm.

Stabilizing hand As per the technique above.

Mobilizing hand The caudal hand explores the anterior diaphragm area with a caudal/lateral glide of the tissues, always looking for the immediate line of tension between the two hands of the therapist. Appropriate depth of tissues is required. The fascia around the rectus abdominis and oblique abdominal muscles may be accessed with this technique if the technique is done superficially. (This would be a technique for the SFL.) However, in order to access the diaphragm, which is part of the DFL, the therapist must first slowly sink into the tissues posterior to the lower ribs and then gently push in a caudal/lateral direction. This technique can be done with either the ipsilateral or the contralateral diaphragm.

Progression The above techniques may be repeated in the same side-lying position but the DFL of fascia is pre-tensed by placing the hips at 0 degrees of extension, the knees flexed at 90 degrees of flexion (Figure 8.6).

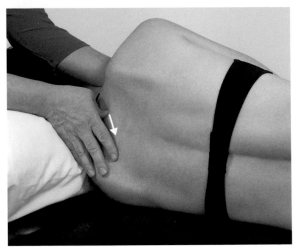

Figure 8.7
MMS A/P C/Thx region

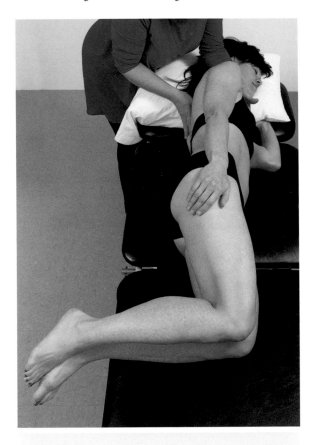

Figure 8.6
MMS A/P Thx with tension on the DFL (hips extended/ knees flexed)

MMS techniques A/P cervicothoracic region (DFL) (Figure 8.7)

The technique above may also be adapted to use with persistent C/Thx dysfunction. When the diaphragm does not function optimally, the patient tends to develop an upper chest breathing pattern. The scalene muscles, in their attempt to compensate, can become overactive and develop trigger points, which may result in referred symptoms similar to the thoracic outlet syndrome and/or the carpal tunnel syndrome. Hypertonic scalene muscles may also maintain pain and dysfunction in the C/Thx region. For this technique, the therapist anchors onto the C/Thx region (C7–T2) via a caudally directed P/A on the right side of the spinous process. The therapist may also explore anchors on the upper ribs, usually at the level of the costotransverse joint. (The technique may also be performed on the left side.) The mobilizing hand explores the pericardial fascia as per the previous technique.

MMS techniques A/P thoracolumbar region (DFL) (Figure 8.8)

The technique above may also be adapted to use with persistent Th/L dysfunction. In an upper chest breathing pattern, the diaphragm does not move downward (shorten). This pattern may result in overactivity of the erector spinae muscles, which may lead to hyperlordosis, with increased tone at the Th/L junction. The lower ribs tend to point upwards rather than remaining in a more caudad position. For this technique, the therapist anchors onto the Th/L region (T11 and T12) via a caudally directed P/A on the right side of the spinous process. (The technique may also be performed on the left side.) The mobilizing hand explores the pericardial fascia as per the previous technique or the anterior diaphragm.

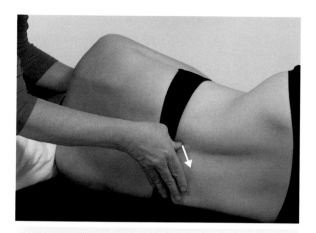

Figure 8.8
MMS A/P Th/Lx region

Case report 8.1 Mac's story*

This 54-year-old musician complained of chronic deep ache in the mid-thoracic region, exacerbated by working at his computer, playing his guitar, and sleeping supine with legs straight. There was no history of trauma and his symptoms had occurred gradually over the past five years. His radiology reports were unremarkable, with mild spondylosis reported. He had previously consulted a chiropractor and an osteopath, with no results. He had also seen a manual physiotherapist who had mobilized the C/Thx and the mid-thoracic regions to improve extension and rotations and had used dry needling to ease tension in the hypertonic extensors of his thoracic spine. This approach improved his symptoms by about 50 percent but then his condition plateaued. He was then seen by a therapist who had received training in the ISM approach. This therapist had noted a ring shift to the right (an intrathoracic torsion left) at ring 4 with thoracic right rotation. This was treated with techniques to release the tension of the muscles maintaining this ring shift as well as muscle reeducation patterns to re-train thoracic rotation. Again he noted improvement in his symptoms but he still had a low-grade ache especially with sleeping supine and at the end of his working day. He was then referred to me for an assessment of the fascial system and the following was noted:

- a pes cavus deformity anteriorly (from birth)

- A/P MMS techniques for the mid-thorax were very tight bilaterally and reproduced his thoracic pain (even with his hips and knees flexed 45 degrees)

- A/P mid-Cx MMS techniques in relation to the DFL (pericardium and diaphragms) also very tight, reproducing cervical pain, an occasional complaint of his (see Chapter 5 for technique)

- A/P C/Thx and Th/L MMS techniques also problematic, although less than the mid-thoracic techniques.

These dysfunctions were treated with MMS techniques in the side-lying position, and later, progressed by placing the hips in 0 degrees of extension, with knees at 90 degrees flexion to increase tension on the DFL. Ultimately, we used suction cups to the area of his pes cavus with movement in a cranio-caudal direction, and combined this with the MMS techniques for A/P mid-thorax in side-lying. This approach solved his long-standing chronic mid-thoracic ache and he could finally sleep supine with his legs straight without bringing on his symptoms. We could then surmise that his work (guitar playing and computer) as well as the pes cavus that he had from childhood, contributed to a tight DFL of fascia. Perhaps the fascial tension between the pericardium and diaphragm areas in relation to the cervical and mid-thoracic spine was a factor that maintained his chronic thoracic ache.

* Please note that the patient's name has been changed to protect his privacy.

MMS techniques iliacus

The diaphragm, psoas, iliacus, and quadratus lumborum (QL) share a fascial connection at the lumbar vertebrae. When proper diaphragmatic breathing is not observed, these muscles are prone to disuse, weakness, and trigger point development – all of which can play a role in back and hip pain (Clifton-Smith & Rowley 2011). These muscles also form a part of the DFL of fascia, but the iliacus also seems to have clinical correlations to the SFL and the Lateral Lines of fascia.

Indications for this technique are the following:

- pain in the area of the abdominal area

- restriction in hip extension – plateau with mobilizations of the hip capsule to increase extension; plateau with techniques to stretch the psoas muscle

- restriction in lumbar extension – plateau with mobilizations to increase extension of the lumbar facet joints

- restriction in hip abduction (due to a tight DFL).

MMS right iliacus with opposite ASIS (SFL) (Figure 8.9)

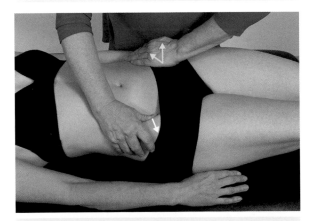

Figure 8.9
MMS right iliacus with opposite ASIS

Stabilizing hand The therapist **gently** places their right thumb on the right iliacus muscle, exploring tension from the ASIS toward the symphysis pubis. The pressure is light and is performed in a mediolateral direction. At times,

there may be so much tension in this area that the therapist feels as though they are on a trampoline. Because the iliacus is a wide muscle that lines the medial aspect of the ilium, several areas may be used as the anchor from which the following techniques are explored and treated.

Mobilizing hand The therapist's left hand explores the opposite ilium, gently moving it toward "outflare" (an osteopathic term that describes a movement of the ilium in a latero-posterior direction), but with the star concept in mind. The therapist looks for the angle where he/she perceives immediate tension in the hand anchoring the right iliacus. If this fascial line is tight, the therapist will feel an increase in tension in the anchoring hand, as if the right iliacus muscle pulls in toward midline. The patient perceives this change as the therapist increasing his/her pressure on the right iliacus. If tension is perceived (quick resistance is felt between the two hands of the therapist), then it can be mobilized as per the approaches outlined in Chapter 4. (The therapist maintains the pressure on the right iliacus to prevent it from moving as he/she performs repeated mobilizations to the left ilium in the direction(s) of most restriction.)

MMS right iliacus with opposite external oblique (SFL)/anterior diaphragm (DFL) (Figure 8.10)

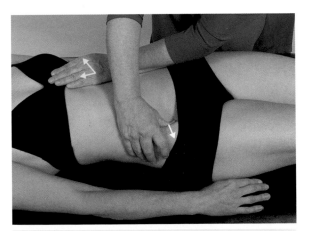

Figure 8.10
MMS right iliacus with opposite EO (SFL)/anterior diaphragm (DFL)

Stabilizing hand As per the technique above.

Mobilizing hand The therapist's left hand explores the area of the left external oblique (for the SFL) and/or the left anterior diaphragm, which has a deeper palpation (for the DFL), gently moving it in a cranio-lateral direction, always with the star concept in mind. The therapist looks for the angle where he/she perceives immediate tension in the hand anchoring the right iliacus. If tension is perceived (quick resistance is felt between the two hands of the therapist), then it can be mobilized as per the approaches outlined in Chapter 4. This technique is also helpful for dysfunctions of the Spiral Line of fascia.

MMS right iliacus with ipsilateral external oblique (SFL)/anterior diaphragm (DFL) (Figure 8.11)

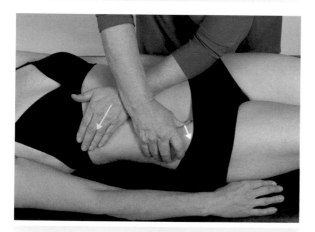

Figure 8.11
MMS right iliacus with ipsilateral EO (SFL)/anterior diaphragm (DFL)

Stabilizing hand As per the technique above.

Mobilizing hand The therapist's left hand explores the area of the right external oblique (for the SFL) and/or the right anterior diaphragm (for the DFL), gently moving it in a cranio-lateral direction, always with the star concept in mind. The therapist looks for the angle where he/she perceives immediate tension in the hand anchoring the right iliacus. If tension is perceived (quick resistance is felt between the two hands of the therapist), then it can

be mobilized as per the approaches outlined in Chapter 4. This technique is also helpful for dysfunctions of the Lateral Line of fascia.

MMS right iliacus with pericardium (DFL) (Figure 8.12)

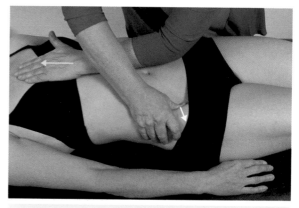

Figure 8.12
MMS right iliacus with pericardium (DFL)

Stabilizing hand As per the technique above.

Mobilizing hand The therapist's left hand explores the area of the pericardium, first by slowly sinking into the tissues posterior to the sternum and then gently pushing them in a cranial direction, all the while maintaining the depth of the fascial line (posterior to the sternum). Using the star concept, the therapist looks for the angle where he/she perceives immediate tension in the hand palpating the right iliacus. That tension may be felt most in a simple cranial direction, or cranial to the right of the client or cranial to the left. Sometimes the tension is most felt when moving the pericardial tissues medio-laterally or in a clockwise/counter-clockwise direction, always maintaining the depth of the tissue. If no tension is perceived, then the DFL of fascia in relation to this muscle is not tight. If this fascial line is tight, the therapist will feel an increase in tension in the anchoring hand, as if the right iliacus muscle pulls in towards the midline and cranially. The patient perceives this as the therapist increasing his/her pressure on the iliacus. Similar concepts for mobilizing this line of fascia apply.

MMS right iliacus with ipsilateral symphysis pubis (SFL) (Figure 8.13)

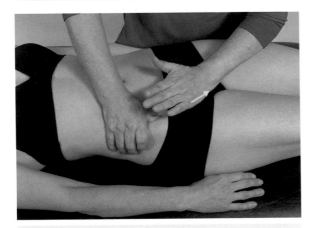

Figure 8.13
MMS right iliacus with ipsilateral symphysis pubis (SFL)

Stabilizing hand As per the technique above.

Mobilizing hand The therapist's left forearm (or heel of the hand) explores the area of the right symphysis pubis, gently moving it in a caudo-medial direction, always with the star concept in mind. The therapist looks for the angle where he/she perceives immediate tension in the hand anchoring the right iliacus. If tension is perceived (quick resistance is felt between the two hands of the therapist), then it can be mobilized as per the approaches outlined in Chapter 4. This technique is also helpful for mobilizing the fascia in the area of the inguinal ligament.

MMS right iliacus with lateral leg/iliotibial band (Lateral Line) (Figure 8.14)

Stabilizing hand As per the technique above.

Mobilizing hand The therapist's left hand explores the right lateral thigh/iliotibial band (ITB), gently moving the tissues in a caudal direction with an internal rotation component, always with the star concept in mind. The therapist looks for the angle and the area(s) on the thigh where he/she perceives

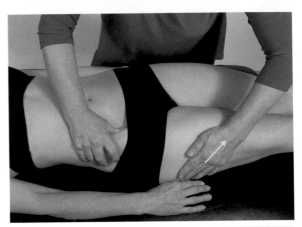

Figure 8.14
MMS right iliacus with lateral leg/ITB

immediate tension in the hand anchoring the right iliacus. Similar concepts for mobilizing this line of fascia apply.

MMS right iliacus with medial leg/adductors (DFL) (Figure 8.15)

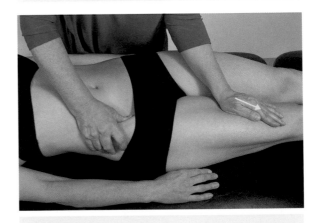

Figure 8.15
MMS right iliacus with medial leg/adductors (DFL)

Stabilizing hand As per technique above.

Mobilizing hand The therapist's left hand explores the right medial thigh/adductors, gently moving the tissues in a caudal direction, often with an external rotation component, always with the star concept in mind. The therapist looks for the angle and the area(s) on the thigh where he/she perceives immediate tension in the hand anchoring the right iliacus. Similar concepts for mobilizing this line of fascia apply.

Note that the iliacus fascia may also be explored in relation to any *abdominal scars* from previous surgeries, including caesarean section scars. The scar itself may be relatively mobile but the scar in relation to the SFL or DFL of fascia is frequently problematic. The anchor is then on the scar rather than the iliacus. Similar techniques may be applied here.

Progressions There are two ways in which these iliacus techniques may be progressed. One is to pre-tense the DFL by asking the patient to actively dorsiflex/evert his ankles as the techniques are repeated. The other is by repeating the techniques with the hips extended/knees flexed, as described below.

MMS right iliacus pre-tensed with hips extended/ knees flexed (Figure 8.16)

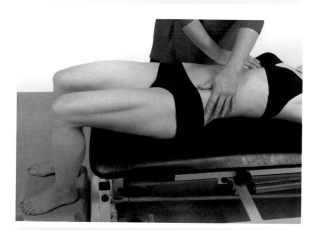

Figure 8.16
MMS right iliacus pre-tensed with hips extended/ knees flexed

All of the techniques above for the iliacus may be repeated with the patient's body placed on the edge of the plinth, hips at 0 degrees of extension and knees at 90 degrees of flexion in order to pre-tense both the SFL and the DFL of fascia.

The therapist must ensure that the patient is comfortable, especially in relation to the lumbar lordosis. A footstool is generally placed to support the patient's legs, and the table must be lowered to the point where the patient is able to comfortably tolerate the lordotic position of the spine.

The quadratus lumborum (QL) muscle is a frequent source of recurrent tension in the area of the lower thoracic and lumbar spine. This muscle may be overactivated if the lateral hip stabilizers are inadequate (primarily gluteus medius). However, tension in the area of the QL may also be maintained if the fascial lines related to this muscle are tight. The QL may be explored in relation to the Lateral Line (upper quadrant technique is described below) and in relation to the DFL (described in Chapter 9).

MMS techniques: right quadratus lumborum in relation to the lateral thorax (Lateral Line – upper quadrant) (Figures 8.17, 8.18)

Stabilizing hand The patient is in left side-lying position with the hips and knees in neutral, the right shoulder flexed. Using the right thumb, the therapist anchors onto the right QL in three areas: the center of the belly of the muscle, its origin at the 12th rib, and its insertion onto the iliac crest. The anchor for the belly of the muscle is in a latero-medial direction (toward the plinth). For the origin of the muscle at the 12th rib, the anchor is also in a latero-medial direction but also angled cranially. For the insertion of the muscle at the iliac crest, the anchor is also in a latero-medial direction but also angled caudally.

Mobilizing hand The therapist's left forearm explores the right lateral ribcage, always with the star concept in mind. The therapist may explore moving the lateral ribcage in a number of possible directions:

- in a cranial direction (toward the patient's head)

- in a cranio-anterior direction (the therapist must adjust their forearm to begin the maneuver slightly posterior to the lateral ribcage), and/or

- in a cranio-posterior direction (the therapist must adjust their forearm to begin the maneuver slightly anterior to the lateral ribcage).

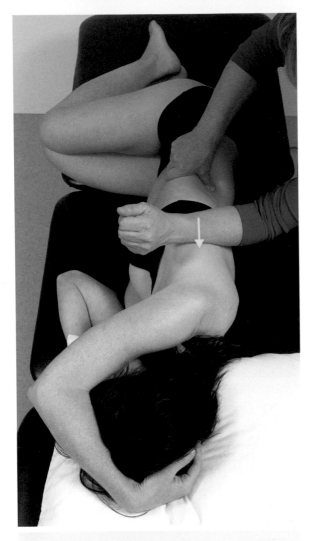

Figure 8.17
MMS right QL with lateral thorax (cranial direction)

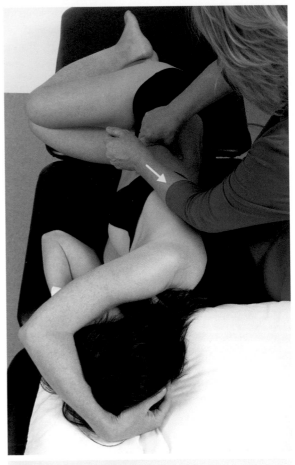

Figure 8.18
MMS right QL with lateral thorax (cranio-posterior direction)

Note that the directions of the mobilizing forearm follow the diamond shape of the intercostal muscles. The ribcage may be explored in this manner, both in the lower thoracic region and the middle thoracic region. This is a general technique although it may also be used in relation to a specific thoracic ring. The therapist looks for the angle and the area(s) on the ribcage where he/she perceives immediate tension in the hand anchor-

ing the right QL. If tension is perceived (quick resistance is felt between the two hands of the therapist), then it can be mobilized as per the approaches outlined in Chapter 4.

Note that the MMS techniques for the right QL in relation to the Lateral Line for the *lower quadrant* are described in Chapter 9.

MMS techniques serratus anterior

The serratus anterior muscle is commonly implicated in dysfunction of the scapula and shoulder complex, with weakness a common feature in scapular dyskinesia, particularly with shoulder flexion. It is also frequently implicated in thoracic ring dysfunction as a hypertonic fascicle of serratus anterior may create a vector that pulls on the thoracic ring and makes it difficult to perform isolated scapular movement independent of the thorax. It therefore impacts the mechanics of the thoracic spine and shoulder girdle function.

If the serratus anterior is found to be problematic, a release with awareness (RWA) approach works well. This is the fourth treatment concept for MMS outlined in Chapter 4.

Release with awareness right serratus anterior (Figure 8.19)

Release with awareness (RWA) is a biofeedback technique developed by Diane Lee and L. J. Lee in which the patient is an active participant. The patient is asked to bring their awareness to the muscle being palpated and various imagery cues are used to facilitate relaxation of the muscle. This engagement of the patient occurs as the therapist is guiding the release with feedback from their hands (Lee & Lee 2011). Please refer to Chapter 4 for a full description of this technique.

Stabilizing hand The patient is in left side-lying position with the hips and knees in neutral, the right arm by the side of the trunk or in a combined shoulder quadrant position, with the patient's hand resting on his/her forehead. (This technique may also be performed in sitting.) Using the fingers of their right hand, the therapist gently palpates the fascicle of serratus anterior that is hypertonic. (Note: there may be more than one fascicle in a given area of the lateral thorax and each fascicle should be explored from its anterior attachment on the rib as far back posteriorly towards the scapula as possible.)

Mobilizing hand The therapist's left hand encompasses the patient's right scapula, guiding it initially toward protraction, followed by retraction. As the therapist provides manual input to the serratus anterior, the patient is instructed to "soften the muscle," "let it go,"

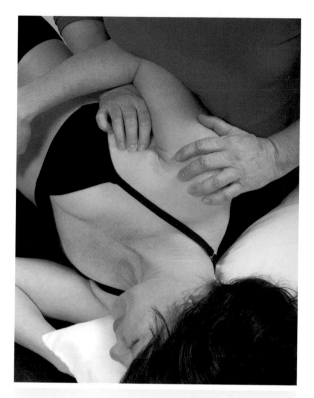

Figure 8.19
MMS right serratus anterior with thorax

"see if you can find a way to allow my fingers to sink into the muscle." At the same time, the therapist moves the scapula to shorten origin and insertion (protraction), diminishing tension on the muscle spindle. The therapist then waits, allowing the patient and his/her system to cue into the release at the same time as the therapist gives manual and verbal cues to let go. The verbal cue "Let your scapula float back towards your spine" usually works well here. Once maximum release is obtained, usually within 10–15 seconds, the muscle is gently taken through a full stretch with scapular retraction, with the therapist listening to its response and avoiding recurrence of overactivity. The therapist may then encourage a release of the muscle fascicle in the direction of scapular retraction, helping to release the "fuzz" of connective tissue that has lost its ability to elongate.

MMS right serratus posterior inferior (Figure 8.20)

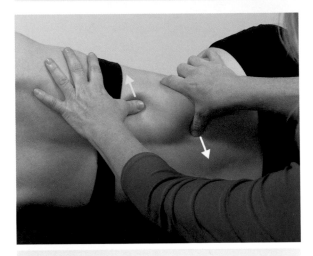

Figure 8.20
MMS right serratus posterior inferior

The serratus posterior inferior muscle is not typically sought out by therapists who look for myofascial restriction that may impact the thorax and/or lumbar spine. The serratus posterior inferior originates on the supraspinal ligament, and the spinous processes of the upper two to three lumbar vertebrae (L1–3) and the lower two thoracic vertebrae (T11–12). It inserts on the lower borders of ribs 9 to 12 (latissimus dorsi lies above this muscle). Functionally, it is an accessory muscle of expiration that helps depress the ribs during exhalation. It may be a factor that limits optimal lateral costal breathing and maintains tension throughout the Th/L area.

Stabilizing hand The patient is in left side-lying position with the hips and knees in neutral. The therapist's right hand stabilizes the spinous processes of T11 to L3 with a caudally directed P/A on the right side of the spinous processes.

Mobilizing hand The therapist's other hand explores the lower thoracic rings, which may extend beyond ribs 9–12 if we consider fascial connections. A release with awareness technique may be performed here, as per the above example.

Another way to release this area is to use the first concept of the MMS approach. In this case, the therapist's right hand explores the area of the lower thoracic ribs, gliding them in a cranio-lateral direction, always with the star concept in mind. The individual ribs may be explored individually but a more global exploration of the lower ribs may also be done. The therapist looks for the angle where he/she perceives immediate tension in the hand anchoring the spinous process. If tension is perceived (quick resistance is felt between the two hands of the therapist), then it can be mobilized as per the approaches outlined in Chapter 4.

Summary

The techniques in this chapter have focused on the myofascial connections in relation to the thoracic region, in particular the pericardium, the diaphragm, iliacus, quadratus lumborum, serratus anterior and serratus posterior inferior muscles. These tissues are frequently problematic in cases of persistent thoracic, C/Thx, Th/L, anterior chest and abdominal pain and should be explored using MMS techniques.

The next chapter will focus on techniques for the lumbopelvic area.

When treating patients with problems in the lumbopelvic area, manual therapists are trained to assess and treat the joints of the lumbar spine, the sacroiliac joint, and the symphysis pubis. In addition, the muscles of the abdominal region, the posterior thoracolumbar and pelvic/hip muscles are assessed and treated for imbalance between hypertonic, tight muscles and weak muscles of the lumbopelvic-hip area. However, mobilizing joints and stretching and strengthening individual muscles can achieve only partial benefits if the fascial system is not taken into consideration.

This chapter will describe the clinical findings of restriction in the following areas of fascial dysfunction:

- the thoracolumbar fascia

- the quadratus lumborum (QL) in relation to the Lateral Line and the DFL

- the lateral sacral fascia in relation to the hip

- the sacrotuberous ligament in relation to the hip, the SBL, and the DFL

- the femoral nerve fascia.

Indications for MMS for this chapter

1. Recurring lumbopelvic-hip pain despite the following treatment approaches:

   - mobilization/manipulation of the lumbar spine, thorax, and sacroiliac joints
   - mobilization of the hip joint capsules
   - stabilization exercises for the thoracolumbar-pelvic-hip area
   - release of trigger points to the thoracolumbar-pelvic-hip muscles with manual or dry needling techniques.

Postural analysis

In an optimal postural alignment, the primary spinal curves should be maintained (i.e., gentle lumbar lordosis, gentle, even thoracic kyphosis and gentle, even cervical lordosis). There

should be no kinks, shifts, hinges, or transverse plane rotations throughout the entire spinal curve (Lee & Lee 2011).

Restrictions in the various fascial lines may contribute to postural dysfunction. If there is restriction of the DFL of fascia, this may help to maintain a forward head posture. This tension can develop as a result of trauma, including surgical scars to the abdominal area. (One may think, for example, of the impact of caesarean section scars, old appendectomy scars, hernia repairs, etc.). In addition, certain activities of daily living, such as excessive time spent in the sitting position for work or leisure activities, can be a factor in creating these fascial lines of tension. Because the pelvic floor muscles form part of the DFL this may also impact the mobility and function of the hip joint. Restriction in the Lateral Line of fascia may create a lateral tilt of the lumbar spine or the pelvis. It may also become a contributing factor for recurring issues with the iliotibial band (ITB).

Position of the pelvic girdle

The pelvic girdle is assessed in the standing position, with the therapist positioned directly behind the patient. Please refer to Diane Lee's and L. J. Lee's book *The Pelvic Girdle* for details on the postural assessment of the pelvic girdle (Lee & Lee 2011). The therapist's hands palpate the anterior aspect of the pelvis bilaterally and the therapist notes the resting position in three body planes (anteroposterior tilt, lateral tilt, transverse plane rotation). The pelvic girdle as a unit should be neutral in all three planes: coronal, sagittal, and transverse. The innominates should not be rotated relative to one another (no intrapelvic torsion (IPT)) and the sacrum should not be rotated.

Active range of motion tests

Lumbar movement testing should be performed before and after MMS techniques, in order to evaluate the impact of the techniques on ROM. These movements include lumbar flexion, extension, rotation and side bending as well as combined movements. The therapist evaluates the quality and quantity of movement as well as reproduction of any symptoms. The emphasis should be on movements that most correspond to the patient's functional problem(s).

Functional tests

Squat test

Assessment of the pelvis with half squat

If the subjective exam points to difficulty with squatting or sitting, then this functional test is required. The squat task may be used to assess control of the foot, knee, hip, lumbar spine, pelvis, or thorax. In this example, it is used to assess intrapelvic control. The therapist palpates the ilium with one hand and the ipsilateral inferior lateral angle (ILA) with the other hand. Note that the therapist's entire hand is palpating as much of the ilium as possible – the therapist avoids using only the thumb at the posterior superior iliac spine (PSIS), as this reduces the reliability of this palpatory test. The ILA is used for palpation of the sacrum as it is more precise than using the depth of the sacral sulcus (which is frequently influenced by atrophy of the sacral multifidus muscle). If there is good strategy with a squat, the two bones should move as a unit and there should be no anterior rotation of the ilium relative to the sacrum. If anterior rotation of the ilium does occur (a relative counternutation of the sacrum), it is termed failed load transfer (FLT) (Lee & Lee 2011). The source of this FLT may be due poor dynamic stability of the lumbopelvic hip complex, but it may also be due to dysfunction above and below this region (ISM model). If the driver is indeed the pelvis, then the pelvis has to be evaluated more thoroughly. (Refer to Diane Lee's and L. J. Lee's book *The Pelvic Girdle* for details on the assessment of the pelvic girdle (Lee & Lee 2011).)

One leg stand test (OLS)

If the subjective exam indicates difficulty with standing, walking, or running, then the functional test of a one leg stand (OLS) is required. The pelvic girdle may be assessed in a similar way as for the squat test, but the functional movement assessed is one in which the patient shifts his/her weight onto one leg and lifts the other off the floor. The weight-bearing side is assessed for FLT. Once again, if there is good strategy with a OLS,

the two bones should move as a unit and there should be no anterior rotation of the ilium relative to the sacrum (Lee & Lee 2011). Failed load transfer (FLT) may once again be due to poor dynamic stability of the lumbopelvic-hip complex, as well as dysfunction above and below this region (ISM model). If the driver is indeed the pelvis, then it has to be evaluated more thoroughly.

These positional and functional tests may be used before and after treatment with the MMS approach. Keep in mind that fascial restrictions may inhibit the dynamic stabilizers of the lumbopelvic-hip complex from working optimally. If the OLS or squat test still shows FLT after releasing tight fascia in this area, then the therapist should assess and treat the muscles that help stabilize this region.

Concepts of treatment using MMS

For this chapter, we will be using primarily the first concept of treatment when using MMS techniques: that is, choose a recurrent articular dysfunction or myofascial trigger point and explore a fascial line in relation to it. The therapist anchors him/herself to a recurrent articular dysfunction or myofascial trigger point and assesses the fascial lines of tension in relation to the anchor, looking for early tension between their two hands.

The following approaches may be used, depending on how the tissues respond:

- work with oscillations (grades III–, III, III+)
- work with sustained pressure
- work with "harmonics" (Dr Laurie Hartman).

Refer to Chapter 4 for further detail on concepts of treatment using MMS.

MMS techniques for the thoracolumbar fascia

The thoracolumbar area is often an area with a tendency towards tightness, perhaps because it is the hub for a number of myofascial tissues, including the diaphragm. Tension in this area can limit thoracic rotation and lumbar side-flexion, especially if a plateau has been reached with mobilizations of the appropriate facet joints and costotransverse joints.

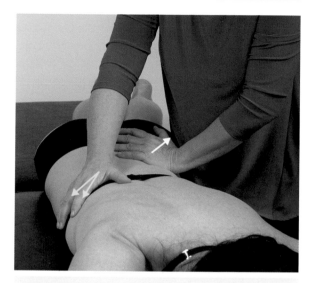

Figure 9.1
MMS for the right Th/L fascia I (Functional Line)

Stabilizing hand The patient is in prone position with the lumbar spine in left side-flexion, the right shoulder in flexion. The therapist stands on the left side of the patient. The therapist anchors onto the area of the patient's left ilium in a caudal/lateral direction, using the star concept to anchor into the area of most tension.

Mobilizing hand Using the right hand, the therapist explores the area of the right lower thorax, gently gliding the Th/L fascia in a craniolateral direction. The tension may be felt most when pushing in the area of the facet joints or the ribs but we must keep in mind that we are not mobilizing joints, but rather the fascia around these structures. Once again, the star concept is a useful approach to determine which vectors pull the most on the stabilizing hand. The tension may be felt most when the Th/L tissues are pushed in a simple cranial direction, or cranial to the right of the client, or cranial to the left. The patient perceives this tension as the therapist pushing harder on the left ilium when, in reality, the therapist is simply preventing the ilium from moving. If no tension is perceived, then this part

of the Th/L fascia is not tight. If tension is perceived (quick resistance is felt between the two hands of the therapist), then it can be mobilized as per the approaches outlined in Chapter 4. (The therapist maintains the anchor on the left ilium to prevent it from moving as he/she performs repeated P/A mobilizations of the thoracolumbar area.)

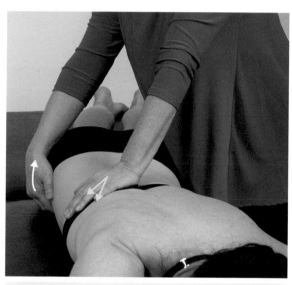

Figure 9.2
MMS for the Th/L fascia II (Lateral Line)

Stabilizing hand The patient is in prone position as per the technique above. The therapist stands on the left side of the patient. The therapist gently anchors onto the area of the patient's right ilium in a caudal/medial direction, as if pulling the ilium into posterior rotation.

Mobilizing hand The therapist explores the area of the right lower thorax with the right hand, gently gliding the Th/L fascia as per the technique above. If this fascial line is tight, the patient perceives this tension as the therapist pulling harder on the right ilium, especially on the anterior portion of the ilium. This technique also commonly reproduces the patient's "sacroiliac" pain. In reality, the therapist is simply preventing the ilium from moving. Similar concepts for mobilizing this line of fascia apply.

Sometimes the patient has tension and restriction in the central lumbar spine. If a plateau is reached using central P/A pressures on the spinous processes, then the following fascial techniques may be explored. The first technique relates to the SBL of fascia. The second technique is a modification of the first, in which the therapist uses various hip movements to pre-tense the fascia.

MMS central sacral/thoracolumbar fascia (SBL) (Figure 9.3)

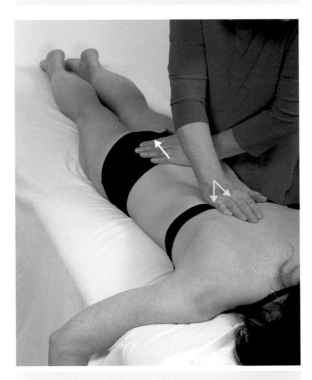

Figure 9.3
MMS central sacral/Th/L fascia (SBL)

Stabilizing hand The patient is in prone position with the lumbar spine in a neutral position. The therapist stands on the either side of the patient. Using the palm of their hand, the therapist anchors onto the area of the patient's sacral base with a P/A pressure in a caudal direction.

Mobilizing hand Using the inferior aspect of the spinous processes as a lever, the therapist explores the central lower thorax and upper lumbar spine with the other hand, gently gliding the tissues in a cranial direction. The therapist may explore the area between L3 and T10 in this manner. (L4 and L5 may be a little more difficult to do in this position because of the lumbar lordosis.) Once again, the star concept is a useful approach to determine which vectors pull the most on the stabilizing hand. The tension may be felt most when the Th/L tissues are pushed in a simple cranial direction, or cranial to the right of the client or cranial to the left. The patient perceives this tension as the therapist pulling harder on the sacrum when, in reality, the therapist is simply preventing the base of the sacrum from moving cranially. If no tension is perceived, then this part of the Th/L fascia is not tight. If tension is perceived (quick resistance is felt between the two hands of the therapist), then it can be mobilized as per the approaches outlined in Chapter 4.

MMS central sacral/thoracolumbar fascia + bilateral hip abduction (Figure 9.4)

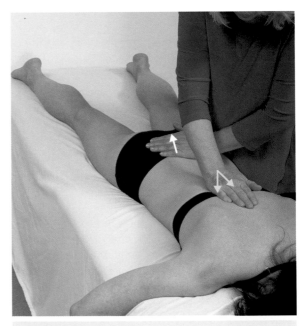

Figure 9.4
MMS central sacral/Th/L fascia + bilateral hip abduction

This is a variation of the technique above, as the therapist explores the placement of the legs in a variety of positions, depending on the patient's functional complaints. In this example, if the patient complains of low back pain with horseback riding, it may be appropriate to add bilateral hip abduction and examine its effect on the central Th/L fascia. It is assessed and treated as per the previous technique.

MMS quadratus lumborum in relation to the Lateral Line

The techniques below are used to release persistent tension in the area of the right quadratus lumborum muscle (QL). They may also be used to release tension in the ITB and/or the lateral lower leg.

MMS right quadratus lumborum + Lateral Line (lower quadrant) 1 (Figure 9.5)

Stabilizing hand The patient is in left side-lying position with the hips and knees in neutral, the right shoulder flexed. Using the left thumb, the therapist anchors onto the right QL in three areas: the center of the belly of the muscle, its origin at the 12th rib, and its insertion onto the iliac crest. The anchor for the belly of the muscle is in a lateromedial direction (toward the plinth), using the star concept to anchor into the area of most tension. For the origin of the muscle at the 12th rib, the anchor is also in a lateromedial direction but it is also angled cranially. For the insertion of the muscle at the iliac crest, the anchor is in a lateromedial direction but it is also angled caudally.

Mobilizing hand The therapist's right hand explores the right lateral thigh/ITB proximally to distally, and always with the star concept in mind. The therapist may explore the lateral thigh in a number of possible directions:

- in a caudal direction (toward the patient's feet)
- in a caudal-anterior direction
- in a caudal-posterior direction.

The therapist looks for the angle and the area(s) on the thigh where he/she perceives immediate tension in the

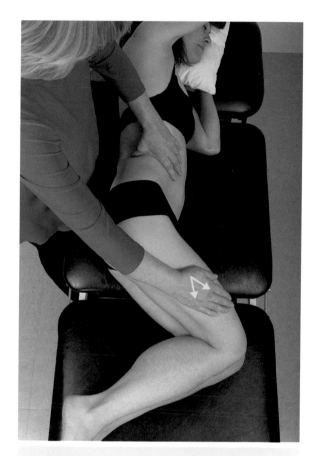

Figure 9.5
MMS right QL + Lateral Line (lower quadrant) I

hand anchoring the right QL. If there is tension in this line of fascia, it will seem like the QL translates laterally before full caudal glide of the thigh fascia can be achieved. The therapist maintains the medial pressure on the QL and simply prevents it from moving laterally. The patient perceives this as the therapist increasing pressure on QL. If tension is perceived (quick resistance is felt between the two hands of the therapist), then it can be mobilized as per the approaches outlined in Chapter 4. (The therapist performs repeated movement of the lateral thigh fascia in the direction(s) of most restriction while maintaining a steady pressure on QL, always to when R1 is perceived. This is repeated until a release is felt between the therapist's two hands and generally requires approximately five to eight cycles.)

MMS right quadratus lumborum + Lateral Line (lower quadrant) 2 (Figure 9.6)

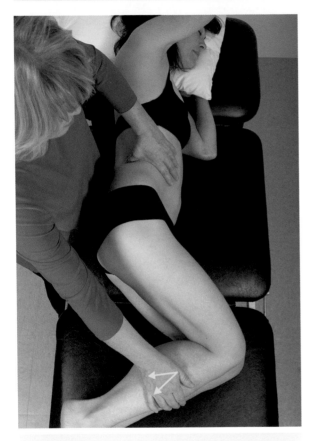

Figure 9.6
MMS right QL + Lateral Line (lower quadrant) II

Stabilizing hand As per the technique above.

Mobilizing hand As per the technique above except that the therapist explores the right lateral lower leg in relation to the right QL.

MMS quadratus lumborum in relation to the Deep Front Line (DFL)

The QL muscle also forms part of the DFL and, as such, may also be explored in relation to this fascial line. This approach is particularly beneficial in situations where lumbar extension and/or hip extension remains limited despite treatment directed towards mobilization of the lumbar or hip joints and/or techniques to lengthen the appropriate muscles (e.g., psoas).

MMS right quadratus lumborum + ipsilateral posterior diaphragm in lumbar spine extension (DFL) (Figure 9.7, 9.8)

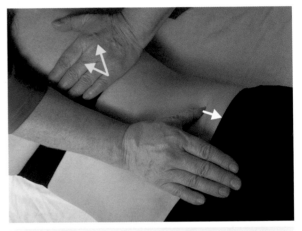

Figure 9.7
MMS right QL in relation to the DFL – hand position

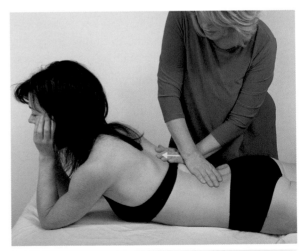

Figure 9.8
MMS right QL + ipsilateral posterior diaphragm in Lx extension (DFL)

Stabilizing hand The patient is in a prone position with the lumbar spine in extension. The patient supports him/herself on the elbows, with the hands cupped under the chin. This position minimizes overactivity of the lumbar extensors. (If there is too much tension in this position, these techniques may initially be performed in the neutral lumbar position, without extension.) The therapist stands on the right side of the patient. Using their right thumb, the therapist anchors onto the right QL, as per the techniques above (Figure 9.7). Each of the techniques below may be repeated with a different anchor on the QL (origin, insertion, and belly of muscle), but the most commonly used anchor is that of the insertion of the QL at the ilium. In that case, the anchor is directed caudally.

Mobilizing hand The therapist explores the area of the right lower thorax with the left hand, gently gliding the area of the posterior diaphragm in a craniolateral direction (Figure 9.8). Once again, the star concept is a useful approach to determine which vectors pull the most on the stabilizing hand. The tension may be felt most when the posterior diaphragm is pushed in a simple cranial direction, or cranial to the right of the client, or cranial to the left. If no tension is perceived, then this part of the DFL is not tight. If there is tension in this line of fascia and the anchor is at the belly of the muscle, it will seem like the QL translates laterally before full craniolateral glide of the posterior diaphragm area can be achieved. The therapist maintains the medial pressure on the QL and simply prevents it from moving laterally. If the anchor of the QL is at the ilium then the therapist will perceive that this area wants to pull up in a cranial direction. In either case, the patient perceives this as the therapist pushing harder on the right QL when, in reality, the therapist is simply preventing the anchor from moving. Similar concepts for mobilizing this line of fascia apply.

> MMS right quadratus lumborum + contralateral posterior diaphragm in lumbar spine extension (DFL) (Figure 9.9)

The technique is similar to the one above except that the therapist explores the contralateral posterior diaphragm area. (Figure 9.9)

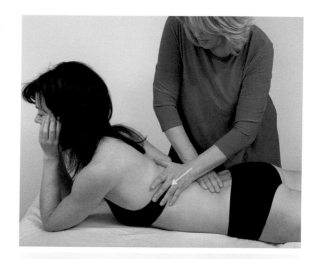

Figure 9.9
MMS right QL + contralateral posterior diaphragm in Lx extension (DFL)

> MMS right quadratus lumborum + central tendon of diaphragm in lumbar spine extension (DFL) (Figure 9.10)

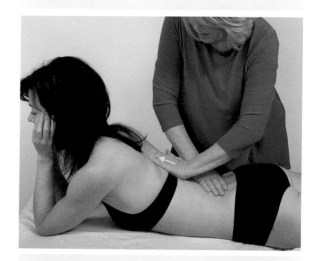

Figure 9.10
MMS right QL + central tendon of diaphragm in Lx extension (DFL)

The technique is similar to the one above except that the therapist explores the area of the central tendon attachments of the diaphragm in the central Th/L region (using central, cranially directed P/A pressures on the spinous processes of T10 to L2) (Figure 9.10).

For the DFL of fascia the therapist may also explore the QL in relation to structures more caudal to it. Adding knee flexion or hip IR are some ways to increase tension on the DFL:

> MMS right quadratus lumborum + ipsilateral knee flex in lumbar spine extension (DFL) (Figure 9.11)

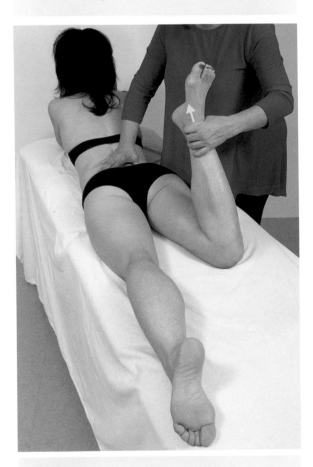

Figure 9.11
MMS right QL + ipsil knee flex in Lx extension (DFL)

The technique is similar to the one above except that the therapist uses passive physiological knee flexion to add tension and explore this part of the DFL. The therapist stops as soon as an increase in tension is perceived in the hand that is anchoring the right QL (to the first resistance

or R1 of Maitland's movement diagram). If there is tension in this line of fascia, it will seem like the QL translates laterally before full knee flexion can be achieved (usually around 120 degrees of flexion). The therapist maintains the medial pressure on the QL and simply prevents it from moving laterally. The patient perceives this as the therapist pushing harder on the right QL when, in reality, the therapist is simply preventing the anchor from moving. Similar concepts for mobilizing this line of fascia apply.

Alternatively, passive physiological hip internal rotation (IR) may be explored with this technique, as the hip external rotators form part of the pelvic floor and hence, the DFL of fascia.

> MMS right quadratus lumborum + ipsilateral hip internal rotation in lumbar spine extension (Figure 9.12)

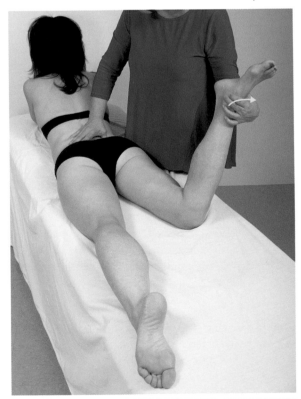

Figure 9.12
MMS right QL + ipsil hip IR in Lx extension (DFL)

The technique is similar to the one above except that the therapist explores IR of the ipsilateral hip.

The DFL fascia in relation to QL may also be explored in relation to the anterior diaphragm, if the technique is done in side-lying with the hips extended.

Stabilizing hand The patient is in left side-lying, with the hips extended at 0 degrees and the knees flexed at 90 degrees. The therapist's left hand anchors onto the right QL.

Mobilizing hand Using the right hand, the therapist explores the area of the right anterior diaphragm, gently gliding it in a cranial direction, using the star concept. The treatment approach is similar to that of the techniques above.

MMS right quadratus lumborum + anterior diaphragm in side-lying (DFL) (Figure 9.13)

MMS right quadratus lumborum + dorsiflexion/eversion in side-lying (DFL) (Figure 9.14)

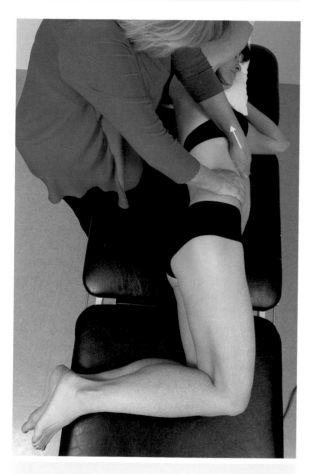

Figure 9.13
MMS right QL + anterior diaphragm in side-lying (DFL)

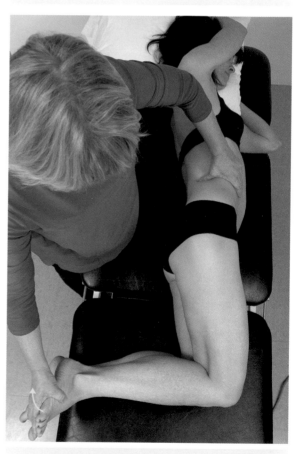

Figure 9.14
MMS Right QL + DF/Ev in side-lying (DFL)

With the patient in the same position as for the technique above, the QL fascia may be further explored by using passive physiological combined ankle dorsiflexion/eversion with the knee flexed, as this maneuver adds tension to the tibialis posterior muscle, the tail end of the DFL. The therapist stops as soon as an increase in tension is perceived in the hand that is anchoring the right QL (to the first resistance or R1 of Maitland's movement diagram). If there is tension in this line of fascia, it will seem as though the QL translates laterally before full combined dorsiflexion/eversion can be achieved. The therapist maintains the medial pressure on the QL and simply prevents it from moving laterally. The patient perceives this as the therapist pushing harder on the right QL when, in reality, the therapist is simply preventing the anchor from moving. If tension is perceived (quick resistance is felt between the two hands of the therapist), then it can be mobilized as per the approaches outlined in Chapter 4. (The therapist performs repeated passive physiological dorsiflexion/eversion while maintaining a steady pressure on QL, always to when R1 is perceived (a grade III– passive physiological movement in Maitland terms). This is repeated until a release is felt between the therapist's two hands and it generally requires approximately five to eight cycles.

Case report 9.1 Elena's story*

This 42-year-old patient had come for therapy with complaints of right low back pain (LBP), especially in standing and sitting positions, and with gym exercises requiring a squat maneuver. She had a history of LBP in the past, successfully treated by another therapist, who used a combination of mobilizations, dry needling, and stabilization exercises. When this latest incident occurred she went back to see her original therapist, who used a similar approach to the one that had been successful in the past, but this time it was not. Elena had also had a right fibular fracture six months prior, from which she recovered well. Her right quadratus lumborum was particularly painful – what she described as "her pain." Dry needling this muscle at this point did not change her pain. Dynamic stability testing of the thoracolumbar-pelvis-hip complex with one leg stand (OLS) and

half squat positions revealed negative findings. Her right foot mechanics were good and the flexibility of the muscles around the foot and ankle was also within normal limits and pain-free. The next area to explore in the assessment of this lady's condition was the mobility of the fascial lines. Using the techniques above, it was noted that there was no tension of QL in relation to the Lateral Line. However, there was considerable tension of QL in relation to the DFL (here was the "Aha!" moment I was looking for). Adding dorsiflexion/eversion to stretch the tibialis posterior in side-lying (technique above), I could feel a definite connection of a shortened fascial line with her right QL. Two treatments later, she was pain-free and once again enjoying her sporting activities.

* Please note that the patient's name has been changed to protect her privacy.

MMS lateral sacral fascia in relation to the hip

A number of muscles (and their corresponding fascia) connect to and/or cross over the posterior aspect of the sacrum. Many patients incorrectly refer to pain in this area as "sacroiliac pain". While the sacroiliac joint (SIJ) could be a factor in their pelvic pain, myofascial tissues are more commonly the source of their complaints. The lateral border of the sacrum is an area where a number of muscles attach, in particular the hip external rotators and the glutei muscles, as well as the longissimus muscles. Overactivity of iliocostalis may also tug on the long dorsal ligament (LDL), causing pain over the SIJ. The techniques below are designed to release the fascia of the lateral border of the sacrum in relation to the hip.

MMS right lateral sacral fascia + hip external rotation (Figure 9.15)

Stabilizing hand The patient is in prone position with the lumbar spine in a neutral position. The therapist stands on the right side of the patient. Using a P/A pressure on the right lateral sacral tissues, the therapist explores areas of tension from S1 toward S5.

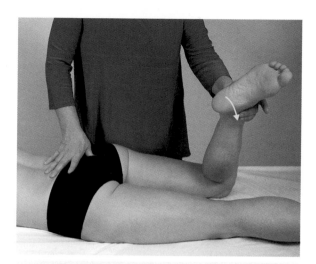

Figure 9.15
MMS lateral sacral fascia + hip ER

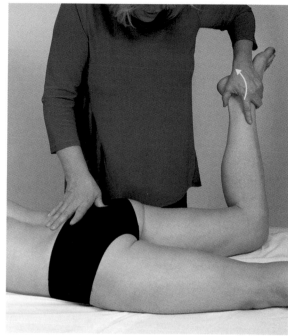

Figure 9.16
MMS lateral sacral fascia + hip IR

Mobilizing hand The therapist's caudal hand supports the right lower extremity at the ankle and performs a passive physiological movement of hip external rotation, stopping as soon as an increase in tension is perceived in the hand palpating the right sacral border (to the first resistance or R1 of Maitland's movement diagram). If there is tension in this line of fascia, it will seem as though the sacrum moves laterally and caudally before full hip external rotation can be achieved (usually around 45–50 degrees of rotation). The patient perceives this as the therapist increasing pressure on the sacrum. The therapist performs repeated passive physiological ER of the hip while maintaining a steady pressure on the sacrum, always to when R1 is perceived (a grade III– passive physiological movement in Maitland terms). This sequence is repeated until a release is felt between the therapist's two hands and generally requires approximately five to eight cycles.

MMS lateral sacral fascia + hip internal rotation (Figure 9.16)

The technique is similar to the one above except that the therapist explores passive physiological hip internal rotation.

MMS lateral sacral fascia + hip extension (Figure 9.17)

The technique is similar to the one above except that the therapist explores passive physiological hip extension.

MMS lateral sacral fascia + hip adduction

Some patients, when lying in a prone position, seem to favor placing their legs in an abducted position. These patients also tend to stand with their legs apart and, when asked to place their legs "underneath their hips" find that this position is uncomfortable. Clinically, I have found that in these cases there is tension between the lateral sacral fascia and the ITB area. In this case, the therapist feels an immediate increase in tension in the hand that is anchoring the lateral

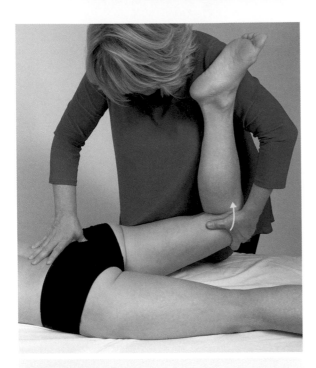

Figure 9.17
MMS lateral sacral fascia + hip extension

sacral region as he/she performs passive hip adduction, starting from an abducted position and moving the thigh towards neutral. The treatment approach is similar to the one above except that the therapist uses passive physiological hip adduction. Ideally, the therapist should be able to attain 20 degrees of hip adduction past neutral before tension is felt in the lateral sacral fascia (technique not pictured).

Sacrotuberous ligament fascia

The sacrotuberous ligament is one of the stabilizers of the sacroiliac joint; sacral nutation increases tension on this ligament (Vleeming et al. 1989). It originates from the medial ischial tuberosity of the ilium and inserts into the posterior superior iliac spine (PSIS), the posterior sacroiliac ligaments (with which it is partly blended), to the lower transverse sacral tubercles and to the lateral margins of the lower sacrum and upper coccyx. Myofascially, it spreads toward a merging with the fascial sheath of the internal pudendal nerves and vessels. The superficial lower

fibers are joined by the tendon of biceps femoris (Vleeming et al. 1989). It also forms part of the SBL of fascia and so must be considered when exploring techniques to improve lumbar flexion or slump. Because of its intimate relationship with the pelvic floor area, it may also be explored in relation to the DFL of fascia. Finally, it must also be considered as a factor in myofascial restrictions in relation to the hip joint and in cases of recurrent hamstring tension.

Sacrotuberous ligament fascia in relation to the SBL

MMS sacrotuberous ligament in relation to the SBL (erector spinae) (Figures 9.18–9.20)

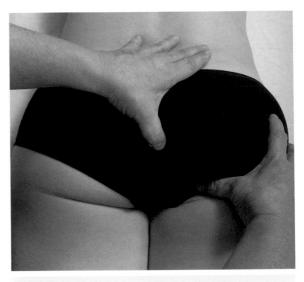

Figure 9.18
MMS sacrotuberous ligament – reference points

Stabilizing hand The patient is in prone position with the lumbar spine in a neutral position. The therapist stands on the left side of the patient. The therapist locates the midpoint of the right sacrotuberous ligament. (The reference points are the ischial tuberosity and the tip of the coccyx.) Using the right thumb, the therapist applies a gentle but firm pressure on the ligament in craniolateral direction

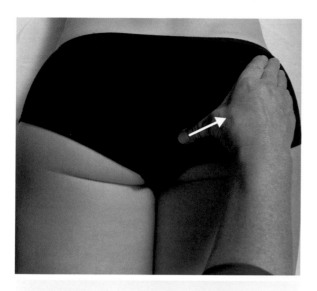

Figure 9.19
MMS sacrotuberous ligament – thumb placement

gliding the fasciae in a cranial direction (Figure 9.20). Once again, the star concept is a useful approach to determine which vectors pull the most on the stabilizing hand. The tension may be felt most when the erector spinae fascia is mobilized in a simple cranial direction, or cranial to the right of the client, or cranial to the left. The patient perceives this tension as the therapist pushing harder on the right sacrotuberous ligament when, in reality, the therapist is simply preventing the anchor from moving. If no tension is perceived, then this part of the SBL is not tight. If tension is perceived (quick resistance is felt between the two hands of the therapist), then it can be mobilized as per the approaches outlined in Chapter 4.

MMS sacrotuberous ligament in relation to the SBL (biceps femoris) (Figure 9.21)

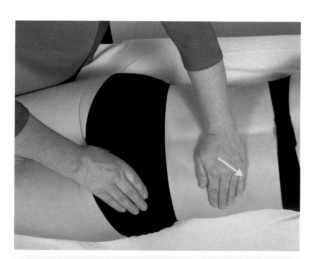

Figure 9.20
MMS sacrotuberous ligament in relation to the SBL (erector spinae)

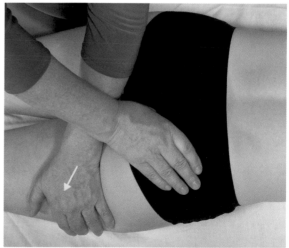

Figure 9.21
MMS sacrotuberous ligament in relation to the SBL (biceps femoris)

(that is, at a 45 degree angle perpendicular to the fibers of the ligament).

Mobilizing hand The therapist's left hand explores the tissues of the SBL above (the fascia of the erector spinae),

The technique is similar to the one above except that the therapist explores the tissues of the SBL below the sacrotuberous ligament, in particular the biceps femoris, usually with a caudally directed motion.

MMS sacrotuberous ligament fascia in relation to the hip

MMS: right sacrotuberous ligament + hip internal rotation (Figure 9.22)

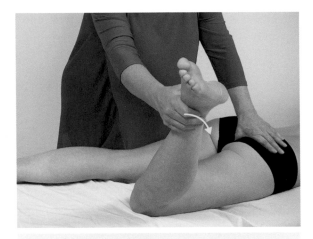

Figure 9.22
MMS sacrotuberous ligament + hip IR

Stabilizing hand As per the technique above except that the therapist uses their left hand to anchor the right sacrotuberous ligament.

Mobilizing hand The therapist's right hand supports the right lower extremity at the ankle and performs a passive physiological movement of hip internal rotation, stopping as soon as an increase in tension is perceived in the hand palpating the sacrotuberous ligament (to the first resistance or R1 of Maitland's movement diagram). If there is tension in this line of fascia, it will seem as though the tension at the sacrotuberous ligament has increased before full hip internal rotation can be achieved (usually around 45 degrees). The patient perceives the therapist increasing his/her pressure on the ligament. The therapist performs repeated passive physiological IR of the hip while maintaining a steady pressure on the ligament, always to when R1 is perceived (a grade III– passive physiological movement in Maitland terms). This is repeated until a release is felt between the therapist's two hands and generally requires approximately five to eight cycles.

MMS sacrotuberous ligament + hip external rotation (Figure 9.23)

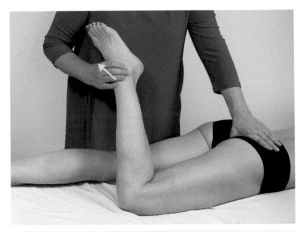

Figure 9.23
MMS sacrotuberous ligament + hip ER

The technique is similar to the one above except that the therapist explores passive physiological hip external rotation.

MMS sacrotuberous ligament + hip extension (Figure 9.24)

The technique is similar to the one above except that the therapist explores passive physiological hip extension.

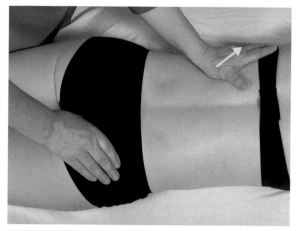

Figure 9.25
MMS sacrotuberous ligament in relation to the DFL (contralateral posterior diaphragm)

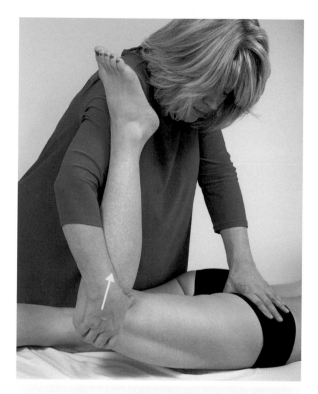

Figure 9.24
MMS sacrotuberous ligament + hip extension

Sacrotuberous ligament fascia in relation to the DFL (Figure 9.25)

Stabilizing hand As per the technique above, except that the lumbar spine is in extension, therefore adding tension to the DFL.

Mobilizing hand The therapist's left hand explores the tissues of the DFL, similar to MMS techniques for the quadratus lumborum (QL) in relation to the DFL. The therapist therefore explores the posterior diaphragm (ipsilateral and contralateral), ipsilateral knee flexion and ipsilateral

dorsiflexion/eversion, all in relation to the sacrotuberous ligament. The example below depicts the technique in relation to the contralateral posterior diaphragm.

MMS modified Butler technique for femoral nerve (Figure 9.26)

For the following techniques, we will be using primarily the third concept of treatment when using MMS techniques; that is, convert a nerve mobilization technique into a fascial technique. (Refer to Chapter 4 for further detail on concepts of treatment using MMS.)

The technique for mobilizing the lumbar interfaces for the femoral nerve is well known (Butler 1991). It generally involves mobilizing the ipsilateral L2–4 facet joints with the lumbar spine in extension, the ipsilateral knee flexed 90 degrees, and the cervical spine flexed. Thinking a little more broadly, with the myofascial tissues in mind, a

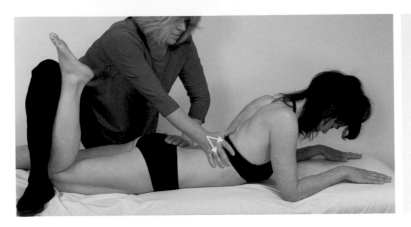

Figure 9.26
MMS modified Butler technique for femoral nerve

therapist may modify this technique by adding a stabilizing hand in the area of the opposite ilium (similar to the technique for the thoracolumbar fascia I at the beginning of this chapter). The therapist may also explore beyond the levels of L2 to L4 to include the levels above and below and to incorporate the thoracolumbar fascia and lower ribs. The concept for treatment remains the same as for other MMS techniques.

Note that the femoral nerve may also be impacted by tension in the area of the inguinal ligament as well. This technique is described in Chapter 11.

Summary

The techniques in this chapter have focused on the myofascial connections in relation to the lumbopelvic area. These include techniques in relation to the thoracolumbar fascia, the quadratus lumborum fascia, the lateral sacral fascia, the fascia of the sacrotuberous ligament and the fascia around the femoral nerve. These tissues are frequently problematic in cases of persistent thoracolumbar, lumbar, and pelvic pain and should be explored using MMS techniques. The following chapter will focus on techniques for the pelvic floor.

The pelvic floor

Why the pelvic floor? Is this not a separate domain in the world of physiotherapy?

The pelvic floor is the home of urologic, obstetric, gynecologic, reproductive, colorectal, and gastrointestinal systems. It is integral to posture, respiration, spinal stability, continence, upper extremity movement, and lymph fluid balance (Hodges et al. 2007; Clifton Smith & Rowley 2011).

Pelvic floor physiotherapists have a wealth of knowledge in this area; however, they too, may become frustrated with the effects of their treatments if they do not consider the body as a whole. The ISM approach (Lee & Lee 2011a) is one way to determine whether the pelvic floor is a "driver" and the source of the patient's meaningful functional problem, or whether, instead, it is the reactor to some other "driver" in the body. This area may be the thorax, the cranium, or the foot.

Another possibility for recurring problems in the area of the pelvic floor/pelvis/hip region is that the muscles of the pelvic floor (accessible either externally or intravaginally) must also be viewed as a part of a fascial line, in particular the DFL. Much can be gained by assessing and treating a tight DFL as it relates to recurrent tension in the pelvic floor muscles.

An additional factor to keep in mind is that the abdominal wall exhibits fascial continuity through to the pelvic floor and the lumbar spine (Stecco C. et al. 2005) (Figure 10.1).

The "double bag" structure that encases the deep abdomen and surrounding structures demonstrates just how each layer is interconnected. This is one reason why women have a tendency to low back pain after pregnancy, especially in caesarean birthing. This has to do with fascial restrictions that alter function, movement, and stability in the pelvic floor. Chapter 8 describes techniques for the abdominal wall that may be helpful for pelvic floor problems because of their connections via this double bag encasing.

This chapter will describe MMS techniques developed to assess and treat myofascial connections between the pelvic floor muscles (extravaginally) and the DFL. Although not shown, pelvic floor therapists may use intravaginal techniques to achieve similar objectives.

The following techniques will be described:

- the obturator internus (OI) muscle in relation to the DFL
- the ischiococcygeus muscle in relation to the DFL
- the obturator externus (OE) muscle in relation to the DFL
- the anterior sacral fascia.

Indications for these techniques include the following:

- pelvic floor pain that has not optimally responded to therapy by trained pelvic floor therapists
- trauma to the pelvic floor (via sport, postpartum)
- a history of abdominal and/or pelvic surgery (caesarean sections, inguinal hernia repairs, etc.)
- persistent hip/groin pain and limitation
- persistent buttock and sacral pain
- when the load and listen test for the hip demonstrates vectors in the area of the pelvic floor (refer to Chapter 11 for a description of this test as it relates to the hip).

Concepts of treatment using MMS

For this chapter, we will be using primarily the first concept of treatment when using MMS techniques; that is, choose a recurrent articular dysfunction or myofascial trigger point

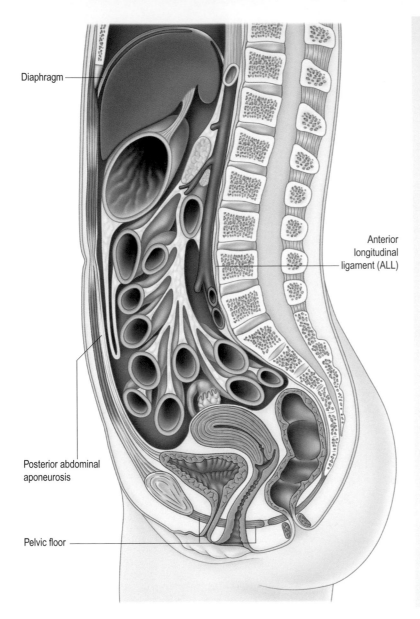

Diaphragm

Posterior abdominal aponeurosis

Pelvic floor

Anterior longitudinal ligament (ALL)

Figure 10.1
The Deep Front Line-pelvic floor fascia connects to the anterior longitudinal ligament, the anterior sacral fascia and the posterior abdominal wall fascia, encompassing both the visceral fascia and the diaphragm

and explore a fascial line in relation to it. The therapist anchors him/herself to a recurrent articular dysfunction or myofascial trigger point and assesses the fascial lines of tension in relation to the anchor, looking for early tension between the two hands.

The following approaches may be used, depending on how the tissues respond:

- work with oscillations (grades III–, III, III+)

- work with sustained pressure

- work with "harmonics" (Dr Laurie Hartman).

Because it is a sensitive area, it would be advisable to use the listening approach to treatment with sustained pressure rather than the oscillatory approach, certainly for the first treatment. Please refer to Chapter 4 for detail on concepts of treatment using MMS.

MMS for the pelvic floor and external rotators of the hip: the DFL

The small hip external rotators (piriformis, obturator internus, obturator externus, gemelli muscles, quadratus femoris) have important implications for optimal functioning of the sacroiliac joint (SIJ), the hip, and the pelvic floor (Figure 10.2).

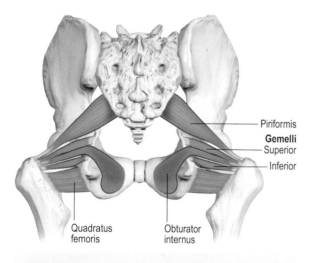

Figure 10.2
Hip external rotators – connecting the pelvic floor and hip

The obturator internus (OI) is a fan-shaped muscle that originates partly from the inner surface of the obturator membrane that covers most of the obturator foramen. Its tendon inserts on the greater trochanter of the proximal femur.

What is less known, however, is the fascial continuity between the OI muscle on the right and the OI on the left, with the pelvic floor connecting the two. This functional sling via the pelvic floor connects one greater trochanter

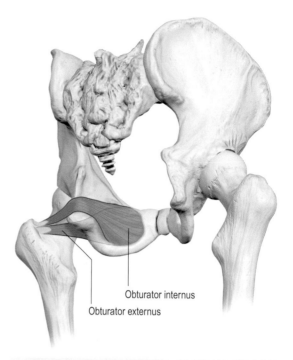

Figure 10.3
Obturator internus (OI) muscles: the left OI muscle is connected to the right OI muscle via a fascial sling through the pelvic floor. This connection also affects the position and function of the hip joints

to the other. So from a fascia perspective, in order to fully explore the right OI fascia, it should be evaluated in relation to both the right and left hip movement, as well as up the chain of the DFL to the diaphragm and beyond (Myers 2014) (Figure 10.3).

MMS right obturator internus fascia: in relation to the pelvis (DFL)

MMS right obturator internus fascia: in relation to ipsilateral sacral base (Figures 10.4–10.7)

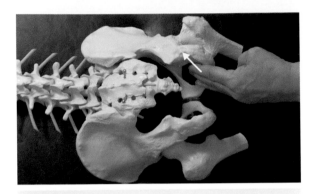

Figure 10.4
MMS anchoring onto right obturator internus (OI)
fascia – hand placement on skeleton

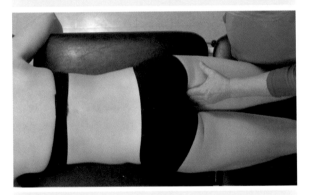

Figure 10.5
MMS anchoring onto right OI fascia – hand
placement on body

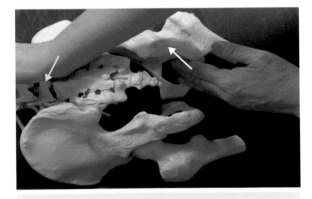

Figure 10.6
MMS right OI fascia in relation to ipsilateral sacral
base – skeleton

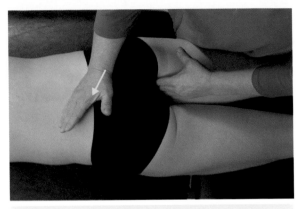

Figure 10.7
MMS right OI fascia in relation to ipsilateral sacral
base – body

Stabilizing hand The patient is in a prone position with
the lumbar spine in neutral. The therapist stands on the
right side of the patient for the right OI technique. Using
the fingers of the left hand, the therapist slowly and gently palpates the muscle at the medial aspect of the ischial
tuberosity, gliding in a cranial and lateral direction.

Mobilizing hand The therapist explores the area of the
right sacral base (S1) with the right hand, using a unilateral
P/A pressure. If this fascial line is tight, the therapist will
feel an increase in tension in the anchoring hand, as if the
OI muscle pushes out medially. The patient will perceive
this tension as the therapist pushing harder on the right
OI when, in reality, the therapist is simply preventing the
anchor from moving. If no tension is perceived, then this
part of the DFL is not tight (with the lumbar spine in neutral position). If tension is perceived (quick resistance is
felt between the two hands of the therapist), then it can
be mobilized as per the approaches outlined in Chapter 4.

Progression Note that all of the techniques of the pelvic
floor may be progressed by repeating them with the lumbar
spine in extension. In this case, the patient supports him/her-
self on the elbows, with hands cupped under the chin. This
position minimizes overactivity of the lumbar extensors.

MMS right obturator internus fascia: in relation to ipsilateral ilium (DFL) (Figures 10.8, 10.9)

The technique is similar to the one above except that the therapist explores the ipsilateral (right) ilium with a P/A pressure along the iliac crest. The star concept is a useful approach to determine which vectors pull the most on the stabilizing hand. The tension may be felt most when the ilium is pushed in a simple anterior direction, as if to produce an anterior rotation of the ilium, or in an anterolateral direction.

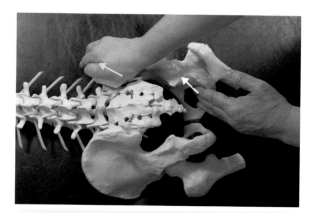

Figure 10.8
MMS right OI fascia in relation to ipsilateral ilium – skeleton

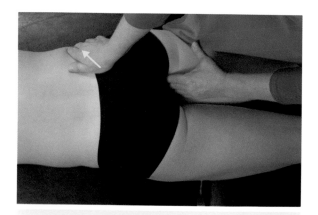

Figure 10.9
MMS right OI fascia in relation to ipsilateral ilium – body

MMS right obturator internus fascia: in relation to contralateral ilium (DFL) (Figure 10.10)

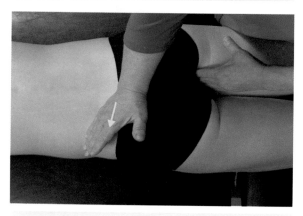

Figure 10.10
MMS right OI fascia – in relation to contralateral ilium

The technique is similar to the one above except that the therapist explores the contralateral (left) ilium with a P/A pressure along the iliac crest. The star concept is a useful approach to determine which vectors pull the most on the stabilizing hand. The tension may be felt most when the ilium is pushed in a simple anterior direction, as if to produce an anterior rotation of the ilium, or in an anterolateral direction.

MMS right obturator internus fascia: in relation to ipsilateral posterior diaphragm (DFL) (Figure 10.11)

The technique is similar to the one above except that the therapist explores the area of the ipsilateral (right) lower thorax with the right hand, gently gliding the area of the posterior diaphragm in a craniolateral direction. The star concept is a useful approach to determine which vectors pull the most on the stabilizing hand. The tension may be felt most when the posterior diaphragm area is pushed in a simple cranial direction, or cranial to the right of the client, or cranial to the left. The patient perceives this tension as the therapist pushing harder on the right OI when, in reality, the therapist is simply preventing the anchor from moving. If no tension is perceived, then this part of the DFL is not tight with the lumbar spine in neutral

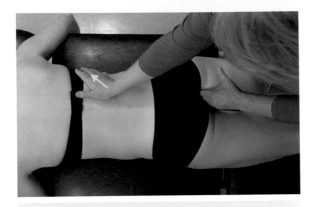

Figure 10.11
MMS right OI fascia – in relation to ipsilateral posterior diaphragm (DFL)

position. It may, however, be explored as a progression, with the lumbar spine in extension (as described above). If tension is perceived (quick resistance is felt between the two hands of the therapist), then it can be mobilized as per the approaches outlined in Chapter 4. (The therapist maintains the pressure on the OI to prevent it from moving as he/she performs repeated P/A mobilizations of the posterior diaphragm in the direction(s) of most restriction.)

MMS right obturator internus fascia: in relation to contralateral posterior diaphragm (DFL) (Figure 10.12)

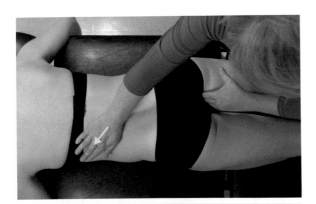

Figure 10.12
MMS right OI fascia – in relation to contralateral posterior diaphragm (DFL)

The technique is similar to the one above except that the therapist explores the area of the contralateral (left) lower thorax with the right hand.

MMS right obturator internus fascia: in relation to central tendon diaphragm (DFL) (Figure 10.13)

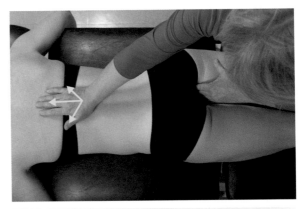

Figure 10.13
MMS right OI fascia – in relation to central tendon diaphragm (DFL)

The technique is similar to the one above except that the therapist explores the area of the central thoracolumbar (Th/L) area. The central tendon of the diaphragm attaches into the lumbar vertebrae L1–3 but the esophageal opening is at T10 and the aortic opening at T12, so it is worthwhile exploring T10–L3 with this technique. The therapist gently glides the area of the Th/L fascia in a cranial direction, using the inferior aspect of the spinous processes as a lever. Once again, the star concept is a useful approach to determine which vectors pull the most on the stabilizing hand. The tension may be felt most when the Th/L tissues are pushed in a simple cranial direction, or cranial to the right of the client, or cranial to the left. The patient perceives this tension as the therapist pushing harder on the OI muscle when, in reality, the therapist is simply preventing it from moving.

MMS right obturator internus fascia: in relation to ipsilateral greater trochanter (Figures 10.14, 10.15)

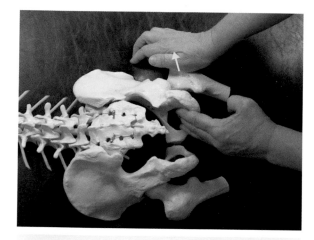

Figure 10.14
MMS right OI fascia in relation to ipsilateral greater trochanter – skeleton

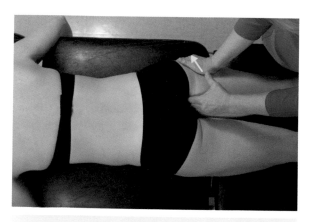

Figure 10.15
MMS right OI fascia in relation to ipsilateral greater trochanter – body

The technique is similar to the one above except that the therapist explores the area of the ipsilateral (right) greater trochanter with the right hand, using a P/A pressure. If this part of the DFL is tight, the patient will perceive this tension as the therapist pushing harder on the right OI when, in reality, the therapist is simply preventing the anchor from moving. If no tension is perceived, then this part of the DFL is not tight with the lumbar spine in neutral position. It may, however, be explored as a progression, with the lumbar spine in extension (described above). If tension is perceived (quick resistance is felt between the two hands of the therapist), then it can be mobilized as per the approaches outlined in Chapter 4.

MMS right obturator internus fascia: in relation to contralateral greater trochanter (Figure 10.16, 10.17)

Because of the sling of fascia between both greater trochanters, it is possible that the right OI fascia may be affected by tension in the left hip. The technique is similar to the one above except that the therapist explores the area of the contralateral greater trochanter.

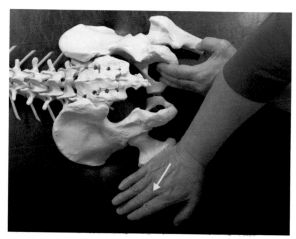

Figure 10.16
MMS right OI fascia in relation to contralateral greater trochanter – skeleton

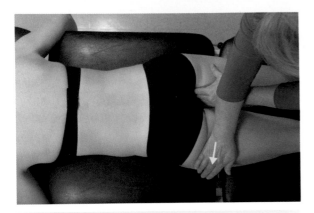

Figure 10.17
MMS right OI fascia in relation to contralateral greater trochanter – body

MMS right obturator internus fascia: in relation to the hip

MMS right obturator internus fascia: in relation to passive physiological hip movement (ipsilateral or contralateral) (Figures 10.18, 10.19)

The technique is similar to the one above except that the therapist uses passive physiological hip movements to add tension and explore this part of the DFL. This may be done with the ipsilateral hip or the contralateral hip. The examples below describe a MMS technique for the right OI in relation to ipsilateral and contralateral hip internal rotation. However, passive physiological hip extension and abduction are also useful to explore the DFL of fascia. In the case of right hip IR, the therapist uses the right hand to support the lower extremity at the ankle and performs a passive physiological movement of hip internal rotation, stopping as soon as an increase in tension is perceived in the hand palpating the OI (to the first resistance or R1 of Maitland's movement diagram). If there is tension in this line of fascia, it will seem like the right OI will push into the therapist's hand before full hip internal rotation can be achieved (usually around 45 degrees of rotation). The patient perceives this as the therapist increasing his/her pressure on the OI. The therapist performs repeated passive physiological IR of the hip while maintaining a steady pressure on the OI, always to when R1

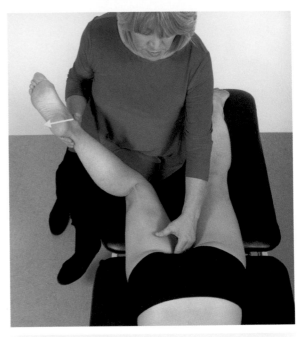

Figure 10.18
MMS right OI fascia – in relation to passive physiological hip IR (ipsilateral)

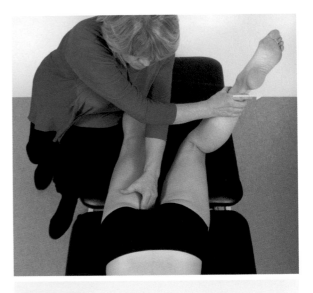

Figure 10.19
MMS right OI fascia – in relation to passive physiological hip IR (DFL) (contralateral)

is perceived (a grade III– passive physiological movement in Maitland terms). This is repeated until a release is felt between the therapist's two hands and generally requires approximately five to eight cycles.

MMS right ischiococcygeus fascia

The ischiococcygeus is a muscle of the pelvic floor located posterior to levator ani and anterior to the sacrospinous ligament. It is a triangular plane of muscular and tendinous fibers, arising from the spine of the ischium and sacrospinous ligament, and inserting into the margin of the coccyx and lower sacrum.

In combination with the levator ani, it forms the pelvic diaphragm (Figure 10.20).

It assists the levator ani and piriformis muscles in closing in the back part of the outlet of the pelvis. In "butt grippers" (those patients who use their hip external rotators excessively in an attempt to stabilize the pelvis/hip region), this muscle is frequently hypertonic (Lee & Lee 2011b). If local treatment to the muscle is insufficient, then the therapist should consider mobilizing this muscle in relation to the DFL of fascia.

MMS right ischiococcygeus fascia: in relation to the hip and DFL (Figure 10.21, 10.22)

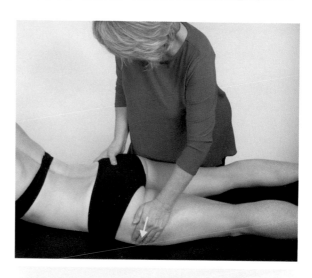

Figure 10.21
MMS right ischiococcygeus fascia – in relation to contralateral greater trochanter

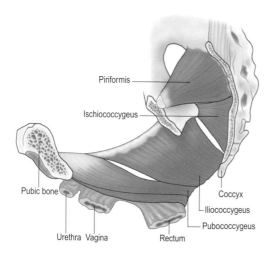

Figure 10.20
Lateral view of the pelvic floor muscles including ischiococcygeus

Piriformis
Ischiococcygeus
Pubic bone
Urethra Vagina
Rectum
Coccyx
Iliococcygeus
Pubococcygeus

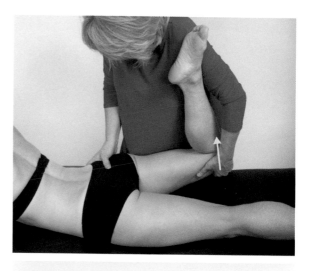

Figure 10.22
MMS right ischiococcygeus fascia – in relation to ipsilateral hip extension

Stabilizing hand The patient is in a prone position with the lumbar spine in neutral. The therapist stands on the right side of the patient for the right ischiococcygeus technique. Using the fingers or thumb of the left hand, the therapist anchors onto the origin of the muscle at the lower sacral border/coccyx area, using a P/A pressure.

Mobilizing hand The therapist explores similar areas of the DFL as described in techniques related to the obturator internus fascia. The examples below depict a MMS technique in relation to the contralateral greater trochanter and in relation to ipsilateral hip extension. However, keep in mind that any passive physiological hip movement may be explored. As well, these techniques may be progressed by repeating them with the lumbar spine in extension.

MMS right obturator externus fascia (Figures 10.23, 10.24)

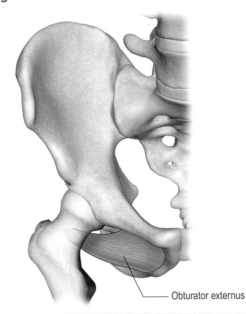

Figure 10.23
Obturator externus muscle – covers the front of the wall of the pelvis and inserts into the back of the hip bone

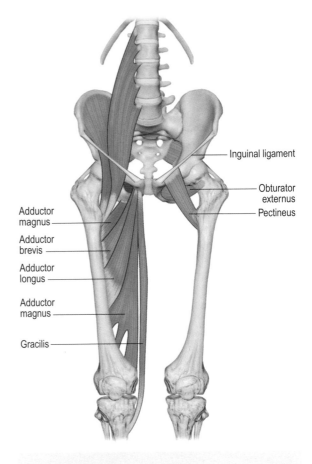

Figure 10.24
Obturator externus in relation to pectineus and the adductor group of muscles

The obturator externus muscle (OE) is a flat, triangular muscle that covers the outer surface of the anterior wall of the pelvis. It originates from the external obturator membrane and the rim of the pubis and ischium and inserts onto the trochanteric fossa on the medial surface of the greater trochanter. It may be palpated in the space between short adductors and the pectineus muscle. It is particularly important to proceed slowly and gently when palpating this muscle, as this is generally a sensitive area.

MMS right obturator externus fascia: thumb placement (Figure 10.25)

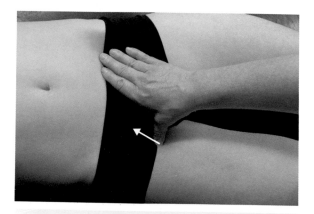

Figure 10.25
MMS right obturator externus (OE) fascia – thumb placement

MMS right obturator externus fascia: in relation to hip adductors (DFL) (Figure 10.26)

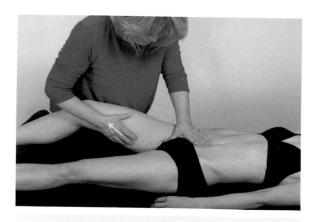

Figure 10.26
MMS right obturator externus (OE) fascia – in relation to hip adductors (DFL)

Stabilizing hand The patient is in a supine position, with the ipsilateral hip in approximately 45 degrees of flexion, supported by the therapist's thigh. The therapist stands on the right side of the patient for the right OE technique. Using the thumb of their right hand, the therapist anchors onto the OE muscle, gently sliding in the space between short adductors and the pectineus muscle.

Mobilizing hand The therapist explores the right hip adductors with the right hand, generally in a caudad direction, using the star concept. The adductor fascia may be explored from the hip to the medial knee. If this part of the DFL is tight, the patient will perceive this tension as the therapist pushing harder on the right OE when, in reality, the therapist is simply preventing the anchor from moving. If no tension is perceived, then this part of the DFL is not tight. If tension is perceived (quick resistance is felt between the two hands of the therapist), then it can be mobilized as per the approaches outlined in Chapter 4. A listening approach is suggested.

MMS right obturator externus fascia: in relation to dorsiflexion/eversion (DFL) (Figure 10.27)

The technique is similar to the one above except that the therapist uses passive physiological ankle dorsiflexion/eversion to add tension to the DFL of fascia.

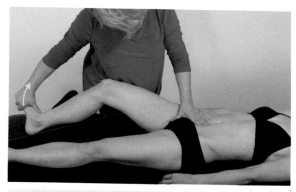

Figure 10.27
MMS right OE fascia – in relation to DF/eversion (DFL)

MMS right obturator externus fascia: in relation to ipsilateral anterior diaphragm (DFL) (Figure 10.28)

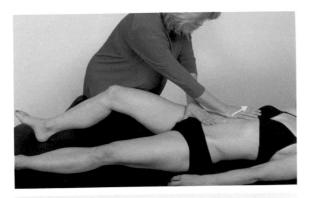

Figure 10.28
MMS right OE fascia – in relation to ipsilateral anterior diaphragm (DFL)

The technique is similar to the one above except that the therapist explores the ipsilateral anterior diaphragm area (using a star concept). Appropriate depth of tissues is important in order to access the DFL of fascia.

MMS right obturator externus fascia – in relation to contralateral anterior diaphragm (DFL) (Figure 10.29)

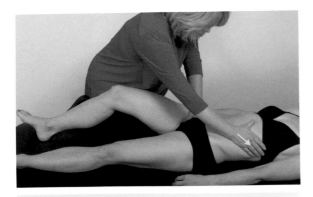

Figure 10.29
MMS right OE fascia – in relation to contralateral anterior diaphragm (DFL)

The technique is similar to the one above except that the therapist explores the contralateral anterior diaphragm area (using a star concept). Appropriate depth of tissues is important in order to access the DFL of fascia.

MMS right obturator externus fascia: in relation to pericardial fascia (DFL) (Figure 10.30)

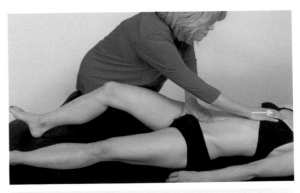

Figure 10.30
MMS right OE fascia – in relation to pericardial fascia (DFL)

The technique is similar to the one above except that the therapist explores the pericardial fascia (using a star concept). Appropriate depth of tissues is important in order to access the DFL of fascia.

MMS anterior sacral fascia

The anterior sacral fascia is innervated and may be the source of pain in the area of the sacrum. One indication that the anterior sacral fascia may be an issue is if the patient complains of pain localized to the sacral area, yet the therapist's palpatory findings in the posterior aspect of the sacrum are negative.

The technique to mobilize the anterior sacral fascia is a modification of the technique in Chapter 7 that is used to balance the occiput with the sacrum. The anterior sacral fascia is accessed indirectly by placing the patient in a side-lying position, with the hips at 0 degrees of extension and the knees flexed 90 degrees. Because extension of the hips and knee flexion add tension to the DFL of fascia, this technique is believed to mobilize the anterior sacral fascia, which is also part of the DFL.

The therapist faces the back of the patient. One hand cups the occiput, with the palm of the hand as close as possible to the base of the occiput. The therapist's other hand cups the sacrum, with the palm of the hand as close as possible to the sacral base (S1) (Figure 10.31). The therapist sinks into the tissues, feeling the myofascial tissue release in the process. The therapist then applies a gentle but firm distraction between their two hands until they feel the connection between the two hands. This technique is best done using sustained pressure. The idea behind a listening approach to treatment is to load the fascial tissues (establish the first resistance in the line of tension), and then wait to see what the body wants to do with this tension. The therapist may

feel the tension increase between their hands, with the body adding small micro-adjustments in multiple directions. The sensation is similar to that of twisted elastic attempting to unwind itself. The therapist follows this unwinding, preventing the tissues either at the sacrum and/or the occiput from going into the direction from which they came. The tension tends to build up gradually and then suddenly releases, often within one minute. This release is accompanied by a fluid-like feel and, often, a therapeutic pulse. The therapist may also modify this technique by anchoring onto the area of S2, S3 or S4 instead of simply using the sacral base (S1).

Case report 10.1 Katherine's story*

Internal pelvic floor muscles and the DFL

Katherine was a 22-year-old student teacher with complaints of left lateral sacral pain, as well as vaginal and coccygeal pain of three years' duration. There was no history of trauma except for a mild cervical strain due to a boating accident that occurred one year prior to the start of her lower quadrant symptoms. She had had a history of headache as a result of grinding her teeth but that was controlled with frictions to the temporomandibular joint (TMJ) muscles and a night splint. Her lower quadrant symptoms began after climbing a large snow bank. She had been diagnosed with piriformis syndrome and had seen other physiotherapists, who had used manual therapy to the sacroiliac (SI) joint and lumbar spine, dry needling for the lumbar and piriformis muscles as well as stabilization exercises, with little change to her symptoms. An MRI of the lumbar pelvis was negative. She had consulted with a number of gynecologists, who could offer no explanations for her pain. She had also seen a physiotherapist who specialized in pelvic floor dysfunctions, and this approach to treatment helped to decrease her symptoms by about 30 percent. Once the pelvic floor therapist reached a plateau with treatment, she referred Katharine to me, asking for a fascial assessment. Katharine's symptoms were increased by walking more than a half hour, using stairs, and doing lunges and squats. This stopped

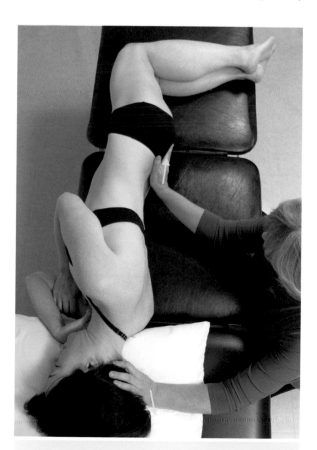

Figure 10.31 MMS anterior sacral fascia

her from playing sports (she was a former track and field athlete), and she was concerned about climbing stairs in the school where she would be starting her new job. In addition, sexual intercourse was painful.

Initial evaluation revealed the following:

- Positional tests of the pelvis demonstrated a transverse plane rotation (TPR) to the right, with an intrapelvic torsion (IPT) to the right.

- Positional tests for the femoral head showed the left femoral head to be anterior in relation to the ilium.

- Positional tests for the thorax demonstrated ring 9 to be laterally shifted to the left (therefore an intrathoracic rotation to the right).

- Normal lumbar active ROM, with pain only at the end of range of extension.

- Passive intervertebral movements (PIVMs) and accessory movement tests (PAVMs) for the lumbar spine were within normal limits.

- Sacroiliac mobility tests were also within normal limits, but the accessory movements in A/P glide had a "gummy" end feel.

- Lumbar instability tests (A/P shears, rotation stability) were negative.

- Positive dynamic instability test with the quarter squat test:
  - the left SIJ demonstrated an "unlocking" (left sacral base counternutated relative to the ilium)
  - the left hip increased its anterior glide
  - the left knee and foot were unremarkable
  - activation of the transversus abdominis muscle did not improve the quarter squat task
  - correction of the thorax ring shift did not correct the SIJ unlocking
  - correction of the hip position improved but did not completely correct the SIJ unlocking (difficulty was noted in achieving full correction of the hip position).

- Left hip ROM test:

- Flex/add 1/3 with anterior groin pain
  - IR in 90 degrees of flexion = 25 degrees, reproducing sacral pain at the end of range
  - ER in 90 degrees of flexion = 45 degrees
  - FABER's test = ½, reproducing sacral, vaginal and coccygeal pain
  - extension = 10 degrees.

- Load and listen test for A/P loading of the hip joint revealed myofascial vectors from the pelvic floor area to begin with, followed by vectors in the iliacus and abdominal area on the left (see Chapter 11).

- Fascia evaluation: DFL restriction especially in relation to the following:
  - left obturator internus in relation to the left and right sacral base, the left and right ilium, both posterior diaphragms, left tibialis posterior (dorsiflexion/eversion); initially with the lumbar spine (Lx) neutral and later, with the Lx in extension
  - left A/P coccyx with the left sacral base, and with dorsiflexion/eversion (refer to Chapter 7)
  - left lateral sacrum with left hip IR, hip extension and hip adduction.

My initial hypothesis was that her left hip was driving the sacral and coccygeal pain, with myofascial vectors in relation to the DFL of fascia mostly responsible for decentralizing the femoral head during a squat maneuver.

- Further fascial evaluation revealed other areas of the DFL that were affected (and subsequently treated):
  - left sacrotuberous ligament with right hip IR (Lx in neutral, then later in extension)
  - left iliacus with the DFL (refer to Chapter 8)
  - left quadratus lumborum (QL) in side-lying with the DFL (refer to Chapter 9)
  - left QL in Lx extension with hip extension and hip adduction (refer to Chapter 9)
  - left obturator externus in relation to the adductors, the psoas, pericardium and the tibialis posterior

(dorsiflexion/eversion). In subsequent treatments, we also used hip FABER as a passive physiological movement in relation to the OE

- – anterior sacral fascia
- – temporalis (R > L) in relation to the DFL (pericardium, diaphragm, tibialis posterior with dorsiflexion/eversion) (refer to Chapter 6)
- – internal pelvic floor (left pubococcygeus) in relation to the bladder, the anterior diaphragm, the pericardium, the adductors, with tibialis posterior (dorsiflexion/eversion). In subsequent treatments, we also used hip FABER as a passive physiological movement in relation to the left pubococcygeus muscles.

As the fascial restrictions began to release, we then followed up with a stabilization program to improve lumbopelvic-hip control in a variety of positions. (Note that in her previous treatments with other practitioners, she had tried stabilization exercise programs but had found them challenging to do and they had had no positive results.) Note that this was not a "quick fix" case as there were many layers to her fascial dysfunction and it took

some time to "peel away" these layers. However, one year later, she was working, climbing stairs without problems, coaching volleyball, playing basketball, and had resumed a pain-free sex life. She thanked me for "giving her life back to her." It is stories like this that keep us going as therapists when we occasionally have a bad day!

* Please note that the patient's name has been changed to protect her privacy.

Summary

The techniques in this chapter have focused on myofascial connections in relation to the lumbopelvic area, specifically in relation to the obturator internus in relation to the DFL and the hip, the ischiococcygeus, the obturator externus in relation to the DFL and the anterior sacral fascia. These tissues are frequently problematic in cases of persistent Th/L, lumbar, pelvic floor, and hip pain and should be explored using MMS techniques. Pelvic floor therapists may also use intravaginal techniques to achieve similar benefits.

The following chapter will focus on techniques for the lower extremity.

The lower extremity

When treating patients with problems of the lower extremity, manual therapists are trained to assess and treat the joints (the hip, tibiofemoral, patellofemoral, superior and inferior tibiofibular joints, and the ankle and foot joints). In addition, the muscles of the lower quadrant are assessed and treated for imbalance between hypertonic and/or tight and weak muscles. The mobility of the nerves of the lower quadrant is also assessed and treated. However, mobilizing joints and nerves and stretching and strengthening individual muscles can achieve only partial benefits if the fascial system is not taken into consideration.

This chapter will focus on the myofascial connections between the hip, thigh, knee, lower leg and ankle/foot. They include the:

- quadriceps fascia in relation to the SFL and DFL
- iliotibial band (ITB) in relation to the Lateral Line (covered in Chapter 9)
- fascia of the biceps femoris and its role in external tibial torsion
- fascia around the inguinal ligament and its role in the pelvic outlet syndrome
- fascia of the adductors in relation to the DFL
- fascia around the knee and superior tib/fib joints (in relation to the SFL and DFL)
- fascia of the lower leg (medial and lateral) in relation to the foot
- plantar fascia and flexor hallucis longus (FHL)
- anterior lower leg fascia in relation to hammer toes (SFL)
- concept of converting joint mobilizations in the lower extremity into fascial techniques
- Release With Awareness techniques for the foot and ankle.

Indications for MMS for this chapter

- Recurring lower extremity pain despite the following treatment approaches:
  - mobilization/manipulation of the joints of the hip, knee, patella, tib/fib joints, ankle and foot
  - release of trigger points to the lower extremity muscles with manual or dry needling techniques
  - stabilization and strengthening exercises for the lower quadrant.

- Quadriceps fascia should be considered when looking for non-articular restrictions of knee flexion.

- Similarly, tight fascia of the lower leg is a common factor that may impact the range of the ankle, especially with dorsiflexion.

- Complete assessment of hammer toes should involve not only an assessment of the foot and toe joints but also an assessment of the fascia of the anterior lower leg and metatarsal fascia.

Postural analysis

Position of the femoral head in relation to the ilium (Figure 11.1)

(photo shows the right side)

A centered femoral head in relation to the acetabulum is a key requirement for a healthy hip. It requires balanced activation of all muscle vectors. The therapist assesses the position of the femoral head of the hip by using the fingers of their right hand to palpate the femoral head midway between the anterior superior iliac spine (ASIS) and the symphysis pubis, just below the inguinal ligament. The therapist's right thumb palpates the posterior edge of the greater trochanter. The therapist then compares the position of the hand that is palpating the femur to the position of their left hand, which encompasses the anterior and

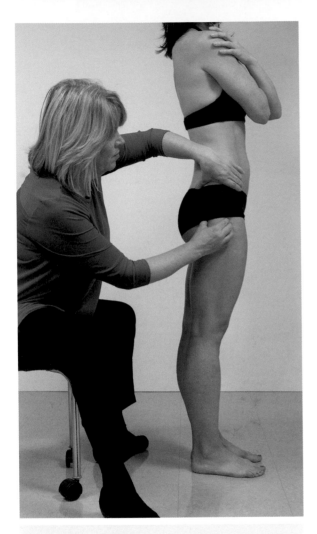

Figure 11.1
Position of hip in relation to the ilium

Position of the foot (Figure 11.2)

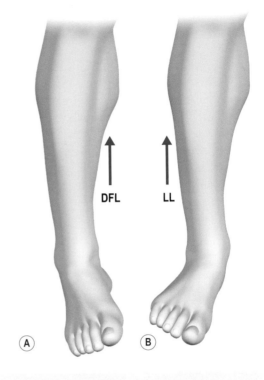

Figure 11.2
Effects of the Deep Front Line and Lateral Line on the foot

In neutral standing posture, the head of the talus should be centered in to the distal tibia/fibula. The position of the talus is assessed by palpating both the medial and the lateral aspects of the dome of the talus. The forefoot should be neither excessively supinated nor pronated, and the lower leg should not be rotated internally or externally (Lee & Lee 2011).

- If there is restriction of the Deep Front Line of fascia, this may have an impact on the foot, in that it may pull the calcaneus into inversion and the forefoot into supination.

- On the other hand, a restriction of the Lateral Line may maintain the calcaneus in eversion, with the talus plantarflexed and adducted, and promote over-pronation of the mid-foot (Figure 11.2).

posterior aspects of the ilium. A patient who stands using a "butt gripping" strategy frequently exhibits overactivation of the deep hip external rotators (including piriformis, obturators, gemelli muscles and quadratus femoris). This strategy tends to pull the greater trochanter posteriorly and "forces" the femoral head anteriorly (Lee & Lee 2011). These muscles may be treated locally by using muscle release techniques (manually or via dry needling) but if tension recurs it would be wise to consider the fascial lines associated with these muscles, in particular the DFL of fascia.

Either extreme will affect the weight-bearing areas of the foot and it may become a "driver" (primary or secondary) for dysfunctions in the rest of the body (ISM approach).

- Imbalance in fascial lines may also have an impact on the knee, maintaining either a valgus or varus position.

- Excessive tension of the biceps femoris and its fascia is frequently a factor that causes excessive external tibial torsion ("duck feet").

Functional tests

Squat test

Assessment of hip with half squat (Figure 11.3)

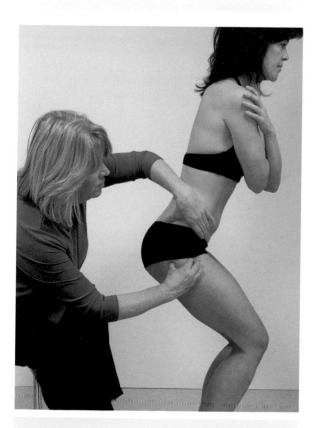

Figure 11.3
Assessment of hip with half squat

If the subjective exam points to difficulty with squatting or sitting, then this functional test is required. The therapist palpates the ilium with one hand and the femoral head with the other hand (as per the positional test). The patient performs a half squat as the therapist assesses if it there is failed load transfer (FLT). If there is a good strategy, the hip starts in a centered position and remains so throughout the squat test. A common pattern with a FLT is that the hip may start in an anterior position and either translate anteriorly more so and/or internally rotate (Lee & Lee 2011). This may be due to weak posterior fibers of gluteus medius, which controls excessive hip internal rotation (IR), but this "weakness" may simply be an inhibited muscle secondary to the myofascial dysfunction present. Repeating the functional test, as well as the manual muscle test, after using the appropriate MMS technique, will let the therapist know if there is true weakness of the gluteus medius.

Assessment of knee with half squat (Figure 11.4)

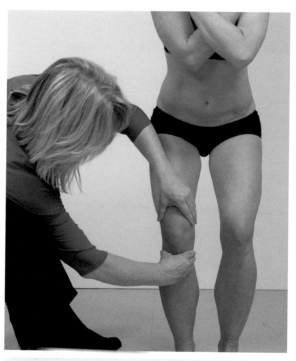

Figure 11.4
Assessment of knee with half squat

The therapist may also assess the knee joint using this test. One hand palpates the distal femur and the other palpates the proximal tibia. Normally, in full extension, the tibia is positioned in slight external rotation relative to the femur. If the strategy for movement is good, with knee flexion we expect to see some internal rotation of the tibia at the start of the squat as the knee de-rotates its "screw home mechanism" of tibial external rotation. The tibia should remain centered relative to the femur throughout the rest of the squat test. If there is FLT, the distal hand will exhibit a torque or twist relative to the femur, usually into external tibial torsion. The therapist must keep in mind that the source of this twist may not be in the knee itself. There may be a driver elsewhere in the foot, hip, pelvis, or thorax, for example (Lee & Lee 2011). The half squat is, however, a good functional test to use for re-assessment.

Assessment of foot with half squat (talus and first ray) (Figures 11.5, 11.6)

The foot may also be assessed for FLT with the squat test. Normal biomechanics for dorsiflexion at the talocrural joint requires an A/P glide of the talus in relation to the inferior tib/fib joint as well as an accessory rocking motion (Maitland A/P tilt). However, dorsiflexion may also be limited by excessive tension in the SBL of the myofascial tissues. If dorsiflexion is limited at the talocrural joint (either because of articular restrictions or fascial restrictions), the common compensatory pattern in the half squat position is for the talus to plantarflex and adduct rather than staying centered under the inferior tib/fib. To do this test the therapist palpates both sides of the dome of the talus in standing and assesses its motion as the patient performs a half squat. Ideally, the talus should remain centered throughout the motion. The therapist may also assess the ability of the first ray of the mid-foot to pronate (navicular, first cuneiform, first metatarsal base). Pronation of the first ray is required for normal biomechanics in weight-bearing dorsiflexion. A common sign of FLT is that the mid-foot stays in a supinated position and fails to pronate during a squat. One of the

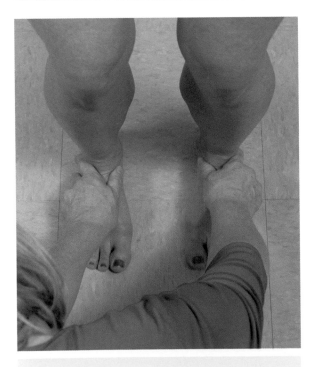

Figure 11.5
Assessment of foot with half squat (talus)

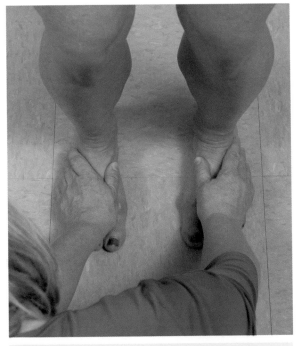

Figure 11.6
Assessment of foot with half squat (navicular)

sources of this dysfunction may, of course, be joint stiffness, but myofascial tension of the anterior lower leg (especially tibialis anterior) and the fascia of the SFL may pull at the joints of the first ray and prevent them from pronating in relation to the hindfoot.

One leg stand test

If the subjective exam indicates difficulty with standing, walking or running, then the functional test of a one leg stand (OLS) is required. The hip, the knee and the foot may be assessed in a similar way as for the squat test but the functional movement assessed is one in which the patient shifts his weight onto one leg and lifts the other off the floor. The weight-bearing side is assessed for FLT (Lee & Lee 2011). The example below shows the test performed for the hip.

Assessment of hip with one leg stand (Figure 11.7)

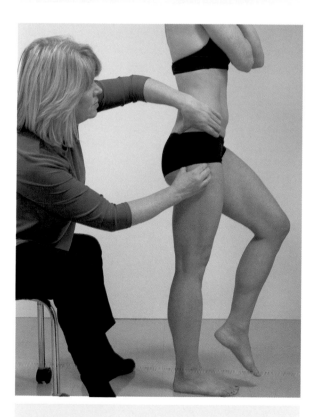

Figure 11.7
Assessment of hip with OLS

For higher load tasks, the therapist may combine functional tests to include a combined OLS with a half squat on the weight-bearing leg (not pictured).

Clinical reasoning using functional dynamic stabilization tests

These positional and functional tests may be used before and after treatment with the MMS approach. For example, if the subjective exam points to a problem with sitting and the patient complains of pain in the sacroiliac (SI) area, it is recommended that the half squat test be used to assess dynamic stability at the SI joint, as well as the thorax, hip, knee and foot and ankle (and sometimes the cervical region or the cranium!) (ISM model). If there is FLT at the SI joint, correction of the non-optimal strategies for the whole body (usually the thorax and the whole lower quadrant) should be performed to see which of these factors has the most positive impact on the dynamic stabilization of the pelvis. If correction of the hip improves the SI joint stabilization strategy (partially or completely), then that points to the hip as a driver or co-driver that is contributing to the SI dysfunction. If the foot correction has the most impact on the SI joint stabilization strategy then the foot may be driving the SI dysfunction. The treatment strategy in this case would be to treat the driver and/or co-drivers and re-assess the impact of this treatment on the dynamic stability of the pelvis. In this way, the therapist can have a test – retest strategy in order to immediately evaluate their hypothesis and effects of their treatment.

"Load and listen" test for the hip (Figures 11.8, 11.9)

If there is failed load transfer (FLT) at the hip during functional tests (and particularly if it is found to be the "driver" in the Integrated System Model) then the next appropriate test to perform would be a load and listen test. This test derives from listening courses developed by Gail Wexler for the Barral Institute. These listening techniques differentiate active and passive listening. Load and listen encompasses both aspects of listening. I find it invaluable in helping to detect the primary myofascial vectors that may be impacting a joint.

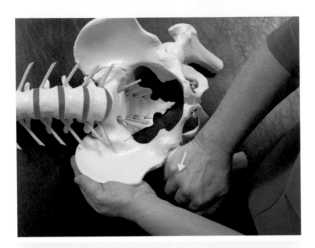

Figure 11.8
Load and listen right hip (skeleton)

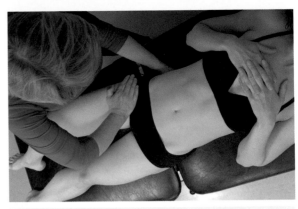

Figure 11.9
Load and listen right hip (body)

The test that is described here is an example in which the hip is held anteriorly, a common finding. The patient is in a supine position, with the leg supported by the therapist's thigh in the position where FLT occurs (often at about 30 degrees of hip flexion). A gentle distraction and posterior glide of the hip joint should be performed. When an accessory movement for a joint is assessed, not only is the resistance of this accessory movement noted, but in this test, particular attention is paid to the release component of the accessory glide.

- In a *healthy hip*, when the therapist glides the femoral head posteriorly, it floats back up to the surface, much like the type of "soap on a rope" that pops back up to the surface of the water after it has been pushed down (Diane Lee, personal communication).

- If the load and listen test points to an *articular restriction*, the therapist will feel that the accessory glide may be stiff with a relatively harder, capsular end-feel. Upon the release of the accessory glide, a small amplitude movement occurs to allow the joint to re-establish its more neutral position.

- If the load and listen test points to a *myofascial restriction*, the therapist may find some limitation in the posterior glide of the hip joint (the loading aspect of the test) but the end feel will not be as hard as

for an articular restriction. More importantly, upon release of the glide (the listening aspect of the test), the therapist will feel a vector that "tugs" on the joint, pulling the femoral head beyond center. This myofascial restriction may be a combination of neuromuscular vectors (increased tone in muscles due to increased neural drive), visceral vectors, muscular and fascial vectors. A myofascial vector is usually a larger amplitude movement than an articular vector.

This test may be used as a "before and after" test, when using any type of release technique. It is particularly useful to use before and after a MMS technique. It guides the therapist as to which myofascial vector(s) have the most impact on a particular joint and encourages exploration of that myofascial vector. Release can be done both locally to the involved muscle and also along its myofascial line (based on Anatomy Trains myofascial meridians).

The following possibilities are some examples that may guide the therapist into determining which neuromuscular vectors may be impacting the hip joint (D. Lee, Course notes from ISM Lumbar/pelvis/hip course):

- A pull of the femoral head into external rotation and in a posterior direction implicates the involvement of the hip external rotators, namely piriformis, quadratus femoris, and the gemelli muscles (see Chapter 10 for MMS sacrum techniques).

- A pull of the femoral head medially toward the center of the body and into ER implicates the obturator muscles (obturator externus and obturator internus) which form part the pelvic floor (see Chapter 10 for MMS techniques).

- A pull of the femoral head in the superomedial direction, without spin, that stops at the pubic ramus, implies the involvement of the adductor muscles (brevis, longus, pectineus) (see MMS technique described in this chapter).

- A pull of the femoral head in the superomedial direction, without spin, that feels like it is beyond the inguinal ligament, implies the involvement of iliacus and psoas muscles (see Chapter 8 for MMS technique).

- A pull of the femoral head into an anterior tilt implies the involvement of rectus femoris muscle (see MMS technique described in this chapter).

All of these neuromuscular vectors may be treated with a number of techniques designed to release muscle hypertonicity, such as contract-relax, strain/counterstrain, release with awareness, dry needling, etc. However, if results of these approaches are difficult to maintain, the therapist should then explore the fascial line(s) related to the muscles involved.

Many of the muscles around the hip are involved with the Deep Front Line (DFL) of fascia. If the DFL is shortened it may maintain dysfunction in and around the pelvis/hip area. Chapter 10 outlines MMS techniques to release the DFL in relation to the pelvic floor. Chapter 8 outlines MMS techniques to release the DFL in relation to the iliacus muscle. After treatment, re-assessment of positional tests, functional tests and the load and listen test for the hip joint are appropriate.

Visceral vectors A pull of the femoral head in the superomedial direction, without spin that feels like it is beyond the inguinal ligament may also imply mobility issues with the fascia of the visceral system. Some examples include:

- the ascending colon, caecum or appendix on the right side

- the sigmoid colon or descending colon on the left

- the bladder or uterus, centrally.

Visceral manipulation techniques would then be appropriate here. Jean-Pierre Barral, a French physiotherapist and osteopath, has developed a comprehensive curriculum for the assessment and treatment of visceral impairments. The reader is referred to the Barral Institute for further information (www.barralinstitute.com). Visceral techniques may be progressed by mobilizing these tissues in relation to the DFL of fascia, using the same concepts as for MMS.

Concepts of treatment using MMS

For this chapter, we will be using primarily the first concept of treatment when using MMS techniques; that is, choose a recurrent articular dysfunction or myofascial trigger point and explore a fascial line in relation to it. The therapist anchors him/herself to a recurrent articular dysfunction or myofascial trigger point and assesses the fascial lines of tension in relation to the anchor, looking for early tension between their two hands.

The following approaches may be used, depending on how the tissues respond:

- work with oscillations (grades III−, III, III+)

- work with sustained pressure

- work with "harmonics" (Dr Laurie Hartman).

Please refer to Chapter 4 for detail on concepts of treatment using MMS.

The fascia around the inguinal ligament and its role in the femoral pelvic outlet syndrome

The inguinal ligament, a band of dense regular fibrous connective tissue in the anterior pelvic region, is rarely addressed by physiotherapists. It should be considered, especially with patients complaining of chronic groin and/or thigh pain. The inguinal ligament may be chronically irritated secondary to an anteriorly positioned femoral head. In this case, a thorough assessment of the hip, including its possible myofascial vectors, is required. If there is fascial thickening of this ligament, it may be a source of impingement for the femoral nerve, artery and vein as they pass through the groin (femoral pelvic outlet syndrome).

MMS right inguinal ligament fascia in relation to the rectus abdominis (SFL) (Figure 11.10)

Stabilizing hand The patient is in supine position, with the leg supported in slight flexion via the therapist's thigh. Using an A/P pressure, the therapist uses their left hand to explore the whole inguinal ligament area from its origin at the symphysis pubis to the ASIS. Both the superior and the inferior aspects of this ligament should be explored. In the following case, the therapist anchors onto the tissues just superior to the ligament.

Mobilizing hand With their right hand, the therapist explores the SFL of fascia, especially the rectus abdominis (RA) (ipsilateral and contralateral) toward its insertion at the 5th to 7th costal cartilages and the xiphoid process of the sternum. The therapist looks for the angle and the

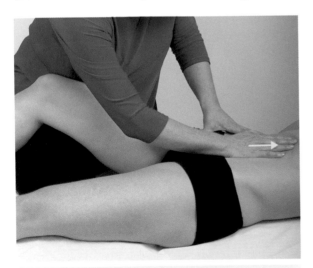

Figure 11.10
MMS right inguinal ligament fascia in relation to the rectus abdominus (SFL)

area(s) on the RA where he/she perceives immediate tension in the hand anchoring the right inguinal ligament. If there is tension in this line of fascia, it will seem as though the inguinal ligament pulls cranially with minimal cranial glide of the mobilizing hand. The therapist maintains the caudal pressure on the inguinal ligament and simply prevents it from moving. The patient perceives this as the therapist increasing his/her pressure on the ligament. If tension is perceived (quick resistance is felt between the two hands of the therapist) then it can be mobilized as per the approaches outlined in Chapter 4. (The therapist performs repeated cranial glides of the RA fascia in the direction(s) of most restriction, while maintaining a steady pressure on the inguinal ligament, always to when R1 is perceived. This is repeated until a release is felt between the therapist's two hands and generally requires approximately five to eight cycles.) The therapist may then explore the SFL a little higher up, toward the fascia on the anterior aspect of the sternum.

MMS right inguinal ligament fascia in relation to the quadriceps (SFL) (Figure 11.11)

Stabilizing hand As per the technique above, except that the therapist anchors the tissues just inferior to the ligament, using a cranial glide if they are exploring the SFL below the ligament.

Mobilizing hand As per the technique above except that the therapist explores the ipsilateral quadriceps fascia all the way to the knee.

MMS right inguinal ligament fascia in relation to the adductors (DFL) (Figure 11.12)

Stabilizing hand As per the technique above.

Mobilizing hand As per the technique above except that the therapist explores the ipsilateral adductor fascia all the way to the knee.

MMS right inguinal ligament fascia in relation to the femoral nerve (Figure 11.13)

The area of the inguinal ligament is one interface of the femoral nerve that is not commonly explored with manual therapy techniques. It may be used if the therapist is considering the possibility the patient may be showing signs of pelvic outlet syndrome.

Stabilizing hand As per the technique above.

Mobilizing hand As per the technique above except that the therapist explores the fascia of the femoral nerve as it

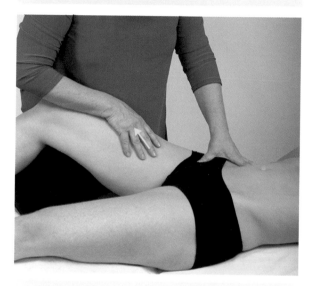

Figure 11.11
MMS right inguinal ligament fascia in relation to the quadriceps (SFL)

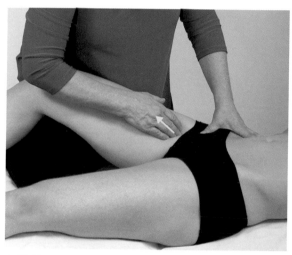

Figure 11.13
MMS right inguinal ligament fascia in relation to the femoral nerve

emerges from under the inguinal ligament to supply the anterior aspect of the thigh and medial leg.

Note that the inguinal ligament may also be explored in relation to the hip movements (hip flexion/extension, abduction/adduction, rotations and combined movement of FABER). If there is fascial tension between the inguinal ligament and the hip, the therapist will feel an increase in tension of the hand that is anchoring the inguinal ligament before full range of motion of the hip is attained. This restriction is usually noted at the beginning of range. For example, the therapist supports the patient's leg at 90 degrees of hip flexion and feels an increase in tension at the inguinal ligament as he/she begins to slowly extend the hip toward the table. The case report illustrates this example.

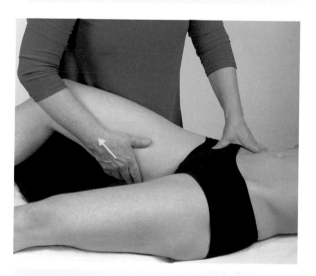

Figure 11.12
MMS right inguinal ligament fascia in relation to the adductors (DFL)

Case report 11.1 Noémie's story*

Noémie was a 45-year-old circus performer with complaints of right anterior abdominal pain and right sacroiliac pain, especially with maneuvers involving standing on the right leg. Symptoms were brought on gradually, with no history of trauma. She had previously been treated by an osteopath, who worked on improving the mobility of the pelvis, the sacrum, and the visceral system, with slight improvement in her condition. She was presently being treated by another physiotherapist, who used mobilizations of the lumbar spine, dry needling for hypertonic lumbosacral muscles, and stabilization exercises to improve right one leg stand (OLS). The therapist had noted that training the lower thoracic deep multifidus muscles had a good impact on the right OLS and half squat strategies. She referred the patient to me to see if there were myofascial vectors that might be impacting the ability of the SI to stabilize. My assessment revealed the following:

- The pelvis was positioned in a left TPR (transverse plane rotation) and a left IPT (intrapelvic torsion).

- The right hip was positioned anteriorly in relation to the ilium.

- The right OLS test revealed FLT of the right SI joint as well as the right hip. The SI stabilization was partially improved with activation of the thoracolumbar stabilizers, but did not affect the dynamic stability of the hip.

- The load and listen test for the right hip revealed a myofascial vector in the area of the right iliacus. Once this vector was released (using the technique in Chapter 8), the second load and listen test revealed a vector in the area of the right inguinal ligament.

- The right iliacus fascia was tight in relation to the right symphysis pubis, the right anterior diaphragm and the right quadriceps, with and without dorsiflexion/eversion of the ankle (see Chapter 8 for MMS technique).

- The right inguinal ligament fascia was tight in relation to the right rectus abdominis, right anterior diaphragm, right thoracic ring 8 and in relation to passive physiological movements of the hip into extension, abduction, and adduction, and later with FABER (see MMS technique above).

Treatment consisted of MMS techniques for both the iliacus and inguinal ligament. After treatment, positional tests for the pelvis and hip were negative. There was no FLT at the pelvis or the hip with the OLS test, even without active recruitment of the thoracolumbar multifidus muscles. Over the next few weeks she reported ease with any circus maneuvers requiring right OLS and her SI pain was considerably decreased.

* Please note that the name of the patient has been changed to protect her privacy.

The quadriceps fascia in relation to the SFL and DFL

The quads fascia may be a factor that limits knee flexion, especially if there has been a history of trauma, including surgery.

MMS right quadriceps – "wiggle/waggle" – medial/lateral (Figure 11.14)

This technique is aptly named (despite it sounding rather unprofessional!) as the therapist literally wiggles the quads fascia in relation to the femur. This technique may be done in a mediolateral direction, or with a clockwise–counterclockwise maneuver.

Stabilizing hand The patient is in supine position with the leg straight. (However, if knee flexion is limited, the quads fascia may be also explored with the knee in various degrees of knee flexion.) The therapist uses both hands to grasp the tissues of the quadriceps muscles and pull them gently in an anterior direction. The quadriceps fascia may be explored centrally, medially, or laterally, both proximally and distally on the thigh.

Mobilizing hand Using a lumbrical grip to maintain the quadriceps fascia away from the femur, the therapist mobilizes the tissue in a mediolateral direction, creating a shearing

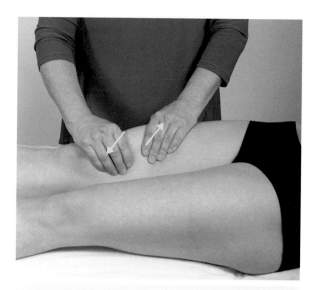

Figure 11.14
MMS right quadriceps "wiggle/waggle" – medial/
lateral

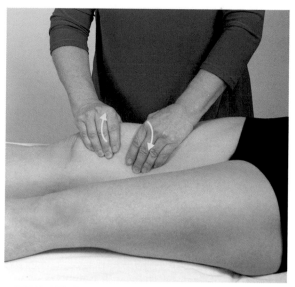

Figure 11.15
MMS right quadriceps "wiggle/waggle" – clockwise/
counterclockwise

moment between their two hands. The therapist looks for tension between the two hands, usually accompanied by some pain. If no tension is perceived, then this part of the quads fascia is not tight. If tension is perceived (quick resistance is felt between the two hands of the therapist), then it can be mobilized as per the approaches outlined in Chapter 4.

MMS right quadriceps – "wiggle/waggle" – clockwise/counterclockwise (Figure 11.15)

Stabilizing hand As per the technique above.

Mobilizing hand As per the technique above except that the therapist explores the quadriceps fascia with both hands moving in a clockwise/counterclockwise maneuver.

The quads fascia may also be explored in relation to the front lines of fascia, namely the SFL and /or the DFL.

MMS right quads + SFL (plantarflexion) (Figure 11.16)

Stabilizing hand The therapist uses the left hand to anchor onto the quadriceps muscles of the thigh (medial, lateral, or central), using a lumbrical grip to pull the quadriceps fascia away from the femur. The group of muscles may be explored both proximally and distally.

Mobilizing hand The therapist uses their right hand to perform a passive physiological movement of the ankle and toes into plantarflexion. The therapist stops as soon as an increase in tension is perceived in the hand that is anchoring the quads (to the first resistance or R1 of Maitland's movement diagram). If no tension is perceived, then the quads fascia in relation to the SFL is not tight.

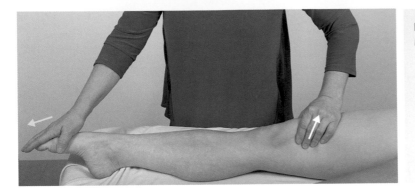

Figure 11.16
MMS right quads + SFL (PF)

If there is tension in this line of fascia, it will seem as though the quad muscles will pull caudally and posteriorly before full plantarflexion of the ankle and toes can be achieved. The therapist maintains the cranially directed anterior pull on the quads and simply prevents it from moving. The patient perceives this as the therapist "pulling harder" on the quads when, in reality, the therapist is simply preventing the anchor from moving. If tension is perceived (quick resistance is felt between the two hands of the therapist), then it can be mobilized as per the approaches outlined in Chapter 4. (The therapist performs repeated passive physiological PF while maintaining a steady pull on quads, always to when R1 is perceived (a grade III– passive physiological movement in Maitland terms). This movement is repeated until a release is felt between the therapist's two hands and it generally requires approximately five to eight cycles.

MMS right quads + DFL (dorsiflexion/eversion) (Figure 11.17)

Stabilizing hand As per the technique above.

Mobilizing hand The quads fascia may finally be further explored by using passive physiological combined ankle dorsiflexion/eversion, as this maneuver adds tension to the tibialis posterior muscle, the tail end of the DFL. The approach to treatment is similar to that of the technique above.

MMS right adductors in relation to the DFL (Figure 11.18)

Recurrent tension in the adductors may be due to overuse of this muscle if the pelvis does not stabilize well. It may also be due to tension of the myofascial line of the adductor muscle, usually the DFL.

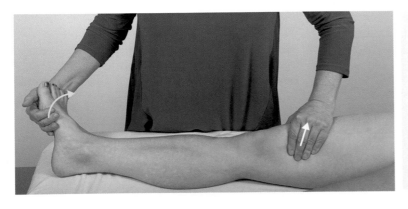

Figure 11.17
MMS right quads + DFL (DF/Ev)

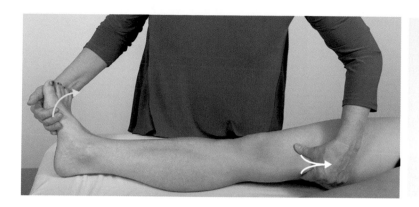

Figure 11.18
MMS right adductors in relation to the DFL (DF/Ev)

Stabilizing hand The patient is in a supine position. The therapist anchors onto the adductors of the thigh, exploring the group of muscles proximally and distally.

Mobilizing hand The therapist explores the tissues of the DFL of fascia, looking for quick resistance between the stabilizing hand and the mobilizing hand. Areas of the DFL that may be explored in this position include the iliacus, the ilium itself, the anterior diaphragms, the pericardium (see Chapter 9) and the tibialis posterior (shown in Figure 11.18 – similar to technique above for quads fascia with the DFL).

The fascia around the tibiofemoral, patellofemoral, and superior tib/fib joints (in relation to the SFL and DFL)

Other problematic areas of the DFL may be explored as outlined in the next section.

MMS right pes anserinus in relation to the DFL (Figure 11.19)

The pes anserinus area is frequently diagnosed as "bursitis." While this may be true in some cases, the area is also the site of fascial restrictions, especially in relation to the DFL, as the adductors form part of this line of fascia.

Stabilizing hand The patient is in a supine position. The therapist anchors onto the area of the pes anserinus distal to the medial knee, exploring this area in its entirety. The anchor is generally done in a cranial direction if the distal aspect of the DFL is explored.

Mobilizing hand The therapist uses their right hand to perform a passive physiological movement of combined DF/eversion. The therapist stops as soon as an increase

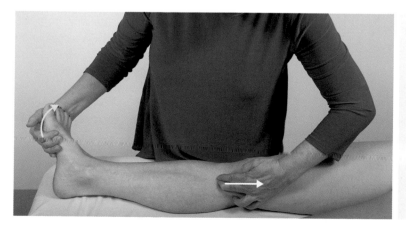

Figure 11.19
MMS right pes anserinus in relation to the DFL

in tension is perceived in the hand that is anchoring the pes anserinus (to the first resistance or R1 of Maitland's movement diagram). If no tension is perceived, then the pes anserinus fascia in relation to the DFL is not tight. If there is tension in this line of fascia, it will seem like the pes anserinus fascia will pull caudally and before full combined dorsiflexion/eversion of the ankle can be achieved. The therapist maintains the cranially directed anterior pull on the pes anserinus and simply prevents it from moving. The patient perceives this as the therapist "pushing harder" on the pes anserinus, when, in reality, the therapist is simply preventing the anchor from moving. If tension is perceived (quick resistance is felt between the two hands of the therapist), then it can be mobilized as per the approaches outlined in Chapter 4. (The therapist performs repeated passive physiological dorsiflexion/eversion while maintaining a steady pull on the pes anserinus, always to when R1 is perceived (a grade III– passive physiological movement in Maitland terms). This is repeated until a release is felt between the therapist's two hands; this generally requires approximately five to eight cycles.

MMS right patellofemoral joint in relation to DFL (Figure 11.20)

With patella-femoral joint dysfunction, the glides of the patella in relation to the femur are frequently restricted. Once the therapist has plateaued with this treatment, he/she should explore the fascial lines in relation to this joint.

Stabilizing hand Using their left hand, the therapist explores the glides of the patellofemoral joint (distraction, cranial, medial, lateral glides, rotations clockwise and counterclockwise, medial and lateral tilts), using the stiffest glide(s) for the anchor.

Mobilizing hand The therapist uses their right hand to perform a passive physiological movement of combined dorsiflexion/eversion. The therapist stops as soon as an increase in tension is perceived in the hand that is anchoring the patella. If there is tension in this fascial line, the therapist will feel an immediate increase in tension of the stabilizing hand as soon as dorsiflexion/eversion is performed. For example, if the therapist is using a patellofem-

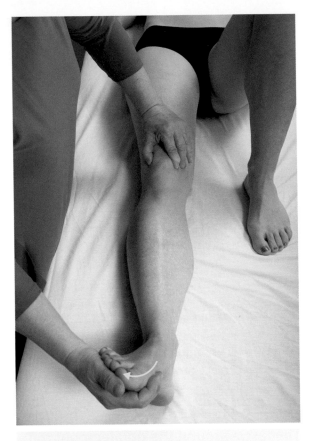

Figure 11.20
MMS right patellofemoral joint in relation to DFL

oral traction as the anchor, restriction of this line will feel like the patella wants to compress towards the femur as soon as DF/eversion is added. Similar concepts for mobilizing this line of fascia apply as per previous techniques.

MMS right tibial tuberosity in relation to DFL (Figure 11.21)

As per the technique above except that the therapist anchors the lateral aspect of the tibial tuberosity, gliding it medially. This technique is particularly useful in patients with chronic Osgood–Schlatter's.

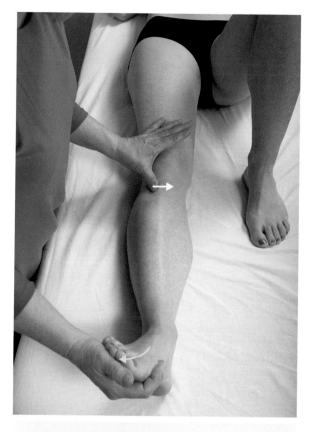

Figure 11.21
MMS right tibial tuberosity in relation to DFL

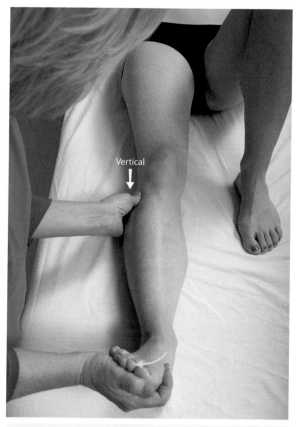

Figure 11.22
MMS right superior tib/fib joint in relation to DFL

MMS right superior tib/fib joint in relation to DFL
(Figure 11.22)

MMS right popliteus in relation to the DFL
(Figure 11.23)

As per the technique above except that the therapist anchors the posterior aspect of the superior tib/fib joint, gliding it anteriorly and cranially. This technique is particularly useful in patients with recurrent or persistent lateral knee pain of myofascial origin.

As per the technique above except that the therapist anchors onto the area of the popliteus muscle on the posterior aspect of the knee, exploring this area in its entirety. This technique is particularly useful in patients with recurrent or persistent posterior knee pain or Baker's cyst.

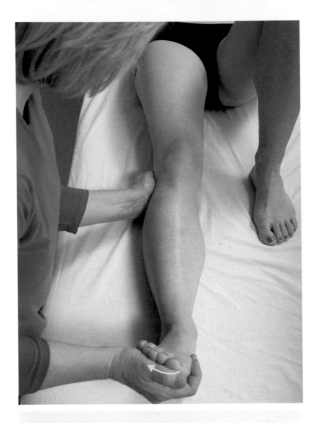

Figure 11.23
MMS right popliteus in relation to the DFL

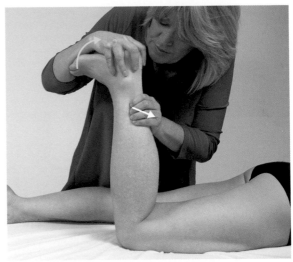

Figure 11.24
MMS right lateral lower leg with IR

The fascia of the lower leg (medial and lateral) in relation to the foot

Tight fascia of the lower leg may impact the range of motion of the ankle, especially dorsiflexion. The techniques below may also be useful to explore with patients complaining of chronic tension in the lower leg and/or difficulty with going down stairs.

MMS right lateral lower leg with internal rotation (Figure 11.24)

Stabilizing hand The patient is in prone position with the knee flexed 90 degrees. The therapist stands on the side of the patient opposite to the leg being treated. Using an A/P pressure, the therapist anchors onto the fascia of the lateral leg muscles, exploring areas of tension, usually in the distal half of the leg.

Mobilizing hand The therapist's right hand supports the heel and lateral foot with the hand and forearm, and performs a passive physiological movement of internal rotation of the lower leg, stopping as soon as an increase in tension is perceived in the stabilizing hand (to the first resistance or R1 of Maitland's movement diagram). If there is tension in this line of fascia, it will seem as though the lateral leg fascia will want to move anteriorly. The patient perceives this as the therapist increasing his/her pressure on the lateral leg. The therapist performs repeated passive physiological internal rotation of the lower leg via the heel and forefoot while maintaining a steady pressure with the stabilizing hand, always to when R1 is perceived (a grade III– passive physiological movement in Maitland terms). This is repeated until a release is felt between the therapist's two hands, which generally requires approximately five to eight cycles.

MMS right lateral lower leg with dorsiflexion (Figure 11.25)

As per the technique above, except that the therapist anchors the lateral aspect of the lower leg fascia in a cranial direction, while the mobilizing hand performs passive physiological ankle DF.

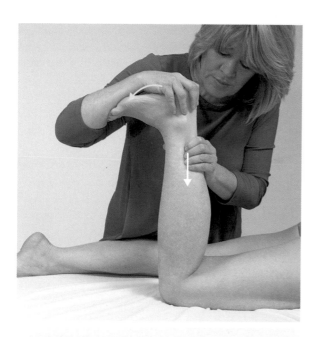

Figure 11.25
MMS right lateral lower leg with DF

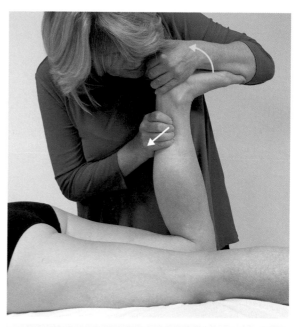

Figure 11.26
MMS right medial lower leg with ER

MMS right medial lower leg with external rotation (Figure 11.26)

Stabilizing hand The patient is in prone position with the knee flexed 90 degrees. The therapist stands on the same side of the leg being treated. Using an A/P pressure, the therapist anchors onto the fascia of the medial leg muscles, exploring areas of tension, usually in the distal half of the leg.

Mobilizing hand The therapist's left hand supports the heel and medial foot of the patient, using their hand and forearm, and performs a passive physiological external rotation movement of the lower leg, stopping as soon as an increase in tension is perceived in the stabilizing hand (to the first resistance or R1 of Maitland's movement diagram). If there is tension in this line of fascia, it will seem like the fascia of tibialis posterior and the toe flexors will want to move anteriorly. The patient perceives this as the therapist increasing his/her pressure on the medial leg. The therapist performs repeated passive physiological external rotation of the lower leg via the heel and forefoot, while maintaining a steady pressure with the stabilizing hand, always to when R1 is perceived (a grade III– passive

physiological movement in Maitland terms). This movement is repeated until a release is felt between the therapist's two hands a generally requires approximately five to eight cycles.

MMS medial lower leg with dorsiflexion (Figure 11.27)

As per the technique above except that the therapist anchors the medial aspect of the lower leg fascia in a cranial direction as the mobilizing hand performs passive physiological ankle dorsiflexion.

The plantar fascia and flexor hallucis longus

Plantar fascia pain has been the bane of therapists, as it is known to be resistant to treatment. The term fasciitis may, in fact, be something of a misnomer, because the disease is actually a degenerative process that occurs with or without inflammatory changes, which may include fibroblastic proliferation (Young 2010). Studies have introduced the etiologic concept of fasciosis as the inciting pathology. Fasciosis, like tendinosis, is defined as a chronic degenerative condition that is characterized

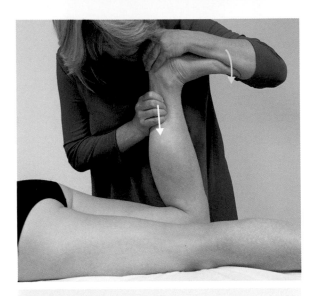

Figure 11.27
MMS right medial lower leg with DF

histologically by fibroblastic hypertrophy, absence of inflammatory cells, disorganized collagen, and chaotic vascular hyperplasia with zones of avascularity (Khan et al. 1999, 2002). These changes suggest a non-inflammatory condition and dysfunctional vasculature, which may be seen on ultrasound (Chen et al. 2013). With reduced vascularity and a compromise in nutritional blood flow through the impaired fascia, it becomes difficult for cells to synthesize the extracellular matrix necessary for repairing and remodeling. With regards to functional risk factors, reduced dorsiflexion has been shown to be an important risk factor for this condition. As well, tightness in the hamstrings, gastrocnemius soleus, and the Achilles tendon are considered risk factors for plantar fasciitis (Bolivar et al. 2013). It is interesting to note that all of these structures form part of the SBL of fascia. In addition, weakness of the gastrocnemius, soleus, and intrinsic foot muscles is also considered a risk factor for plantar fasciitis.

Treatment approach varies. Some people will respond better to heat, though more will respond positively to ice in terms of pain reduction, especially in the acute phase. A hydrocortisone injection can be helpful if it is done precisely at the site of inflammation but this approach will be ineffective if there is no "fasciitis." It is important

to work out the proper foot and ankle mechanics, so appropriate manual therapy directed toward joint mobility and muscle imbalance issues is essential here. Rolling gently/slowly on a ball before sleep and on waking may reduce the pain and stimulate blood circulation. From a fascia point of view, the therapist must consider the SBL, especially in chronic cases and/or if working directly on the plantar fascia has negative effects. Plantar fasciitis is often the result of tension in the Achilles complex, the hamstrings, or even up at the suboccipital muscles. The techniques below may also be useful to explore with patients complaining of chronic plantar fascia pain (Myers 2015).

> **MMS right plantar fascia with forefoot adduction +/– knee flexion (Figure 11.28)**

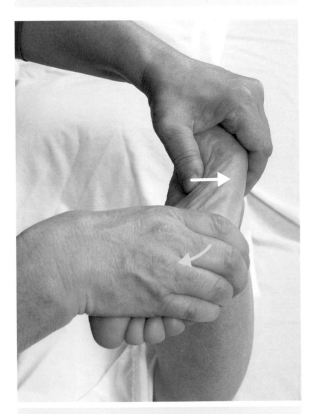

Figure 11.28
MMS right plantar fascia with forefoot adduction +/- knee flexion

Stabilizing hand The patient is in prone position with the knee flexed 90 degrees. The therapist stands on the side of the patient opposite to the leg being treated. Using a medial to lateral pressure, the therapist anchors onto the plantar fascia, exploring areas of tension, from its origin at the tuberosity of the calcaneus toward the heads of the metatarsal bones. The lateral band should also be explored in a similar way.

Mobilizing hand The therapist's right hand performs a passive physiological movement of forefoot adduction, stopping as soon as an increase in tension is perceived in the stabilizing hand (to the first resistance or R1 of Maitland's movement diagram). The therapist must keep the ankle in a neutral position of about 0 degrees of dorsiflexion and the forefoot in a neutral position between pronation and supination throughout this technique. If there is tension in this line of fascia, it will seem like the thumb that is anchoring the plantar fascia will want to move medially. The patient perceives this as the therapist increasing his/her pressure on the plantar fascia. The therapist performs repeated passive physiological forefoot adduction while maintaining a steady pressure with the stabilizing hand, always to when R1 is perceived (a grade III– passive physiological movement in Maitland terms). This is repeated until a release is felt between the therapist's two hands and generally requires approximately five to eight cycles.

Progression Once tension has been released throughout the whole plantar fascia, the technique may be progressed by adding passive knee flexion. While doing so may seem contrary to what should be done to release the SBL, clinically it is very applicable. Perhaps an element of the plantar fascia and the flexor hallucis longus involves the DFL of fascia, which could explain why knee flexion seems to increase tension.

MMS flexor hallucis longus in the plantar aspect of the foot (Figure 11.29)

Because the flexor hallucis longus (FHL) muscle is small, injuries associated with this muscle and its tendon are often overlooked. What is perceived as plantar fascia pain can frequently be a problem with the mobility of the FHL and its fascia. The technique for this muscle is similar to the technique above except that the therapist anchors the FHL tendon at various points on the plantar aspect of the foot while the mobilizing hand of the therapist hooks

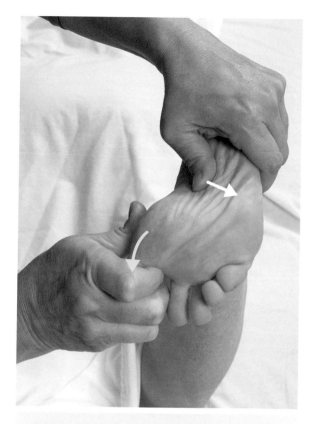

Figure 11.29
MMS right FHL in the plantar aspect of the foot

around the first toe and performs passive physiological dorsiflexion of the first metatarsophalangeal (MTP) joint, making sure to maintain dorsiflexion of the ankle with the forefoot in neutral position for pronation/supination and abduction/adduction.

MMS flexor hallucis longus in relation to the inferior tib/fib joint

Tension of this muscle and its fascia is also a factor that can "push" the medial tibia anteriorly in relation to the fibula at the inferior tibiofibular joint. This is one element that may contribute to external tibial torsion. The therapist can modify the technique above to perform the same movements of the first toe with the foot in the same position, but the patient is in a high sitting position instead of the prone position. The therapist uses an A/P pressure on the medial tibia as their anchor (not pictured).

Anterior lower leg fascia in relation to hammer toes

Complete assessment of hammer toes should involve not only an assessment of the foot and toe joints, but also an assessment of the flexibility of the toe extensors and the fascia of the anterior lower leg and metatarsals. Besides the problem of finding proper shoes to accommodate the hammer toes, patients with this issue also complain of pain in the plantar aspect of the base of the metatarsal joints since these joints must "live" in dorsiflexion, secondary to the abnormal tension of the dorsal muscles and fascia.

MMS anterior lower leg in relation to hammer toes (Figure 11.30)

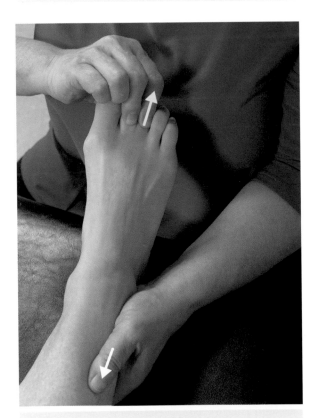

Figure 11.30
MMS right anterior lower leg in relation to hammer toes

Stabilizing hand The patient is in a supine position. The therapist anchors onto the area of the fascia of the tibialis anterior, the extensor hallucis longus (EHL) and/or the extensor digitorum longus (EDL), anchoring the myofascial tissues in the A/P, cranial direction.

Mobilizing hand The therapist's caudal hand performs a passive physiological movement of toe flexion, stopping as soon as an increase in tension is perceived in the stabilizing hand (to the first resistance or R1 of Maitland's movement diagram). If there is tension in this line of fascia, it will seem like the thumb that is anchoring the anterior lower leg fascia will want to move caudally. The patient perceives this as the therapist increasing his/her pressure on the anterior lower leg. The therapist performs repeated passive physiological flexion of the toes (individually or together as a group), always to when R1 is perceived (a grade III– passive physiological movement in Maitland terms). This technique is repeated until a release is felt between the therapist's two hands and generally requires approximately five to eight cycles. Note that the second and third toes are frequently the most problematic.

Progression The technique above may be progressed by repeating it with the ankle in full plantarflexion.

MMS dorsal metatarsal fascia in relation to hammer toes (Figure 11.31)

The technique above may be modified to explore and release the dorsal intermetatarsal fascia. The stabilizing hand (in this case, the left hand of the therapist) seeks out the intermetatarsal fascia, anchoring these tissues with an A/P glide directed cranially and diagonally. The mobilizing hand repeats the same technique as above. Once again, the area of the second and third metatarsals is frequently problematic.

The fascia of the biceps femoris

Recurrent tension in the biceps femoris muscle may be due to overuse of this muscle if the pelvis does not stabilize well. It may also be due to tension of the myofascial line of this hamstring muscle, usually the SBL.

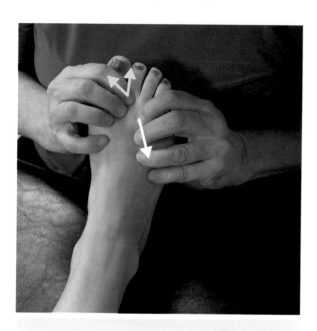

Figure 11.31
MMS right dorsal metatarsal fascia in relation to hammer toes

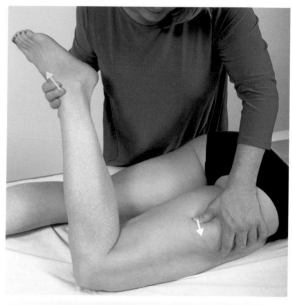

Figure 11.32
MMS right biceps femoris fascia with hip ER

MMS right biceps femoris fascia with hip external rotation (Figure 11.32)

Stabilizing hand The patient is in prone position with the lumbar spine in a neutral position. The therapist stands on the left side of the patient. Using a P/A pressure directed laterally, the therapist anchors onto the biceps femoris fascia, exploring areas of tension from its proximal attachment just below the greater trochanter to its distal attachment toward the lateral knee.

Mobilizing hand The therapist's caudal hand supports the lower extremity at the ankle and performs a passive physiological movement of hip external rotation, stopping as soon as an increase in tension is perceived in the hand palpating the biceps femoris (to the first resistance or R1 of Maitland's movement diagram). If there is tension in this line of fascia, it will seem like the lateral hamstrings move medially before full hip external rotation can be achieved (usually around 45–50 degrees of rotation). The patient perceives this as the therapist increasing his/her pressure on the lateral thigh. The therapist performs repeated passive physiological external rotation of the hip while maintaining a steady pressure with the stabilizing hand, always to when R1 is perceived (a grade III– passive physiological movement in Maitland terms). This is repeated until a release is felt between the therapist's two hands and generally requires approximately five to eight cycles.

Note that this technique may also be performed in the same position, but using passive physiological knee flexion/extension as the exploratory movement (not pictured).

Biceps femoris/vastus lateralis in relation to tibial torsion (duck foot) (Figure 11.33)

One of the myofascial vectors that may be causing excessive external tibial torsion is the fascia of the lateral thigh, in particular the biceps femoris, vastus lateralis, and the posterior aspect of the iliotibial band (ITB) (Aguilar 2015).

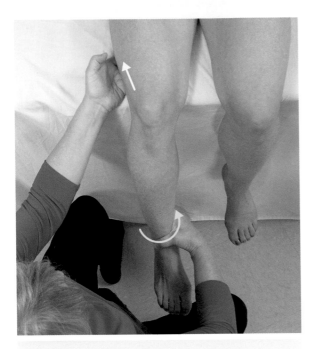

Figure 11.33
Right biceps femoris in relation to tibial torsion
(duck foot)

In his video, Aguilar demonstrates a home exercise program using a ball in the seated position to anchor the affected fascia. This approach may also be used as a technique to perform in clinic.

Stabilizing hand The patient is in a seated position, with their weight shifted toward the affected leg. The therapist palpates the distal half of the lateral thigh, anchoring the fascia with a lateral/cranial pull of the tissues. The therapist may explore these tissues caudally toward the knee.

Mobilizing hand The therapist maintains internal rotation of the tibia as he/she passively extends the patient's knee, stopping as soon as an increase in tension is perceived in the hand palpating the biceps femoris (to the first resistance, or R1 of Maitland's movement diagram). If there is tension in this line of fascia, it will seem as though the lateral hamstrings move medially and caudally before full knee extension can be achieved. The patient perceives this as the therapist increasing his/her pressure on the lateral thigh. The therapist performs repeated passive

physiological extension of the knee while maintaining a steady pressure with the stabilizing hand, always to when R1 is perceived (a grade III– passive physiological movement in Maitland terms). This technique is repeated until a release is felt between the therapist's two hands and generally requires approximately five to eight cycles.

Joint mobilizations converted to MMS techniques

The second concept of treatment using MMS techniques is that any joint mobilization may be converted into a fascial technique. This approach is particularly useful when the therapist has reached a plateau with treatment using joint mobilizations and/or manipulations. The following examples may be used for the lower quadrant.

MMS A/P talus in slump +/– cervical flexion (Figure 11.34)

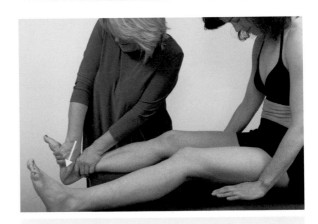

Figure 11.34
MMS right A/P talus in slump +/– Cx flexion

The therapist performs an A/P glide of the talocrural joint with the patient lying supine and compares this glide to one that is performed with the patient sitting in a slump position (lumbar, thoracic, and cervical spine flexed, legs extended). This slump position adds tension not only to the posterior neural structures but also the fascia of the SBL. The A/P glide of the talus is repeated until the therapist no longer perceives a difference with the A/P glide performed in supine (usually within one minute). Test/re-test maneuvers may include a SLR test, ankle dorsiflexion, and/or the slump test itself. Care must be used when the neural structures are irritated and when the condition is deemed to be irritable.

MMS P/A superior tib/fib in straight leg raise/plantarflexion (Figure 11.35)

The superior tib/fib joint is a common interface problem for mobility of the superficial peroneal nerve. The clinical test most commonly used to test the mobility of this nerve is straight leg raise (SLR) combined with plantarflexion and inversion. Indications for this technique are patients who complain of tension in the posterolateral knee area that has not changed with localized treatment and/or patients with decreased mobility of the superficial peroneal nerve.

The therapist performs a P/A glide of the proximal fibula with the patient in crook lying position. He/she compares this glide to one that is performed with the patient in side-lying, with the affected leg "up" and positioned in SLR/plantarflexion. The P/A glide of the superior tib/fib joint is repeated until the therapist no longer perceives a difference with the P/A glide performed in crook lying position (usually within one minute). Test/re-test maneuvers may include a SLR test with ankle plantarflexion/inversion, and/or the slump test performed with plantarflexion/inversion. Care must be used when the neural

structures are irritated and when the condition is deemed to be irritable.

MMS A/P superior tib/fib in slump (Figure 11.36)

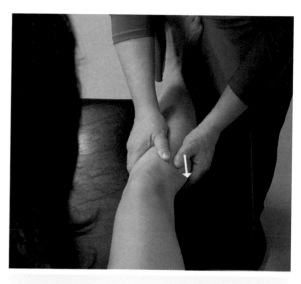

Figure 11.36
MMS right A/P superior tib/fib in slump

This technique is similar to the one above except that an A/P glide is assessed in crook lying and compared to the same glide in slump position.

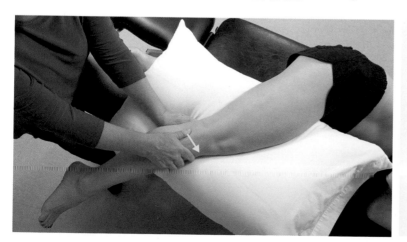

Figure 11.35
MMS right P/A superior tib/fib in SLR/PF

Release with awareness techniques for the foot and ankle (RWA) (Figures 11.37–11.39)

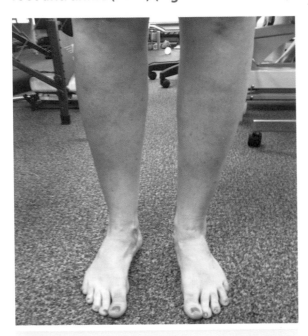

Figure 11.37
Patient 1 position of feet in standing

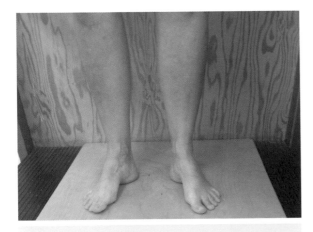

Figure 11.38
Patient 2 right foot before RWA

This is the third concept of treatment using MMS techniques and is described in Chapter 4. A common pattern

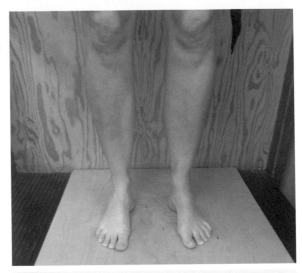

Figure 11.39
Patient 2 right foot after RWA

of ankle and foot dysfunction is one in which is depicted in Figure 11.37) (Patient 1). The patient was instructed to stand with the feet as parallel as possible. Focus on the left foot:

- the talus is plantarflexed and adducted in relation to the tibia
- the navicular is externally rotated (more supinated) in relation to the talus
- the medial cuneiform is externally rotated in relation to the navicular and
- the base of the first metatarsal is also more externally rotated in relation to the medial cuneiform.

Note that the right foot is also problematic, but in this case, the first ray is positioned in such extreme supination that the forefoot is unable to adduct in relation to the hindfoot and the patient stands with the leg in external tibial torsion.

A full assessment of the joint mobility of the entire foot and ankle should be carried out and appropriate treatment done. However, in many cases a plateau is quickly reached with treatment using joint mobilizations and/or manipulation. We must consider the fascial element of these restrictions. This situation is one in which the technique of release with awareness (RWA) is particularly useful.

RWA is a biofeedback technique developed by Diane Lee and L. J. Lee (Lee & Lee 2011) in which the patient is an active participant. The patient is asked to bring their awareness to the muscle being palpated and various imagery cues are used to facilitate relaxation of the muscle. The patient's participation is elicited at the same time that the therapist is guiding the release with feedback from their hands. I have found this technique to be very useful clinically. Involving the patient in the release seems to create a longer-lasting effect and carry-over from one treatment to the next is excellent.

Figures 11.38 and 11.39 show Patient 2 before and directly after one treatment to the right foot and ankle, using RWA. Note that Patient 2's left foot also requires work!

It is important to address the whole foot when using this approach; so all of the following techniques must be used within a same treatment in order to achieve optimal outcomes.

RWA right A/P talus + fascia on medial aspect of lower leg (Figure 11.40)

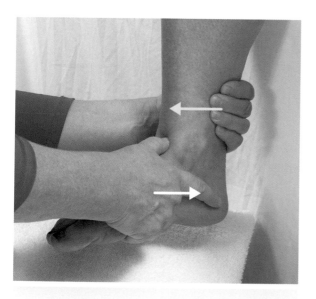

Figure 11.40
RWA right A/P talus + fascia on medial aspect of lower leg

In order to achieve full ankle dorsiflexion, the talocrural joint requires mobility in the posterior glide of the talus and in an A/P rock or tilt. The posterior glide usually responds to mobilizations and/or manipulation but if a plateau is reached with this approach, the following technique may be used. From a fascial perspective, there is commonly a neuromuscular vector in the medial gastrocnemius that prevents the talus from rocking posteriorly to allow full dorsiflexion to occur.

Stabilizing hand The therapist performs an accessory movement of an A/P rock to the talus with one hand and maintains it at the point where initial resistance to the movement is felt.

Exploring hand At the same time, the therapist palpates and monitors the area of the gastrocnemius muscle that has most connection with the restricted A/P rock of the talus; that is, an area where a gentle pressure and stretch of the medial gastrocnemius in a cranial direction has an almost immediate impact on the accessory movement at the talus, giving the therapist the sensation that the talus is being pushed anteriorly. As the therapist provides manual input to the gastrocnemius, the patient is instructed to "soften the muscle," "let it go," "see if you can find a way to allow my fingers to sink into the muscle." At the same time, the therapist moves the joint or muscle to shorten origin and insertion, diminishing tension on the muscle spindle. The therapist then waits, allowing the patient and his/her system to cue into the release at the same time as the therapist gives manual and verbal cues to let go. Once maximum release is obtained, usually within 10–15 seconds, the muscle is gently taken through a full stretch, with the therapist listening to its response and avoiding recurrence of overactivity. A full A/P rocking movement is encouraged, using a sustained movement at the ankle. At the same time, the therapist may encourage a release of the muscle fascicle in a cranial direction, helping to release the "fuzz" of connective tissue that has lost its ability to elongate. Once the tissue releases, the therapist may seek and explore other areas of the calf that may be limiting this accessory movement. (There is usually more than one area.)

RWA pronation right first ray with tibialis anterior (Figure 11.41)

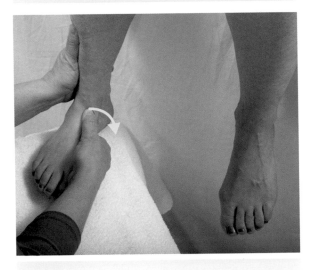

Figure 11.41
RWA pronation right first ray with tibialis anterior

Stabilizing hand With this technique, the therapist performs an accessory movement of a P/A glide of the navicular into pronation in relation to the talus, with the ankle in neutral position for dorsiflexion/plantarflexion.

Exploring hand At the same time the therapist palpates and monitors the area of the tibialis anterior muscle that has most connection with the restricted navicular bone; that is, an area where a gentle pressure and stretch of the tibialis anterior cranially and laterally has an almost immediate impact on the accessory movement at the talonavicular joint, giving the therapist the sensation that the navicular is being pulled dorsally into external rotation. As the therapist provides manual input to the tibialis anterior, the patient is instructed to "soften the muscle." The therapist shortens the origin and insertion, waits a few seconds to allow the patient and his/her system to cue into the release, and then takes the muscle through a full stretch

as the hand on the navicular bone moves into internal rotation/pronation, using a sustained pressure (as per the technique above). Once the area is released, the therapist may seek and explore other areas of the lateral lower leg that may be limiting this accessory movement.

Progression This technique may be progressed by placing the ankle in full dorsiflexion and repeating the technique.

This technique is also used to release the rest of the first ray (medial cuneiform in relation to the talus, and the base of the first metatarsal in relation to the medial cuneiform), if they are restricted.

RWA right inter-metatarsal fascia + A/P talus (Figure 11.42)

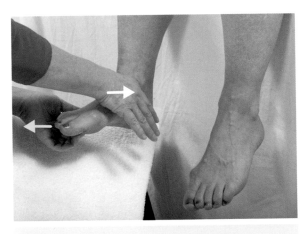

Figure 11.42
RWA right intermetatarsal fascia + A/P talus

Last, but not least, the plantar aspect of the foot is explored as the therapist maintains the ankle in full dorsiflexion, with the first ray in a more neutral position (i.e., not supinated). The therapist explores the inter-metatarsal area or the insertion of peroneus longus on the base of the first metatarsal, using a caudal/distal glide. The hand under the foot is the anchoring hand.

Similar concepts of releasing from within are used, at the same time as the therapist promotes full ankle dorsiflexion, using the web of their hand on the dome of the talus.

Release with awareness (RWA) techniques for the foot and ankle (as described above) help restore optimal biomechanics in the foot and ankle, and if the foot is a driver in relation to other parts of the body, this technique may also improve dynamic stability of the knee, hip, sacroiliac joint (SIJ), thorax, and neck.

Summary

The techniques in this chapter have focused on the myofascial connections in relation to the hip, the thigh, the knee, the lower leg, and the ankle/foot. The concept of converting joint mobilizations in the lower extremity into fascial techniques was also covered. Release with awareness techniques may be used throughout the body but are particularly useful to release neuromuscular and fascial vectors that may be impacting the foot and ankle. The next chapter will focus on techniques for the shoulder girdle.

When treating patients with problems in the shoulder girdle area, manual therapists are trained to assess and treat the sternoclavicular (SC), acromioclavicular (AC), and glenohumeral (GH) joints. In addition, the muscles of the upper quadrant are assessed and treated for imbalance between hypertonic and/or tight and weak muscles. However, mobilizing joints and stretching and strengthening individual muscles can achieve only partial benefits if the fascial system is not taken into consideration.

This chapter will focus on the myofascial connections between the clavicle, sternum, manubrium, cervical, scapula and GH joints. These include:

1. The sternoclavicular fascia in relation to the:
   – manubrium
   – anterior cervical spine/scalenes/sternocleidomastoid (SCM)
   – occiput and mastoid process of the temporal bone
   – C/Thx (cervicothoracic) and/or mid-Thx (thoracic spine) region
   – scapula
   – ipsilateral or contralateral thoracic ring.

2. The clavicle fascia in relation to the:
   – GH joint
   – deltoid, pectoralis major muscles
   – ipsilateral sternoclavicular joint
   – anterior cervical spine
   – occiput and mastoid process of the temporal bone
   – neural tissues of the upper extremity.

Indications for MMS for this chapter

Recurring shoulder girdle or cervical pain and dysfunction despite the following treatment approaches:

- mobilization/manipulation of the joints of the SC, AC, and GH joints

- release of trigger points to the muscles of the shoulder girdle area with manual or dry needling techniques

- stabilization and strengthening exercises for the upper quadrant.

Positional tests for the shoulder girdle

For this section, particular attention is paid to the following:

Position of glenohumeral joint in relation to the scapula (Figure 12.1)

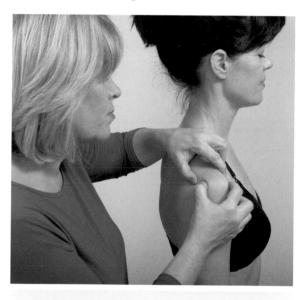

Figure 12.1
Position of GH in relation to the scapula

From the side, the therapist can assess the humeral head position relative to the acromion. For the right shoulder, the therapist palpates the anterior and posterior aspects of the lateral acromion with the left index finger on the anterior aspect and the thumb on the posterior aspect of the acromion. The right hand palpates the anterior humeral head with the right index finger and the thumb is placed over the posterior humeral head. Traditionally, it is has been taught that one third of the humeral head should be anterior to the acromion but the reliability of this supposition is questionable. The therapist should also assess if the humeral head is positioned inferiorly in relation to the acromion (Watson 2013; Konieczka et al. 2017).

Position of the scapulae in relation to the thorax (Figure 12.2)

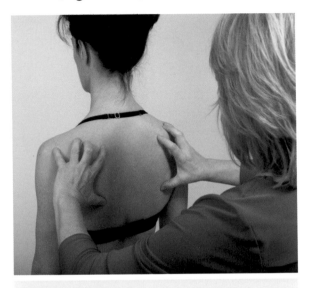

Figure 12.2
Position of the scapulae in relation to the thorax

From the back of the patient, the therapist can assess the resting position of the scapulae for elevation/depression, upward or downward rotation, internal or external rotation. The symmetry of scapulae is noted as well as muscle bulk/wasting of shoulder external rotators, winging of the scapula (implying serratus anterior weakness), prominence of inferior angle of the scapula (implying pectoralis minor tightness) (Green et al. 2013; Watson 2013).

Position of the clavicles: palpation for intra-shoulder girdle torsion

The shoulder girdle involves the SC joint, clavicles, manubrium, and scapulae. Ideally, with the patient in the sitting or standing position, both clavicles should be in a relatively neutral position with regards to anterior or posterior rotation, and there should be a sense of space between the clavicles and the manubrium. An intra-shoulder girdle torsion (ISGT) is considered undesirable as this twist may

contribute to cranial, scapular, cervical, and/or thoracic dysfunction (Lee 2018).

In this discussion of ISGT, a brief review of SC joint biomechanics provides important context. Because the SC joint has a fibrocartilaginous disc, the joint has both a medial joint (between the manubrium and the disc) and a lateral joint (between the disc and the medial end of the clavicle).

The biomechanics of the SC joint are as follows:

- With scapular elevation there is normally an inferior glide at the lateral joint as well as an anterior rotation at the medial joint.

- With combined elevation and protraction, the clavicle should rotate anteriorly.

- Anterior rotation of both clavicles should occur with cervical flexion.

- With cervical right rotation the right clavicle posteriorly rotates, the left clavicle anteriorly rotates, the first thoracic ring rotates and sideflexes to the right (the manubrium right rotates and sideflexes as part of this), the right temporal bone posteriorly rotates, the left temporal bone anteriorly rotates and the cervical vertebrae right rotate and sideflex. The opposite occurs for cervical left rotation. In either case, there should be no excessive medial translation of the clavicle (either right or left), as this suggests there are horizontal compressive factors (Lee 2018).

In order to palpate for positional tests related to this torsion, the therapist places him/herself behind the patient (Figure 12.3). The therapist places their index and middle fingers on the superior and inferior aspect of each of the patient's clavicles, in order to determine their relative position in space.

The model in Figure 12.3 demonstrates an ISGT to the left. If there is an ISGT to the left, the clavicles "live" in a position where the left clavicle is posteriorly rotated, the right clavicle is anteriorly rotated and there is increased medial compression of the right SC joint. If there is an ISGT to the left and the right SC joint is compressed medially,

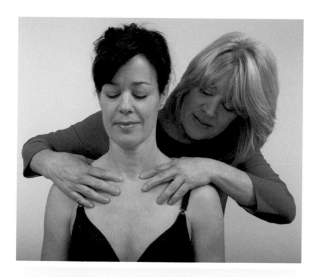

Figure 12.3
Position of the clavicles – palpation for ISGT

then the inferior glide of the right SC joint becomes quite limited. The joint may be compressed medially by articular dysfunction but more often, there are myofascial vectors that can compress this joint. For example, the upper fibers of trapezius (UFT), scalenes, or subclavius muscles may create excessive medial compression of the SC joint. If the shoulder girdle is unable to come out of this position, it may impact not only the cervical range of motion in right rotation but also the mobility of the thorax, scapulae, and shoulders, especially if the ISGT is deemed to be a primary driver of dysfunction.

Functional tests: sitting arm lift test

The sitting arm lift (SAL) test is similar to the active straight leg raise test but is used for the upper quadrant. The test assesses if there is a difference in effort required to lift the arm to 90 degrees of shoulder flexion. The arm that the patient perceives as more difficult to lift is then re-tested with other areas of the body corrected. For example, with a positive SAL test on the right, the therapist corrects the positional faults noted in certain areas, in order to evaluate its impact on the SAL test. Common areas for correction include the cervical spine, the thoracic spine (including the thoracic rings), the scapula, the GH joint

and the position of the clavicles and SC joints (correction of an ISGT) (Lee 2003).

If the correction of an ISGT has most positive impact on the SAL test, then the load and listen test is used in order to determine the vector(s) that may impact the mobility of the SC joints. (Note that there is frequently more than one vector.)

Load and listen test for sternoclavicular joints

The accessory movements for the SC joint may be performed with the patient in a supine position. If the restriction is articular, the end feel of the accessory movement will be hard and fibrotic. However, if there is a myofascial restriction, the therapist feels the resistance to the accessory movement but the end feel will be softer and more "rubbery." The therapist should then have the patient sit or stand and try to correct the ISGT. For an ISGT to the left, the therapist should decompress the right SC joint through the clavicle and then de-rotate the clavicles gently and gradually, using both hands at the same time. In this example, the therapist would guide the right clavicle into posterior rotation and the left clavicle into anterior rotation, while continuing to create space between the two clavicles. A certain resistance will be felt with this correction but much valuable information will be gleaned if the therapist pays attention to the release component of this test, listening (passively) for vectors that are "tugging" on the clavicles and SC joints. In this example, particular attention is paid to the vectors that affect the right SC joint. Vectors may be long or short, pull in a cranial or caudal direction, and may feel either superficial of deep.

There may be a combination of neuromuscular vectors (increased tone in muscles due to increased neural drive), visceral vectors, muscular, and fascial vectors. The therapist pays attention to where the first pull is felt, be it on the right or the left clavicle, and then tries to determine the direction of pull. Once this is first vector released, then the therapist seeks a second vector on a repeat load and listen test, and so on until no further tension is felt on the release component of the load and listen test. At this point, positional tests for the ISGT should also be negative.

The possibilities for vectors are varied but the most frequent are outlined below:

- The right SC joint is pulled medially and caudally toward the manubrium/sternum (this could be joint restriction at the sternomanubrial junction or a deeper pericardial fascial pull).

- The right SC joint is pulled toward the right anterior cervical spine (uncovertebral joints, scalene muscles, or the SCM).

- The right SC joint is pulled higher up, toward the right occiput or the right mastoid process of the temporal bone.

- The right SC joint is pulled posteriorly toward the C/Thx and /or the mid-Thx regions (this implies tension in the fascial planes in between the anterior and the posterior thorax).

- The right SC joint may be pulled toward the first rib on the right (subclavius).

- Either SC joint may be pulled toward a particular ring in the thorax (ipsilaterally or contralaterally).

- The right SC joint may be pulled toward the symphysis pubis (SFL of fascia).

All of these neuromuscular vectors may be treated with a number of techniques designed to release muscle hypertonicity, such as contract-relax, strain/counterstrain, release with awareness, dry needling, etc. However, if results of these approaches are difficult to maintain, the therapist should then explore the fascial line(s) related to the muscles involved.

After treatment, re-assessment of positional tests, functional tests, and the load and listen test for the clavicles is recommended.

Concepts of treatment using MMS

For this chapter, we will be using primarily the first concept of treatment when using MMS techniques; that is, choose a recurrent articular dysfunction or myofascial trigger point and explore a fascial line in relation to it. The therapist anchors him/herself to a recurrent articular dysfunction and assesses the fascial lines of tension in relation to the anchor, looking for early tension between their two hands.

The following approaches may be used, depending on how the tissues respond:

- work with oscillations (grades III−, III, III+)

- work with sustained pressure

- work with "harmonics" (Dr Laurie Hartman).

Release with awareness (RWA) techniques also work quite well for the techniques in this chapter (concept 3 for treatment using MMS).

Please refer to Chapter 4 for detail on concepts of treatment using MMS.

Sternoclavicular joint fascia

The following techniques are suggested for exploring and treating fascial dysfunction in relation to the sternoclavicular joints. The technique(s) used will be determined by the load and listen test when correcting an ISGT (described above).

> **MMS right sternoclavicular joint in relation to ipsilateral scalenes (Figure 12.4)**

Stabilizing hand The patient is in sitting or supine position. The therapist uses their left thumb to anchor onto the right SC joint (a laterally and caudally directed decompression glide).

Mobilizing hand The therapist explores the area of the right scalenes with the fingers of their right hand, gently gliding the anterior cervical spine and scalenes in a craniolateral direction. Several levels of the cervical spine may be explored with this technique. If this fascial line is tight, the therapist will feel an immediate increase in tension in the anchoring hand, as if the right SC joint pulls medially and cranially. The patient perceives this as the therapist increasing his/her pressure on the SC joint. If no tension is perceived, then the SFL of fascia in relation to this region is not tight. If tension is perceived

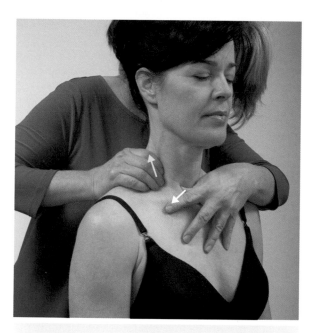

Figure 12.4
MMS right SC joint in relation to ipsilateral scalenes

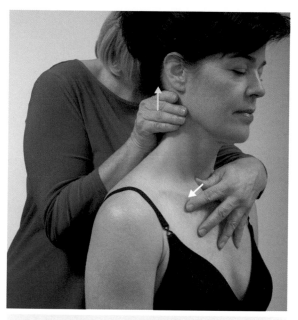

Figure 12.5
MMS right SC joint in relation to ipsilateral occiput

(quick resistance is felt between the two hands of the therapist), then it can be mobilized as per the approaches outlined in Chapter 4. (The therapist maintains the caudal and lateral pressure to the right SC joint as he/she performs repeated A/P mobilizations of the scalene muscles in the direction(s) of most restriction.) Alternatively, the therapist may want to use a release with awareness (RWA) technique.

MMS right sternoclavicular joint in relation to ipsilateral occiput (Figure 12.5)

Stabilizing hand As per the technique above.

Mobilizing hand The therapist explores the right occiput, using a cranially directed P/A on the right side of the occiput. An area about 2 cm square may be explored at the occiput using this technique. The concepts for release are similar to the technique above. Cues for lengthening may be something along the lines of "allow your neck to grow long."

MMS right sternoclavicular joint in relation to the cervicothoracic region (Figure 12.6)

Stabilizing hand As per the technique above.

Mobilizing hand The therapist explores the cervicothoracic (C/Thx) region posteriorly, using the star concept to seek and release tension between their two hands. The tension may be felt most when the C/Thx region is mobilized in a simple caudal direction, or caudal to the right or left of the client, or with a clockwise or counterclockwise twist. The patient perceives this tension as the therapist pushing harder on the right SC joint when, in reality, the therapist is simply preventing the right medial clavicle from moving. If no tension is perceived, then the fascia between the clavicle and the C/Thx area is not tight. If tension is perceived (quick resistance is felt between the two hands of the therapist), then it can be mobilized as per the approaches outlined in Chapter 4.

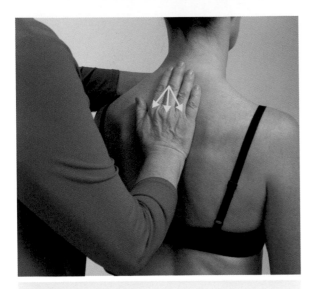

Figure 12.6
MMS right SC joint in relation to C/Thx region

MMS right sternoclavicular joint in relation to mid-thoracic region (Figure 12.7)

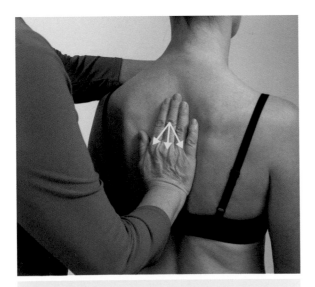

Figure 12.7
MMS right SC joint in relation to mid-Thx region

Stabilizing hand As per the technique above.

Mobilizing hand As per the technique above except that the therapist explores the mid-thoracic region posteriorly. This technique addresses the anteroposterior fascia between the SC joint and the mid-thoracic region, which also includes the pericardial fascia.

MMS right sternoclavicular joint in relation to ipsilateral scapula (Figure 12.8)

Stabilizing hand As per the technique above.

Mobilizing hand As per the technique above except that the therapist explores the right scapula in all its directions (elevation, depression, medial and lateral slide, upward and downward rotation), looking for an immediate increase in tension of the stabilizing hand on the SC joint as the scapula is moved. The concepts for release are similar to the technique above.

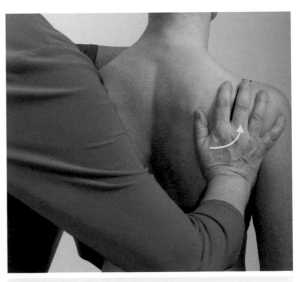

Figure 12.8
MMS right SC joint in relation to ipsilateral scapula

MMS right sternoclavicular joint in relation to manubrium (Figure 12.9)

Stabilizing hand The patient is in supine position. The therapist uses their right thumb to anchor onto the right SC joint with a laterally directed decompression glide, as he/she encourages posterior rotation of the right clavicle.

Mobilizing hand The therapist explores the area of the manubrium with the palm of their left hand, gently gliding the manubrium to the left and caudally. As with all MMS techniques, the star concept is a used to determine which vectors pull the most on the stabilizing hand. The tension may be felt most when the manubrium is pushed in a simple caudal direction, or to the left of the client, or with a clockwise or counterclockwise twist. The patient perceives this tension as the therapist pushing harder on the right SC joint when, in reality, the therapist is simply preventing the right medial clavicle from moving. If no tension is perceived, then this part of the fascia is not tight. If tension is perceived (quick resistance is felt between the two hands of the therapist), then it can be mobilized as per the approaches outlined in Chapter 4.

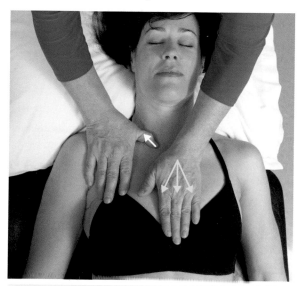

Figure 12.9
MMS right SC joint in relation to manubrium

Fascial twists and their impact on the vascular and neural systems (thoracic inlet)

In the upper quadrant, the jugular vein drains into the subclavius vein and the brachiocephalic veins merge to become the superior vena cava behind the second thoracic ring. Flow of venous drainage may therefore be disturbed secondary to cranial dysfunction, to tension in the pectoralis minor, the serratus anterior muscles, the clavicles and the upper rings (ring 1 to ring 4), and in fascial twists in relation to these areas.

In addition to the vascular system, the neural system may also be impacted by such fascial twists. The nerves that are particularly affected in the region of the thoracic inlet are the phrenic nerve, the vagus nerve and the sympathetic trunks. Phrenic nerve irritation may lead to overactivation of the diaphragm and therefore affect its function. The vagus nerve has many functions, in particular its role in the parasympathetic control of the heart (improving heart rate variability), the bronchi and the gastrointestinal tract. Fascial twists may therefore have wide impact on these systems (Lee 2018).

The following techniques can be used if there is a fascial hold between the sternoclavicular joint and the upper thoracic rings.

MMS right sternoclavicular joint in relation to ipsilateral ring (Figure 12.10)

Stabilizing hand As per the technique above.

Mobilizing hand As per the technique above except that the therapist explores the ipsilateral thoracic ring, looking for an immediate increase in tension of the stabilizing hand as the ring is mobilized. For example, if the second thoracic ring is shifted right and rotated left, the second ring on the right will seem to be positioned anteriorly in relation to the ring above and/or below it. In this case, if fascia between the right SC joint and the second ring is an issue, the therapist will feel an immediate increase in tension of the hand anchoring the right SC joint as the therapist attempts to move the

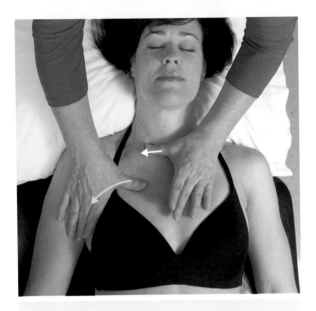

Figure 12.10
MMS right SC joint in relation to ipsilateral ring

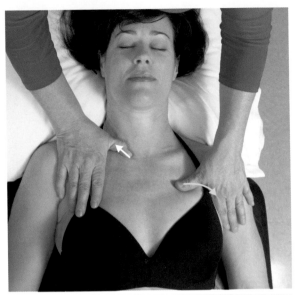

Figure 12.11
MMS right SC joint in relation to contralateral ring

right second ring posteriorly and to the right around the thorax, so as to de-rotate the ring. The concepts for release are similar to the technique above.

MMS right sternoclavicular joint in relation to contralateral ring (Figure 12.11)

A similar approach to the technique used above is used here except that the therapist explores the contralateral ring. In this case, the correction would be to move the ring posteriorly and to the left around the thorax and evaluate the impact of this maneuver on the right SC joint.

MMS clavicular fascia

A number of muscles attach to the clavicle. These include the upper fibers of trapezius (UFT), the sternocleidomastoid (SCM), deltoid, pectoralis major, subclavius, and sterno-hyoid muscles. These muscles can impact the mobility of the clavicle and therefore affect its biomechanics. The clavicle is also the hub for a number of fascial connections

(Figure 12.12). The clavipectoral fascia is a thick, bilateral connective tissue structure deep to pectoralis major muscle. It extends superiorly from the clavicle, medially from the costochondral joints, and superolaterally from the coracoid process.

It converges in the axilla, where it acts as a protective structure over the neurovascular structures of the axilla. The sheath reunites at the inferior border of subclavius muscle and forms a well-defined thickening called the costocoracoid ligament, spanning the distance between the coracoid process and the first costochondral joint. The fascia continues loosely downward until it divides again at the superior border of pectoralis minor and encloses the muscle. The fascia thickens to become the suspensory ligament of the axilla. Here, the suspensory ligament of the axilla is attached to the axillary fascia that forms floor of the axilla. There is an opening through which two structures enter and leave the deep compartment of the pectoral girdle:

1. The cephalic vein enters from the arm to join the axillary vein.

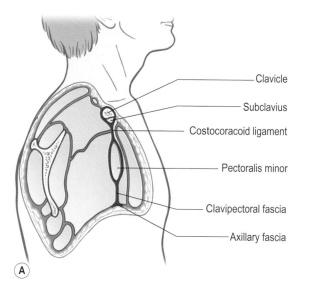

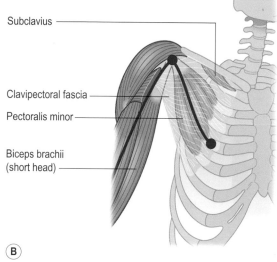

Figure 12.12
The clavipectoral fascia in relation to the Deep Front Arm Line. Reproduced from Tom Myers, *Anatomy Trains: Myofascial Meridians for Manual and Movement Therapists*, 3rd edition. With kind permission from Elsevier

2. The lymphatic vessels from the infraclavicular nodes pass through the hiatus to join the apical nodes of the axilla (KenHub 2017; Volker, 2017).

Fascial twists in the area of the clavipectoral fascia may then impact the function of the vascular and lymphatic systems.

The supraclavicular space (superior to the clavicle) contains the supraclavicular nerves and the external jugular vein. It also has connections to the deep cervical fascia.

A number of MMS techniques related to clavicular fascia have been developed. Indications for these techniques include:

- persistent pain/tension in the shoulder girdle and shoulder

- persistent pain/tension in the cervical spine

- persistent pain/tension in the thorax

- post fracture of the clavicle to encourage optimal alignment.

MMS right clavicle + glenohumeral traction (Figures 12.13, 12.14)

Stabilizing hand The patient is in supine position. The therapist uses their right hand with a gentle lumbrical grip to anchor onto the posterior-lateral edge of the clavicle, guiding and anchoring it into anterior rotation.

Mobilizing hand The therapist uses their left hand to encompass the anterior and posterior aspects of the right GH head, gently adding a traction maneuver to the joint in a lateral and inferior direction (through the axis of the humeral head). As always, the therapist is looking for the immediate line of tension between the two hands, which indicates fascial tension. The patient perceives this tension

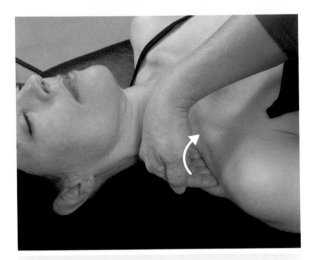

Figure 12.13
MMS position on anterior clavicle

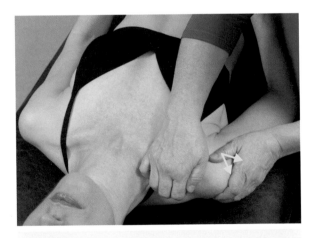

Figure 12.14
MMS right clavicle + G/H traction

MMS clavicle + deltoid (Figure 12.15)

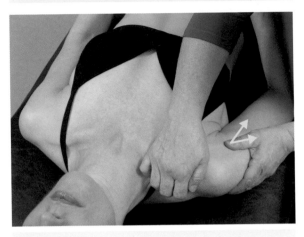

Figure 12.15
MMS clavicle + deltoid

Stabilizing hand As per the technique above.

Mobilizing hand As per the technique above, except that the therapist explores the deltoid muscle, gliding the anterior portion of the deltoid caudally and laterally. The anterior deltoid is explored proximally to distally, toward the deltoid insertion, an area that is fascially rich.

MMS clavicle + pectoralis major (Figure 12.16)

Stabilizing hand As per the technique above. Keep in mind that the anchor may also be explored with a star concept, depending on the direction of the mobilizing hand. In this case, because the fascial tissues of the pectoralis major will be explored in a medial direction, the stabilizing hand should incorporate a lateral glide component.

Mobilizing hand As per the technique above, except that the therapist explores the pectoralis major muscle, gliding the tissues in a medial/caudal direction, away from the clavicle and as always, using the star concept to seek out the fascial line with most tension.

as the therapist pulling harder on the right clavicle when, in reality, the therapist is simply preventing the clavicle from moving as he/she performs a traction to the GH joint. If no tension is perceived, then this part of the fascia is not tight. If tension is perceived (quick resistance is felt between the two hands of the therapist), then it can be mobilized as per the approaches outlined in Chapter 4. This technique may be used with any accessory movement of the GH joint.

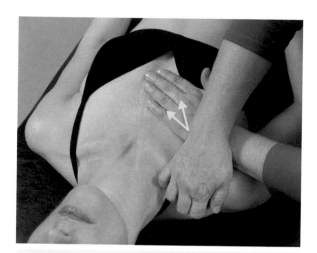

Figure 12.16
MMS clavicle + pectoralis major

MMS clavicle + ipsilateral sternoclavicular joint (Figure 12.17)

Stabilizing hand As per the technique above.

Mobilizing hand As per the technique above, except that the therapist explores the ipsilateral SC joint, gliding it medially, away from the hand that is anchoring the lateral aspect of the clavicle. This particular technique, in addition to mobilizing the subclavius fascia, is also useful to treat the fascia of the clavicle bone itself. If we consider bone to be very dense fascia, it too can be mobilized to stimulate optimal alignment, especially post fracture, once the bone has healed (see Case report 12.1, Michael's story).

MMS clavicle + A/P cervical spine (Figure 12.18)

Stabilizing hand As per the technique above.

Mobilizing hand As per the technique above, except that the therapist explores the tissues superior to the clavicle; in this case, the anterior aspect of the cervical spine, which includes the scalene muscles as well as the uncovertebral joints. The therapist performs an A/P glide in a cranial direction and may explore several levels of the cervical spine in this manner. Clinically, the

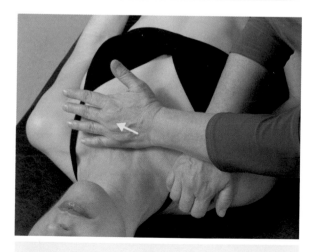

Figure 12.17
MMS clavicle + ipsilateral SC joint

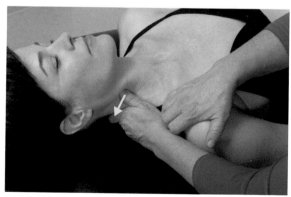

Figure 12.18
MMS clavicle + A/P Cx

mid-cervical spine, especially C4, is often implicated with this technique. If no tension is perceived, then this part of the fascia is not tight. If tension is perceived (quick resistance is felt between the two hands of the therapist), then it can be mobilized as per the approaches outlined in Chapter 4.

MMS clavicle + A/P C1 (Figure 12.19)

Stabilizing hand As per the technique above.

Mobilizing hand As per the technique above; Figure 12.19 demonstrates the technique of an A/P at C1. If the craniovertebral region is chronically tight despite mobilizations and/or manipulation of the upper cervical joints, it is worth exploring the fascia that attaches to the levels involved – in this case, the anterior aspect of C1.

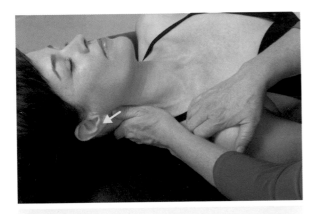

Figure 12.19
MMS clavicle + A/P C1

MMS clavicle + A/P mastoid process (Figure 12.20)

Stabilizing hand As per the technique above.

Mobilizing hand As per the technique above, except that the therapist explores the mastoid process of the temporal bone with an A/P glide. A number of muscles attach to the mastoid process, such as the sternocleidomastoid (SCM), the posterior belly of the digastric muscle and the splenius capitis. The SCM and its fascia are of particular interest for

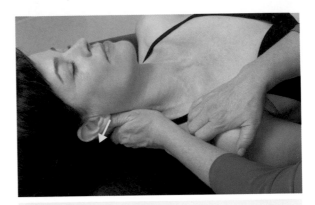

Figure 12.20
MMS clavicle + A/P mastoid process

recurring cranial dysfunctions, as tension from the SCM and its fascia may contribute to posterior rotation and/or internal rotation of the temporal bone.

MMS clavicle + flexion occiput (Figure 12.21)

Stabilizing hand As per the technique above.

Mobilizing hand As per the technique above except that the therapist explores the occiput, pulling it into flexion. Recurring tension in the craniovertebral (Cr/V) region, especially a tendency toward a limitation in Cr/V flexion, is an indication for exploring this fascial technique.

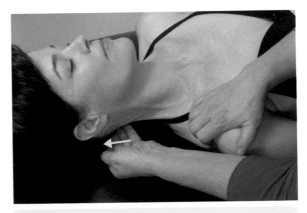

Figure 12.21
MMS clavicle + flexion occiput

MMS right clavicle + glenohumeral abduction (Figure 12.22)

Note that in this example GH abduction is demonstrated but all passive movements of the GH joint may be explored with this technique.

Stabilizing hand As per the technique above.

Mobilizing hand The therapist's left hand supports the patient's upper arm and performs a passive physiological movement of the GH joint into abduction, stopping as soon as an increase in tension is perceived in the hand palpating the clavicle (to the first resistance or R1 of Maitland's movement diagram). If there is tension in this line of fascia, it will seem like the tension on the clavicle increases before full GH abduction can be achieved (usually around 90–100 degrees of abduction). The therapist maintains the anchor on the lateral clavicle as he/she performs repeated passive physiological abduction of the shoulder, always to when R1 is perceived (a grade III– passive physiological movement in Maitland terms). This is repeated until a release is felt between the therapist's two hands and generally requires approximately five to eight cycles.

MMS right clavicle + glenohumeral lock (Figure 12.23)

Stabilizing hand As per the technique above.

Mobilizing hand As per the technique above, except that the therapist explores the GH lock position (Maitland technique to mobilize the periarticular tissues in combined abduction, horizontal extension, and slight internal rotation).

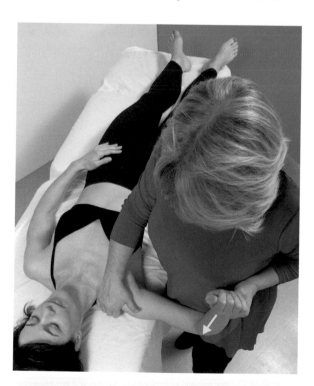

Figure 12.22
MMS right clavicle + GH abduction

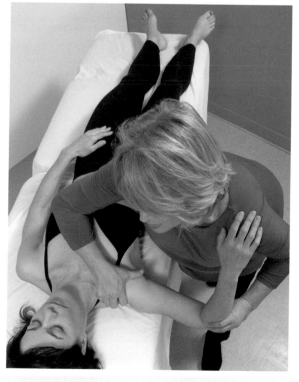

Figure 12.23
MMS right clavicle + GH lock

MMS right clavicle + glenohumeral quadrant
(Figure 12.24)

Stabilizing hand As per the technique above.

Mobilizing hand As per the technique above, except that the therapist explores the GH quadrant position (Maitland technique to mobilize the periarticular tissues in combined flexion, abduction, and internal or external rotation).

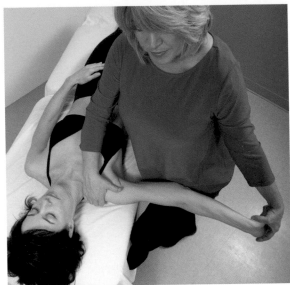

Figure 12.25
MMS right clavicle + ULNT1

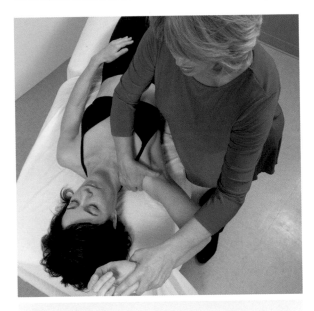

Figure 12.24
MMS right clavicle + GH quadrant

MMS right clavicle + upper limb neural tension test 1 (ULNT1) (Figure 12.25)

Stabilizing hand As per the technique above.

Mobilizing hand As per the technique above, except that the therapist performs the test for mobility of the neural tissues of the upper quadrant (ULNT1). Other neural mobility tests may also be explored with this technique. For this technique, the therapist must compare the ULNT1 test on its own and re-evaluate it with the anchor at the clavicle. Traditionally, the typical interfaces for this nerve are in the area of the mid-cervical spine or the flexor retinaculum at the wrist. Because the clavicle is intimately related to the clavipectoral fascia and the supraclavicular fascia, it too must be considered when exploring interfaces that may impact the mobility of the neural tissues in the upper quadrant. In this test, the therapist will use the component of the test that adds an immediate increase in tension at the hand anchoring the clavicle. Once that component is released (similar concepts of using passive physiological movement as per technique above), then the next component of the ULNT1 may be explored and treated until the patient has equal mobility of the test with or without the anchor at the clavicle.

Case report 12.1 Michael's story

This case hits close to home as it involves my son Michael, who is presently 25 years old. When he was 14 years old, he fell skateboarding and sustained a severe fracture of his left clavicle – it had fractured into three pieces, with the middle portion angled vertically. He was initially placed in a sling and told to go home – the assumption was that the bone would heal on its own. Lyn Watson, a shoulder specialist in Melbourne, Australia, whom I consulted, stated that, in Australia, they would operate on such a case. Needless to say, I made sure to go with Michael to his follow-up appointment. I had a number of concerns about the long-term function of his shoulder girdle, including the possibility that it would heal in a shortened position and forever impact his upper quadrant function. Unfortunately, I could not convince the chief orthopedic doctor to perform surgery. He assured me that healing was coming along and I should just allow nature to take its course. Knowing that bone was essentially dense fascia, I proceeded to remodel the clavicular fascia, initially with a listening approach and later, as healing progressed, with a more directive, MMS mobilization approach. The clavicle fascia was tight in a number of directions (see techniques above), particularly in relation to the SFL (clavicle in relation to the pectoral muscles and rectus abdominis) and the anterior functional line of fascia (left clavicle with right ilium). The intraclavicular fascia also was remodeled to encourage healing in the most lengthened position possible. This work was followed up with a strengthening program to his scapular upward rotators. Initial treatment was performed weekly, and then periodically over the next year, as bone (and fascia) remodeling took place. Throughout his growth spurt, Michael could feel the need for more fascial release and periodically through the years, as his system adjusted to a new gym program. Today, he is fully functional and grateful that his mother is a physiotherapist with skills in MMS!

Summary

The techniques in this chapter have focused on myofascial connections in relation to the shoulder girdle, including those in relation to the sternoclavicular joint as well as the clavicle itself. These tissues are frequently problematic in cases of persistent shoulder girdle, cervical, thoracic, or head pain, depending on the vectors that may be impacting this area. The following chapter will focus on techniques for the upper extremity.

The upper extremity

When treating patients with problems of the upper extremity, manual therapists are trained to assess and treat the joints (the glenohumeral, humeroulnar, superior and inferior radioulnar joints, and the wrist, finger, and thumb joints). In addition, the muscles of the upper quadrant are assessed and treated for imbalance between hypertonic, tight muscles and weak muscles. The mobility of the nerves of the upper quadrant is also assessed and treated. However, mobilizing joints and nerves, and stretching and strengthening individual muscles can achieve only partial benefits if the fascial system is not taken into consideration.

This chapter will describe the clinical findings of restriction in the following fascial dysfunctions:

- deltoid fascia
- supraspinatus fascia in relation to the SFL and the DFL
- fascia of the long head of biceps
- brachialis fascia
- forearm fascia
- flexor retinaculum fascia
- fascia in relation to Dupuytren's contracture
- fascia in relation to de Quervain's tenosynovitis
- fascia in relation to the distal radius (post-Colles' fracture)

Indications for MMS for this chapter

- Recurring upper extremity pain despite the following treatment approaches:
  - mobilization/manipulation of the joints of the shoulder, elbow, forearm, wrist, and hand
  - release of trigger points to the upper extremity muscles with manual or dry needling techniques
  - stabilization and strengthening exercises for the upper quadrant.

Superficial Front Arm Line (SFAL)

The Superficial Front Arm Line (SFAL) involves the following structures: pectoralis major, latissimus dorsi, medial intermuscular septum, flexor group of muscles, carpal tunnel. (Please refer to Chapter 2 for a full description and illustration of this line of fascia.)

Clinical implications

- This line extends above and beyond the territory of the median nerve distribution. In treating problems of mobility for the *median nerve*, we may consider looking at interfaces that include the pectoral muscles and latissimus dorsi in addition to the flexor retinaculum and the anterior cervical spine. (See MMS flexor retinaculum with shoulder abduction.)

- The rotator cuff muscles are considered part of the DBAL, but the *insertion of supraspinatus* anteriorly may clinically be considered as part of the SFAL. It is also often affected by tension in the SFL and the DFL of the trunk. This tension can contribute to an anterior position of the humeral head in relation to the acromion and to forward head posture in general. (See Supraspinatus in relation to the contralateral shoulder (SFL) and to the pericardium and diaphragm (DFL).)

- *Dupuytren's contracture* does not simply involve the finger flexor tendons in the hand. There are also strong fascial connections to the SFAL that may contribute to this dysfunction. (See MMS Dupuytren's in relation to the long head of biceps (SFAL) and MMS Dupuytren's in relation to the contralateral shoulder (SFAL with the trunk SFL.)

Deep Front Arm Line (DFAL)

The Deep Front Arm Line (DFAL) involves the following structures: pectoralis minor, the clavipectoral fascia, biceps, radial periosteum and thenar muscles. (Refer to Chapter 2 for a full description and illustration of this line of fascia.)

Clinical implications

- Adding wrist extension and ulnar deviation can help release the fascial line associated with tightness of *pectoralis minor*, a muscle that commonly contributes to an anterior tilt of the scapula and therefore may affect shoulder girdle function. Tightness of this fascial line may also maintain a forward head posture. (See MMS pectoralis minor in relation to the DFAL.)

- Releasing the *fascia around the clavicle* can have a positive effect on improving shoulder mobility and promoting an axially extended posture. (Refer to Chapter 12 for clavicle fascia techniques.)

- If periosteum is to be considered "dense fascia," then (after the appropriate healing time has occurred), the site of a *clavicular fracture* may benefit from fascial release of the clavipectoral fascia (see Chapter 12 for MMS technique) in order to minimize the effects of shortening of the clavicle on the upper quadrant.

- The attachment of the *long head of biceps* is commonly affected by tension in the SFL and the DFL of the trunk. This tension can pull the humeral head anteriorly in relation to the acromion and contribute to a forward head posture. (See MMS long head of biceps with contralateral rectus abdominis (SFL).) Tension of the DFAL may also contribute to a flexed position of the elbow in a standing posture, as the body attempts to offload the glenohumeral head. Adding wrist flexion to a stretch of the biceps (elbow extension, pronation) also converts this into a fascial technique. (See MMS long head of biceps with elbow extension/pronation/wrist flexion.)

- Treatment of *De Quervain's tenosynovitis* may extend beyond the use of transverse frictions of the retinaculum with the thumb in the Finkelstein position (thumb adduction, with wrist ulnar deviation) if we consider this fascial line to include the biceps, clavipectoral fascia and pectoralis minor. (See MMS Finkelstein's in relation to the shoulder (DFAL.)

Superficial Back Arm Line (SBAL)

The Superficial Back Arm Line (SBAL) involves the following structures: trapezius muscles (upper, middle, and lower), deltoid, brachialis, lateral intermuscular septum, extensor muscles of wrist and fingers. (Refer to Chapter 2 for a full description and illustration of this line of fascia.)

Clinical implications

- This line extends above and beyond the territory of the radial nerve distribution. In treating problems of mobility for the *radial nerve*, we may consider looking at interfaces that include the trapezii, deltoid, and the cervicothoracic region in addition to the area of the radial head and the anterior cervical spine. (See MMS P/A radial head with elbow extension/pronation/wrist flexion for an example.)

- The deltoid, brachialis, and wrist extensor muscle group all have a fascial connection through the SBAL. Deltoid fascia should be considered when looking for non-articular restrictions of the shoulder. (See MMS anterior deltoid with glenohumeral internal rotation and MMS posterior deltoid with glenohumeral external rotation.)

- Persistent pain and tension in the lateral elbow region may be due to tension in relation to the SBAL of fascia. Releasing this fascia is frequently helpful with recalcitrant problems of *lateral epicondylosis*. (See MMS lateral brachialis with elbow extension/pronation.)

- If periosteum is to be considered "dense fascia," then (after the appropriate healing time has occurred) the site of a *Colles' fracture* may benefit from fascial release of the distal radius in relation to the SBAL in order to optimize wrist mobility. (See MMS Colles' fracture fascia in relation to the SBAL.)

Deep Back Arm Line (DBAL)

The Deep Back Arm Line (DBAL) involves the following structures: rectus capitis lateralis, rhomboids, levator scapula, rotator cuff muscles, triceps, ulnar periosteum, hypothenar muscles. (Refer to Chapter 2 for a full description and illustration of this line of fascia.)

Clinical implications

- This line extends above and beyond the territory of the *ulnar nerve* distribution. In treating problems of mobility for the ulnar nerve, we may consider looking at interfaces that include the rotator cuff and the levator scapula in addition to the area of the tunnel of Guyon at the wrist and the anterior cervical spine.

Postural analysis for the upper quadrant

- Position of the humeral head in relation to the acromion.
- Position of the scapulae in relation to the thorax.
- Position of the clavicles.

Please refer to Chapter 12 for details of postural analysis as it pertains to the upper extremity.

Load and listen test for the shoulder

The load and listen test is useful for detecting myofascial vectors that may have an impact on the position and therefore the function of a joint. The test is described in detail for the hip joint in Chapter 11, but a similar approach can be used in relation to the glenohumeral (GH) joint.

If the patient presents with an anteriorly positioned GH head in relation to the acromion, the therapist may perform an A/P glide of the GH joint in a supine or seated position. If the restriction is articular, the end feel of the posterior glide (for example) will be hard and fibrotic. However, if there is a myofascial restriction, the therapist will feel the resistance to the accessory movement with an end feel that is softer. A certain resistance will be felt with this correction but valuable information will be gleaned if the therapist pays attention to the release component of the test, listening (passively) for vectors that are "tugging" on the GH joint. Vectors may be long or short, pull in a cranial, caudal, or medial direction, and may feel either superficial or deep.

There may be a combination of neuromuscular vectors (increased tone in muscles due to increased neural drive), visceral vectors, muscular, and fascial vectors. The therapist pays attention to where the first pull is felt and then tries to determine the direction of pull. Once this first vector is released, then the therapist seeks a second vector on a repeat load and listen test, and so on until no further tension is felt on the release

component of the load and listen test. At this point, positional tests for the GH joint should also be negative. The possibilities for vectors are varied but the most frequent are outlined below:

- A pull of the humeral head inferiorly and anteriorly implies the involvement of the long head of biceps.
- A pull of the humeral head in the supero-antero-medial direction may imply the involvement of the coracobrachialis, subclavius, or clavicle.
- A pull of the humeral head in the anteromedial direction may imply the involvement of the pectoralis major muscle and/or the fascia of the SFL of the trunk. If the vector feels deep it may also involve visceral fascia, such as that of the lungs and pericardium.

All of these neuromuscular vectors may be treated with a number of techniques designed to release muscle hypertonicity, such as contract–relax, strain/counterstrain, release with awareness, dry needling, etc. However, if results of these approaches are difficult to maintain, the therapist should then explore the fascial line(s) related to the muscles involved.

Concepts of treatment using MMS

For this chapter, we will be using primarily the first concept of treatment when using MMS techniques; that is, choose a recurrent articular dysfunction or myofascial trigger point and explore a fascial line in relation to it. The therapist anchors him/herself to a recurrent articular dysfunction or myofascial trigger point and assesses the fascial lines of tension in relation to the anchor, looking for early tension between the two hands.

The following approaches may be used, depending on how the tissues respond:

- work with oscillations (grades III−, III, III+)
- work with sustained pressure
- work with "harmonics" (Dr Laurie Hartman).

Please refer to Chapter 4 for detail on concepts of treatment using MMS.

MMS pectoralis minor fascia

> MMS right pectoralis minor in relation to the DFAL (Figure 13.1)

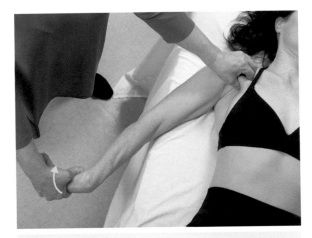

Figure 13.1
MMS pectoralis minor in relation to the DFAL

The pectoralis minor muscle is frequently hypertonic and facilitated. Dry needling may help restore a more normal tone to this muscle; however, tight fascia around this muscle may contribute to its tendency to be recalcitrant. The pectoralis minor is part of Tom Myers's Deep Front Arm Line (DFAL), and as such, may be put under tension with the addition of wrist ulnar deviation, with wrist and finger flexion.

The patient is in supine position. The therapist uses their left hand to "pinch" the pectoralis minor between the thumb and fingers, especially in the area of recurring trigger points. The muscle may be explored along its length for tension.

Mobilizing hand With the patient's arm in pronation with the elbow extended, the therapist performs ulnar deviation of the wrist and flexes the patient's wrist and fingers, stopping as soon as an increase in tension is perceived in the hand that is anchoring the pectoralis minor. If there is tension in this line of fascia, it will seem like the tension in the pectoralis minor increases before full wrist and finger flexion can be achieved. The therapist main-

tains the pinch of the pectoralis minor and simply prevents the tissues from gliding laterally and caudally. The patient perceives this as the therapist increasing his/her pressure on the muscle. The therapist performs repeated movement of the wrist into flexion and ulnar deviation while maintaining a steady pressure on the pectoralis minor, always to the point when R1 is perceived. This action is repeated until a release is felt between the therapist's two hands and generally requires approximately five to eight cycles.

MMS deltoid fascia

> MMS right anterior deltoid with glenohumeral internal rotation (Figure 13.2)

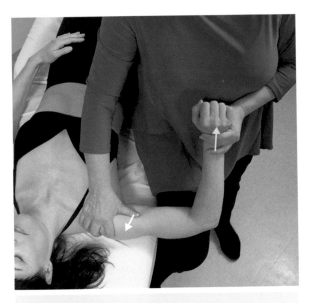

Figure 13.2
MMS right anterior deltoid with GH IR

The fascia of the anterior deltoid may be a limiting factor to gaining range of shoulder internal rotation.

Stabilizing hand The patient is in supine position. The therapist uses their right hand to anchor the anterior deltoid into external rotation. The muscle may be explored along its length, towards the deltoid insertion (an area rich in fascia).

Mobilizing hand The therapist's left hand supports the patient's wrist and forearm and performs a passive physiological movement of the glenohumeral joint into internal rotation (IR), stopping as soon as an increase in tension is perceived in the hand palpating the anterior deltoid (to the first resistance, or R1 of Maitland's movement diagram). If there is tension in this line of fascia, it will seem as though the tissues of the anterior deltoid will push into the therapist's thumb before full glenohumeral internal rotation can be achieved (usually around 70 degrees of IR). The patient perceives this as the therapist increasing his/her pressure on the anterior deltoid. The therapist performs repeated passive physiological IR of the shoulder while maintaining a steady pressure on the anterior deltoid, always to when R1 is perceived (a grade III– passive physiological movement in Maitland terms). This technique is repeated until a release is felt between the therapist's two hands and generally requires approximately five to eight cycles.

The fascia of the posterior deltoid may be a limiting factor to gaining range of shoulder external rotation. This technique may be useful to regain this ROM.

Stabilizing hand The patient is in supine position. The therapist uses their left hand to anchor the posterior deltoid into internal rotation. The muscle may be explored along its length, toward the deltoid insertion.

Mobilizing hand The therapist's left hand supports the patient's wrist and forearm and performs a passive physiological movement of the glenohumeral joint into external rotation (ER), stopping as soon as an increase in tension is perceived in the hand palpating the posterior deltoid (to the first resistance, or R1 of Maitland's movement diagram). The approach to treatment is the same as for the technique above.

MMS Supraspinatus fascia in relation to the SFL and the DFL

MMS right posterior deltoid with glenohumeral external rotation (Figure 13.3)

MMS right supraspinatus in relation to the contralateral shoulder (SFL) (Figure 13.4)

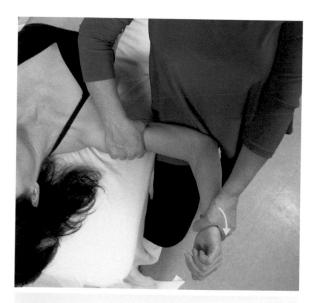

Figure 13.3
MMS right posterior deltoid with GH ER

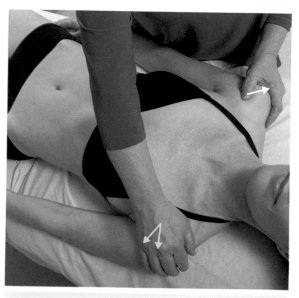

Figure 13.4
MMS right supraspinatus in relation to the contralateral shoulder (SFL)

Stabilizing hand The patient is in supine position. Using a craniolateral hold, the therapist uses their left hand to anchor the insertion of the supraspinatus at the greater tubercle of the humerus on the right side.

Mobilizing hand With the star concept in mind, the therapist's right hand explores the left shoulder and shoulder girdle area with an anteroposterior caudal glide of the tissues in the area of the lateral clavicle and/or the glenohumeral joint, always looking for the immediate line of tension in relation to the hand that is anchoring the supraspinatus. If this fascial line is tight, the therapist will feel an increase in tension in the anchoring hand, as if the tissues of the supraspinatus were being pulled medially towards the center of the body. The patient perceives this action as the therapist increasing his/her pressure on supraspinatus. If tension is perceived (quick resistance is felt between the two hands of the therapist), then it can be mobilized as per the approaches outlined in Chapter 4.

MMS right supraspinatus in relation to the pericardium (DFL) (Figure 13.5)

Stabilizing hand As per the technique above.

Mobilizing hand The therapist explores the area of the pericardium, first by slowly sinking into the tissues posterior to the sternum and then gently pushing in a caudal direction, all the while maintaining the depth of the fascial line posterior to the sternum. The therapist looks for the angle where he/she perceives immediate tension in the hand anchoring the supraspinatus. That tension may be felt most in the pericardial area in a simple caudal direction, or caudal to the left of the client. Sometimes the tension is most felt when moving the pericardial tissues mediolaterally or in a clockwise/counterclockwise direction, always maintaining the depth of the tissue. If no tension is perceived, then the DFL of fascia in relation to this muscle is not tight. If tension is perceived (quick resistance is felt between the two hands of the therapist), then it can be mobilized as per the approaches outlined in Chapter 4.

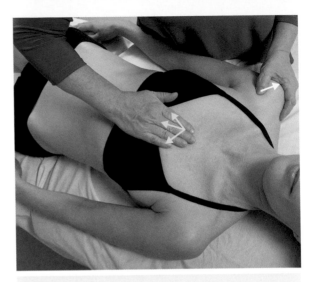

Figure 13.5
MMS right supraspinatus in relation to the pericardium (DFL)

MMS right supraspinatus in relation to the contralateral diaphragm (DFL) (Figure 13.6)

Stabilizing hand As per the technique above.

Mobilizing hand The caudal hand explores the anterior diaphragm on the patient's left side with a caudal/lateral glide of the tissues, always looking for the immediate line of tension between the two hands. Appropriate depth of tissues is required. The fascia around the rectus abdominis and oblique abdominal muscles may be accessed with this technique if the technique is done superficially (this would be a technique for the SFL). However, in order to access the diaphragm, which is part of the DFL, the therapist must first slowly sink into the tissues posterior to the lower ribs and then gently push in a caudal/lateral direction. This technique can be done with either the ipsilateral or the contralateral diaphragm.

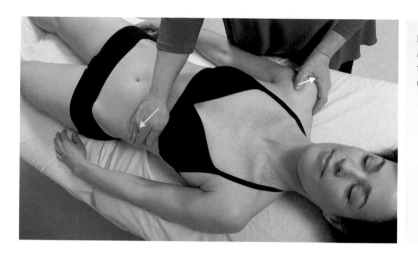

Figure 13.6
MMS right supraspinatus in relation to the contralateral diaphragm (DFL)

MMS right supraspinatus in relation to the contralateral iliacus (DFL) (Figure 13.7)

MMS right long head of biceps with elbow extension/pronation/wrist flexion (DFAL) (Figure 13.8)

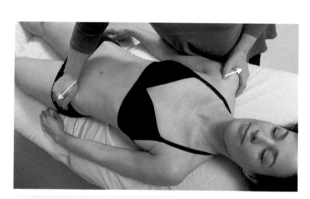

Figure 13.7
MMS right supraspinatus in relation to the contralateral iliacus (DFL)

Stabilizing hand As per the technique above.

Mobilizing hand The caudal hand explores the contralateral iliacus, either similar to the iliacus position outlined in Chapter 8 or using the ilium to explore posterior and anterior rotations, using a star concept. This technique may also be performed for the ipsilateral iliacus.

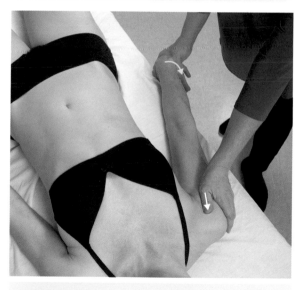

Figure 13.8
MMS right long head of biceps with elbow extension/pronation/wrist flexion (DFAL)

The long head of biceps (LHB), because of its attachment to the superior portion of the glenoid labrum and the anterosuperior capsule of the glenohumeral joint, may cause the humeral head to displace anteriorly in relation to the acromion. The fascia of the long head of biceps should be explored, both in relation to the elbow and in relation to the SFL of the trunk.

Stabilizing hand The patient is in supine position. Using a craniolateral hold, the therapist uses their left hand to anchor the long head of biceps (LHB) in the bicipetal groove. An area of approximately 5 cm may be explored in this way.

Mobilizing hand The right hand of the therapist performs passive physiological elbow extension, with the forearm pronated and the wrist flexed, stopping as soon as an increase in tension is perceived in the hand palpating the LHB (to the first resistance or R1 of Maitland's movement diagram). If there is tension in this line of fascia, it will seem as though the tissues of the LHB will push into the therapist's thumb before full elbow extension in pronation can be achieved. The patient perceives this as the therapist increasing his/her pressure on the LHB. The therapist performs repeated passive physiological extension of the elbow with the forearm pronated and the wrist flexed while maintaining a steady pressure on the LHB, always to when R1 is perceived (a grade III– passive physiological movement in Maitland terms). This action is repeated until a release is felt between the therapist's two hands; this generally requires approximately five to eight cycles.

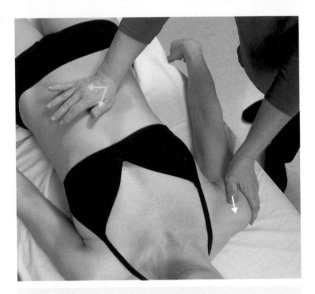

Figure 13.9
MMS right long head of biceps with RA (DFAL with SFL of trunk)

pressure on the LHB. If tension is perceived (quick resistance is felt between the two hands of the therapist), then it can be mobilized as per the approaches outlined in Chapter 4.

MMS right lateral brachialis with elbow extension/ pronation (SBAL) (Figure 13.10)

Lateral elbow pain may have several sources, but one common source of tension is commonly found in the lateral brachialis area.

Stabilizing hand The patient is in supine position. Using a craniolateral hold, the therapist uses their left hand to anchor the lateral brachialis muscle, located posterior to the biceps. An area of approximately 4 cm may be explored in this way.

Mobilizing hand Same as per the MMS for the long head of biceps with elbow extension/pronation/wrist flexion. The technique may be explored by starting with the forearm supinated, then progressed to neutral, and then finally to full pronation.

MMS right long head of biceps with rectus abdominis (DFAL with SFL of trunk) (Figure 13.9)

Stabilizing hand As per the technique above.

Mobilizing hand With the star concept in mind, the right hand of the therapist explores the rectus abdominis area (contralaterally and ipsilaterally all the way down to the symphysis pubis) with an anteroposterior caudal glide of the tissues, always looking for the immediate line of tension in relation to the hand that is anchoring the LHB. If this fascial line is tight, the therapist will feel an increase in tension in the anchoring hand, as if the tissues of the LHB were being pulled caudally and medially towards the center of the body. The patient perceives this as the therapist increasing his/her

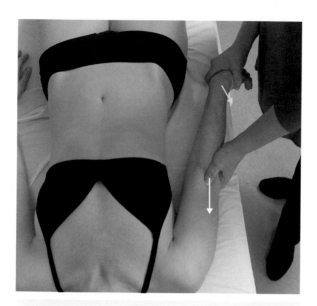

Figure 13.10
MMS right lateral brachialis with elbow extension/
pronation (SBAL)

MMS P/A right radial head with elbow extension/
pronation/wrist flexion (Figure 13.11)

Another source of lateral elbow pain is tension of the fascia around the head of the radius. It is also a common interface for problems with mobility of the radial nerve.

Stabilizing hand The patient is in supine position. A P/A pressure of the radial head is performed as the anchoring maneuver.

Mobilizing hand Same as per the MMS for the long head of biceps with elbow extension/pronation/wrist flexion.

The following MMS techniques may be used to explore tension and decreased range of motion in the forearm (pronation/supination) and the wrist and fingers (flexion/ extension, radial and ulnar deviation), particularly if a plateau in treatment has been reached with mobilization of the affected joints. The first three techniques will involve MMS techniques in relation to the anterior aspect of the wrist extensors (Figures 13.12 to 13.14). This will be

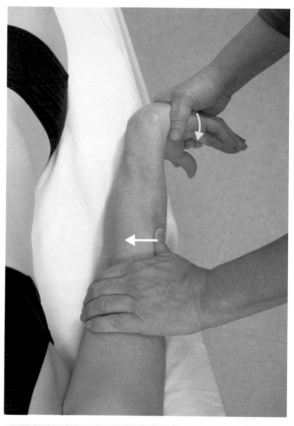

Figure 13.11
MMS P/A right radial head with elbow extension/
pronation/wrist flexion

followed by MMS techniques in relation to the posterior aspect of the wrist extensors (Figures 13.15 and 13.16).

MMS anterior aspect of right wrist extensors with
elbow extension/pronation/wrist flexion (SBAL)
(Figure 13.12)

Stabilizing hand The patient is in supine position. Using their left hand, the anterior portion of the wrist extensor muscle group is explored and anchored with a cranial/lateral glide.

Mobilizing hand Same as per the MMS for the long head of biceps with elbow extension/pronation/wrist flexion.

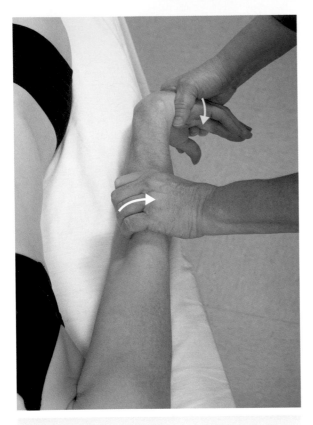

Figure 13.12
MMS anterior aspect of right wrist extensors with
elbow extension/pronation/wrist flexion (SBAL)

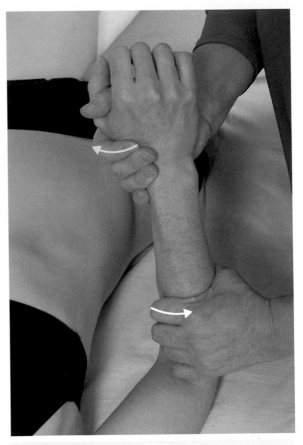

Figure 13.13
MMS anterior aspect of right wrist extensors with
pronation

MMS anterior aspect of right wrist extensors with pronation (Figure 13.13)

Stabilizing hand The patient is in supine position with the elbow flexed. The anterior portion of the wrist extensor muscle group is explored and anchored by the therapist's left hand, with a "glide" of the tissues into supination. An area of approximately 4 cm may be explored in this way.

Mobilizing hand The therapist's right hand grips the radial aspect of the patient's wrist and hand, with their thumb between the patient's thumb and index finger. The therapist performs passive physiological pronation of the forearm, stopping as soon as an increase in tension is perceived in the hand palpating the anterior aspect of the

wrist extensors (to the first resistance or R1 of Maitland's movement diagram). If there is tension in this line of fascia, it will seem as though the anterior portion of the wrist extensors will push into the therapist's fingers before full pronation can be achieved. The patient perceives this as the therapist increasing his/her pressure on the anterior aspect of the wrist extensors. The therapist performs repeated passive physiological forearm pronation while maintaining a steady pressure on the wrist extensor group, always to the point when R1 is perceived (a grade III– passive physiological movement in Maitland terms). This sequence is repeated until a release is felt between the therapist's two hands and generally requires approximately five to eight cycles.

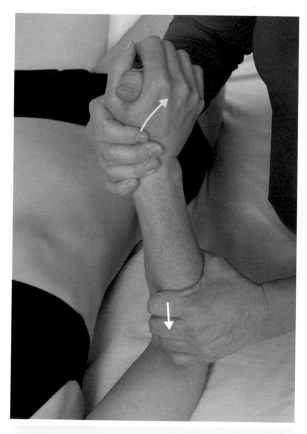

Figure 13.14
MMS anterior aspect of right wrist extensors with ulnar deviation

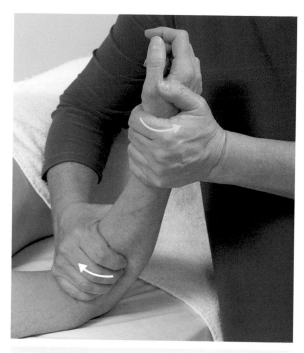

Figure 13.15
MMS posterior aspect of right wrist extensors with supination

MMS anterior aspect of right wrist extensors with ulnar deviation (Figure 13.14)

Stabilizing hand As per the MMS technique above, except that the therapist anchors the anterior aspect of the wrist extensors with a cranial glide of the tissues.

Mobilizing hand As per the MMS technique above, except that the therapist performs passive physiological wrist ulnar deviation.

MMS posterior aspect of right wrist extensors with supination (Figure 13.15)

Stabilizing hand As per the technique above except that the therapist explores the dorsal aspect of the wrist extensor muscle group with their right hand and anchors it with a "glide" of the tissues into pronation. An area of approximately 4 cm may be explored in this way.

Mobilizing hand As per the technique above except that the therapist uses their left hand to perform passive physiological forearm supination.

MMS posterior aspect of right wrist extensors with ulnar deviation (Figure 13.16)

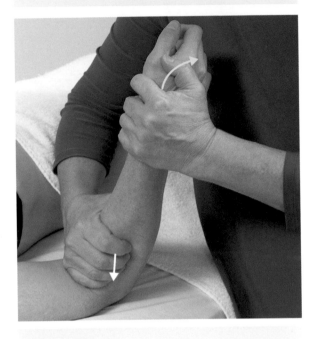

Figure 13.16
MMS posterior aspect of right wrist extensors with ulnar deviation

Stabilizing hand As per the MMS technique above, except that the therapist anchors the dorsal aspect of the wrist extensors with a cranial glide of the tissues.

Mobilizing hand As per the technique above, except that the therapist performs passive physiological wrist ulnar deviation.

MMS right interosseous membrane with ulnar deviation (Figure 13.17)

Stabilizing hand The therapist anchors the interosseous membrane between the radius and ulna on the dorsal aspect of the forearm, using a cranial anchor.

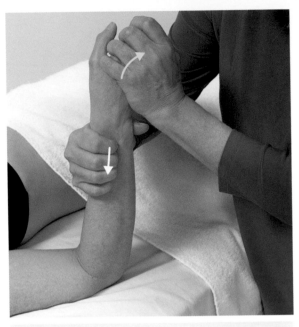

Figure 13.17
MMS interosseous membrane with ulnar deviation

Mobilizing hand As per the technique above.

Flexor retinaculum

The flexor retinaculum is a fascia that forms the roof of the carpal tunnel and is considered part of the SFAL of fascia. It originates from the distal radius and ulna and continues distally to attach to the scaphoid tubercle and trapezium laterally and the pisiform and hook of the hamate medially. It is a common interface for problems with mobility of the median and ulnar nerves as the tunnel tends to become narrow, with the hamate/pisiform and scaphoid/trapezium approaching each other to increase the arch of the wrist. It can be mobilized locally and in relation to the median and ulnar nerves by adding shoulder abduction, a maneuver that increases tension to both nerves.

MMS flexor retinaculum (SFAL), with and without shoulder abduction (Figure 13.18)

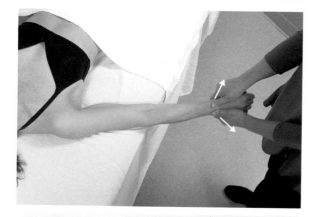

Figure 13.18
MMS right flexor retinaculum with shoulder abduction (SFAL)

MMS technique Using both thumbs, the therapist stabilizes the dorsal aspect of the distal radius and ulna. He/she then uses their third digits to explore the fascia in the area of the pisiform/hamate and scaphoid/trapezium, gently pulling the fingers apart. If there is sufficient mobility in the flexor retinaculum there should be some "give" in the tissues when trying to pull them gently apart. If there is tension, it may be felt in a straight medial/lateral direction or in a diagonal direction (e.g., between the pisiform/hamate and the radius).

The therapist may use either the mobilization approach with MMS, or a more sustained pressure until tension is perceived to lessen between the therapist's two hands. This technique may be progressed by adding passive wrist and finger flexion/extension while maintaining a stretch on the retinaculum. The flexor retinaculum technique may also be performed in positions that increase tension on the median and/or ulnar nerve (e.g., shoulder abduction).

Dupuytren's contracture

There are strong fascial connections between the finger flexors and the SFAL of fascia, as well as the fascia of the anterior trunk (SFL). Dupuytren's usually begins as small hard nodules just under the skin of the palm, most commonly affecting the 4th, the 5th and the 3rd digits. Treatment with fascial techniques can minimize signs and symptoms, especially if treated before contractures start to interfere with the function of the hand.

MMS anchor for Dupuytren's (Figure 13.19)

Stabilizing hand The therapist uses their thumb to anchor the nodular fascial tissue, exploring the tendon itself, as well as either side of the tendon. The direction of the anchor depends on where the mobilizing hand will explore. The anchor is in a distal/ulnar direction if the other hand explores the radial aspect of the hand. The

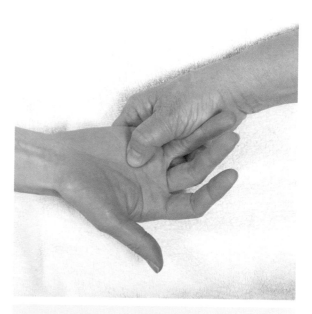

Figure 13.19
MMS anchor for Dupuytren's

anchor is in a distal direction (always with the star concept in mind) if the other hand explores more proximal areas in relation to the hand.

MMS right Dupuytren's in relation to hand fascia (SFAL) (Figure 13.20)

Mobilizing hand The therapist's left hand explores the fascia on the radial aspect of the hand, either distally or proximally in relation to the nodule. The therapist may also use passive physiological movement of flexion/extension of all of the fingers of the hand (not only the finger most involved). If this fascial line is tight, the therapist will feel an increase in tension in the anchoring hand, as if the tissues of the nodule were being pulled proximally and medially towards the center of the hand. The patient perceives this as the therapist increasing his/her pressure

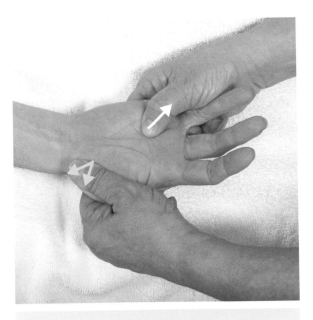

Figure 13.20
MMS right Dupuytren's in relation to hand fascia (SFAL)

on the affected digit. If tension is perceived (quick resistance is felt between the two hands of the therapist), then it can be mobilized as per the approaches outlined in Chapter 4.

MMS right Dupuytren's in relation to the long head of biceps (DFAL) (Figure 13.21)

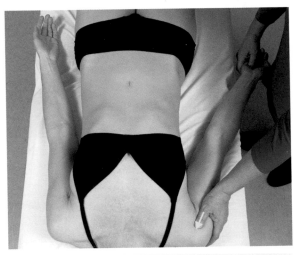

Figure 13.21
MMS right Dupuytren's in relation to the ipsilateral shoulder/LHB (DFAL)

Stabilizing hand As per the technique above.

Mobilizing hand The therapist's left hand explores the area of the ipsilateral glenohumeral joint and long head of biceps with an A/P glide directed cranially, but also with the star concept in mind. If this fascial line is tight, the therapist will feel an increase in tension in the anchoring hand, as if the tissues of the nodule were being pulled proximally. The patient perceives this action as the therapist increasing his/her pressure on the affected digit. Similar concepts for mobilizing this line of fascia apply as per previous techniques.

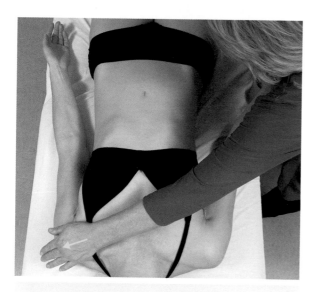

Figure 13.22
MMS right Dupuytren's in relation to the contralateral shoulder (SFAL with SFL of the trunk)

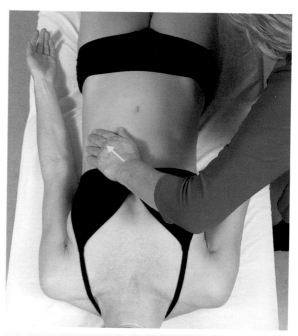

Figure 13.23
MMS right Dupuytren's in relation to the contralateral diaphragm (SFAL with DFL of the trunk)

MMS right Dupuytren's in relation to the contralateral shoulder (SFAL with SFL of the trunk) (Figure 13.22)

Stabilizing hand As per the technique above.

Mobilizing hand This technique explores the links between the SFAL and the SFL of the trunk. This time the therapist's left hand explores the area of the contralateral shoulder and scapula. A more laterally directed glide of the shoulder/scapula usually creates the most tension with this technique.

MMS right Dupuytren's in relation to the contralateral diaphragm (SFAL with DFL of the trunk) (Figure 13.23)

Stabilizing hand As per the technique above.

Mobilizing hand This technique explores the link between the SFAL and the DFL of the trunk, anterior fascia that is deeper than the SFL of the trunk. The therapist's left hand explores the area of the diaphragm or the iliacus, either ipsilaterally or contralaterally, using the same concepts as for the techniques above.

De Quervain's

De Quervain's tenosynovitis is a condition that may be difficult to treat unless the therapist considers factors besides overuse that may contribute to this pathology. For example, an abduction lesion of the elbow (secondary to a fall on the outstretched hand) can alter the biomechanics of the forearm and the wrist and therefore increase the load on the thumb muscles. (This condition is generally treated with a manipulation to restore optimal biomechanics.) Once the acute stage starts to settle, the therapist traditionally performs deep transverse frictions to the group of thumb tendons. This technique is usually performed in the Finkelstein position (thumb flexion and adduction with wrist ulnar deviation), which increases tension on the retinaculum surrounding the tendons. The therapist should also explore the fascia in relation to these tendons, usually in relation to the DFAL (Figure 13.24).

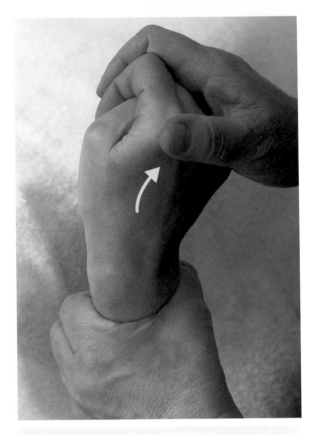

Figure 13.24
MMS positioning the right wrist in Finklestein's test

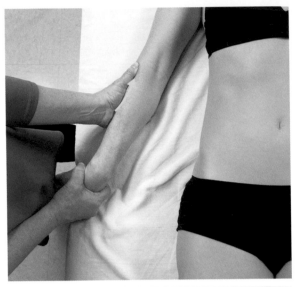

Figure 13.25
MMS Finklestein's in relation to DFAL

MMS Finklestein's in relation to the DFAL (Figures 13.25, 13.26)

Stabilizing hand The therapist holds the thumb and wrist in the Finkelstein position (see above). If there is pain associated with this test, the therapist should stop just short of the start of painful symptoms.

Mobilizing hand The therapist's left hand explores the fascia of the DFAL (radial periosteum, biceps, clavipectoral fascia, pectoralis minor), usually in a cranial direction, but always with the star concept in mind. If there is tension in this line of fascia, it will seem like the hand holding the wrist will want to go into radial deviation. The patient perceives this action as the therapist increasing his/her pressure on the wrist. The therapist performs repeated passive physiological cranial glides of the affected fascia while maintaining the wrist and thumb in Finkelstein's position. This sequence is repeated until a release is felt between the therapist's two hands and generally requires approximately five to eight cycles.

MMS techniques post Colles' fracture

If we consider bone as dense fascia, then we can understand how fascial techniques may be used to regain optimal range of motion and function of the wrist and forearm post-fracture. Of course, the therapist should wait until the bone has had sufficient healing time (minimum six weeks) before beginning these techniques. It is also wise to start gently, using listening techniques at first to see what the body can tolerate (see Chapter 4). With time, the approach can become firmer and more directive, if needed. The fact that the anchoring hand is stabilizing the site of fracture also helps to make these techniques safe.

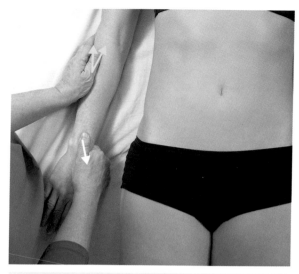

Figure 13.27
MMS right Colles' fracture fascia in relation to the forearm (SBAL)

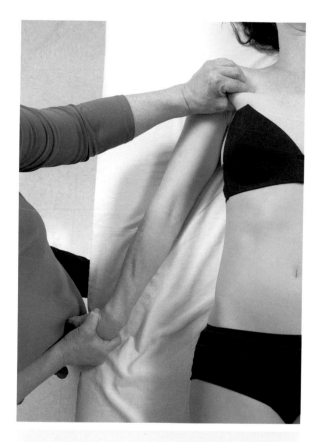

Figure 13.26
MMS Finklestein's in relation to the pectoralis minor (DFAL)

MMS right Colles' fracture fascia in relation to the SBAL (Figures 13.27, 13.28)

Stabilizing hand The therapist uses the thenar eminence of their right hand to stabilize the dorsal aspect of the distal radius (site of fracture) with a broad anchor. With time,

this technique may become more specific by anchoring the distal radius with a smaller, firmer hold (e.g., using the thumb).

Mobilizing hand The therapist's left hand explores the fascia of the SBAL (extensor muscles of wrist and fingers, brachialis, deltoid, trapezii muscles), usually in a cranial direction, but always with the star concept in mind. If there is tension in this line of fascia, it will seem like the hand holding the distal radius will want to move dorsally and cranially. The patient perceives this as the therapist increasing his/her pressure on the radius. The therapist performs repeated passive physiological cranial glides of the affected fascia while maintaining the anchor on the radius. This is repeated until a release is felt between the therapist's two hands and generally requires approximately five to eight cycles.

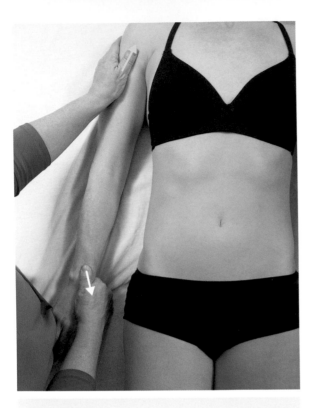

Figure 13.28
MMS right Colles' fracture fascia in relation to the deltoid (SBAL)

Summary

The techniques in this chapter have focused on the myofascial connections in relation to the upper quadrant, namely the shoulder, elbow, forearm, wrist and hand. The next chapter will discuss a more active treatment approach to help maintain the effects of treatment with MMS.

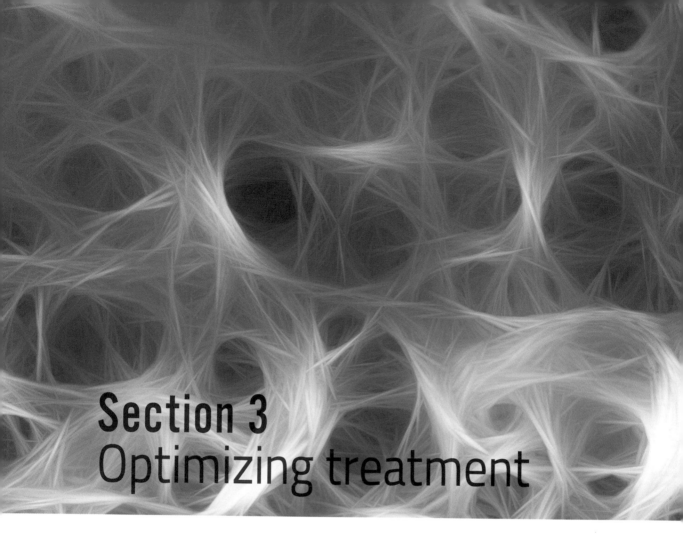

Section 3
Optimizing treatment

Movement and fascia

The overall goal of any physical therapy is to move well. It is difficult to feel well if one is unable to move well. Sometimes the ability to move well is inhibited by restrictions of certain tissues in the body, whether it is due to a hypomobile joint or a tight myofascial line. Appropriate intervention by skilled therapists can facilitate a pathway to enable the body to move more freely. However, manual therapy of any kind is a passive treatment. In order to achieve optimal therapeutic results, manual therapy must be followed by active movement. Complementary forms of movement could include a specific stretch exercise to maintain the effects of treatment and/or retraining movement patterns that relate to the patient's meaningful task. The oft-repeated line that "Neurons that fire together wire together" (Hebb 1949) applies in these situations. Therapists draw on the concept of neuroplasticity to help create new neural networks for function and performance. For such neurological remapping to occur, the patient's body and brain needs new and novel experiences, not simple rote exercises done in front of the television. Optimal movement requires focused attention. Adopting new strategies for movement may be even more challenging for those patients who are taking neuropathic pain medications, such as gabapentin, as these medications have a tendency to desensitize the nervous system. Nevertheless, movement needs to be a primary goal of therapy.

With regards to maintaining fascial mobility, Tom Myers (in his blogs on Anatomy Trains) summarizes current thoughts about the critical role of movement in that process:

- New discoveries in fascia research hold tremendous implications for changing not just human form but also behavior and emotional patterns.

- The emerging understanding of the central role played by the fascia in bodily health puts new emphasis on the role of movement therapies in healing. Myers predicts a medicine of the future in which the emphasis on movement as therapy will play a central role.

- New discoveries in fascia research imply that traditional isolated approaches to exercise can be counterproductive – more holistic movement forms such as yoga may be far more useful for training the fascia.

Stretching

If we look to research for evidence of the benefits of stretching, the results are mixed and not as universally promising as some advocates maintain. As Tom Myers observes,

On the surface, stretching seems like a great warm-up activity, a pre-game or pre-run stretch. It 'wrings out' the tissue, refreshing the water, breaks up any adhesions, and prepares the body to move quickly without injury. Doesn't it? No, it doesn't – research has fairly consistently shown no benefit in terms of muscle soreness, injury prevention, and it may reduce strength or sport performance from 5% to 20% (Herbert et al. 2011). A second argument against stretching as a form of human maintenance is that we do not do a lot of movement in our daily life at the end range of motion. Stretching, as it is commonly practiced in many yoga classes, sports prep, and even rehabilitation involves taking the stretch to the end-range of motion. It has simply not been shown that exploring the end-range of motion with active or passive stretches improves the quality of movements in daily life. Finally, all the research points to training being very highly specific – when you train a motion, you train for that motion only. It does not bleed over into other motions so easily or so generally as we have supposed. If you are training yourself in a twisting stretch, you are 'training' for that specific stretch, and it may not translate into more or better motion in daily life. (Myers 2015)

There are better arguments for stretching at the end of activity rather than at the start of activity: The warmed muscles and fascia are more amenable to change, so perhaps more increase in ROM can be obtained by stretching after exercise. Even the stretched out yogi who can put their hands on the floor can have areas of the hamstrings that are painful and held very tight. Everything around that tight spot is loose and limber to allow the movement in the joint, but the careful 'combing through' the tissue I do as a body-worker reveals these islands of supreme tension within the ocean of availability. (Myers 2015)

Myers also suggests the following:

1. Do self myofascial release (SMR) yourself – with a ball or a roller. Find the places that you feel are stuck or dense, and roll over them with your body weight, moving very slowly and with awareness to get into the worst of it and open it up to hydration. In his blog on foam rollers and self myofascial release he does, however, state a few precautions about their use (Myers April 2015).

2. Find a good body-worker, osteopath, or even experienced yoga teacher who can help you find the stuck places you don't know about. (This author would add physiotherapist to that list!) You work the stuck places you do know about. Other spots may be just as stuck, but not producing pain or being obviously limiting (Myers 2015).

Other integrative therapies

There are a number of integrative therapies that are complementary to the treatment approaches by various professionals (physiotherapists, osteopaths, massage therapists, etc.). The following list is not exhaustive but includes some complementary treatments that incorporate movement:

• Feldenkrais approach (Moishe Feldenkrais)

• Alexander technique (F. M. Alexander)

• Tai-Chi

• Chi-Gong

• Pilates (Elizabeth Larkam, *Fascia in Motion: Fascia-focused Movement for Pilates, 2017*)

• MELT method (Sue Hitzmann)

• Resistance flexibility (Bob Cooley, Dr Christiane Northrup)

• Fascial stretch therapy (Ann and Chris Frederick)

• Fascial fitness (Robert Schleip and Johanna Bayer)

• Medical therapeutic yoga (Dr Ginger Garner)

Ginger Garner's book *Medical Therapeutic Yoga: Biopsychosocial Rehabilitation and Wellness Care* (Handspring Publishing) is highly recommended reading. Dr Garner has developed a biomechanically safe yoga practice that involves a functional movement assessment algorithm and requires kinesthetic awareness and respiration. She states: "Healthy movement is dictated not by the amount of movement you have, but how well you can control your available movement. Controlled flexibility is a tenet of my approach to using yoga therapeutically in any condition where human movement is required" (Garner 2016).

The focus in this chapter will be on stretches and yoga poses for each the fascial lines described by Tom Myers. A note of caution, however. Yoga is a wonderful tool but it is not for everyone and there are injuries that can occur from doing "bad yoga." As therapists, we must be careful not to take the yoga asanas out of context for the sole purpose of fascial lengthening. My suggestion to therapists who are not familiar with yoga is to find a qualified yoga therapist who understands the proper form and alignment of these postures and try a number of classes first before you prescribe these asanas for your patients. The body needs some preparation in order for the fascial tissue to react more efficiently – a body that is not warmed up will not react the same way as one that is warm. Taking a whole yoga class that is progressively building is not the same as choosing the odd asana.

Before launching into a description of these poses, the question that begs to be answered is "What is the optimal time to hold a yoga pose?" In his blog (September 13, 2016), Tom Myers responds to this question:

1. Suggested times holding a pose vary from for five to 10 minutes, although Iyengar recommended three minutes. Individual variation is what is important, as there isn't a number that works for everyone. For some, the physiological changes may be done in a shorter time, for others, it might be rewarding and delicious to hold the pose for a half hour.

2. Myotatic reflex release: when a muscle is first stretched, the myotatic reflex is released; that is, its own stretch reflex tries to re-contract the muscle back to its original length. If the stretch is maintained, the reflex gives up after a time and the muscle lengthens. Again, that time varies with the person, but mostly with the training. After a certain time in the pose, there's an 'Ah!' feeling as the body relaxes into the pose. That moment will come sooner for the trained yogi and will take longer for the neophyte. The deep fascia within the muscle does not begin to stretch until this relaxation occurs, suggesting that new students should hold the pose longer – say, three minutes from the 'Ah'.

3. Move within poses. The ability of the tissue to plastically/visco-elastically deform will depend on local hydration of the specific tissue – not how much water one drinks, but how "wet" is the specific fascia that is being challenged to stretch. By not going into the ultimate stretch position, i.e., by only going to 75 percent of stretch capacity, you may look like the stiffest person in the room in terms of the form of the asana, but you will be able to move within the pose, rather than holding still for the full ten minutes. While there may be some value in disciplining yourself to stay still, your body will thank you for the extra hydration gained by moving around within the pose.

The stretches and yoga poses described below offer ways to maintain flexibility in each of the fascial lines. The stretches and poses for each line of fascia are arranged in order of difficulty. The easier poses are described first, followed by more advances poses that require more flexibility and motor control.

Precautions and contraindications

These poses are contraindicated in cases of acute joint pain. Precautions to be aware of are excessive hip anteversion (positive Craig's test) and femoroacetabular impingement (FAI), especially where "hip openers" are concerned. The thoracic spine should be monitored and corrected for any ring shifts, in particular for any poses involving thoracic rotation. Any poses involving extension should be done in a manner that avoids abnormal shearing at any particular

level of the lumbar or cervical spine. The sacroiliac joint (SIJ) should maintain its neutral position in nutation of the sacrum unless the pose calls for full flexion of the spine (as in the cat part of the cat/cow pose).

Across all poses, there are some common concepts for the practitioner of these poses to keep in mind. These are common themes taught by most yoga therapists and articulated beautifully by Melissa Kreiger, yoga therapist (Kreiger 2018):

- Breath moves in, breath moves out – keep using breath throughout your practice, breathing into the area of perceived tightness to create more space.

- Maintain a sense of softness and space in the body.

- It's OK if stretches are strong – it's not OK if stretches hurt; everything should feel safe and comfortable.

- It's not about getting low – it's about creating length and space through the body.

Superficial Back Line stretches

Supine hamstring stretches (Figure 14.1)

The spine is neutral, the hands are gently clasped together behind the knee; active knee extension is performed, keeping the foot in neutral position. The spine stays long and the knee does not have to straighten completely. This stretch can be done with or without extension of the opposite leg. The pull is easier if the opposite leg is flexed and is more challenging if the opposite leg is extended on the floor.

Supine hamstring stretch with active ankle dorsiflexion (Figure 14.2)

This variation adds more tension to the SBL of fascia. Active dorsiflexion of the ankle may be added to the stretch above, in an on/off fashion or in a more sustained manner.

Supine hamstring stretch with active ankle plantarflexion/inversion (Figure 14.3)

This variation adds more tension to the Spiral Line of fascia because it involves the lateral myofascial structures. It also mobilizes the superficial peroneal nerve.

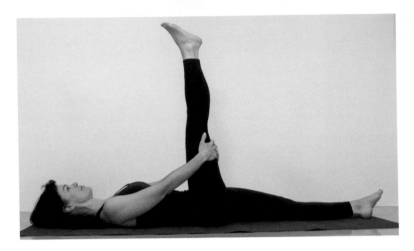

Figure 14.1
Supine hamstring stretch

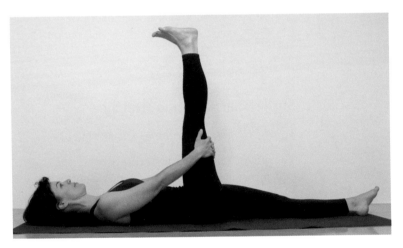

Figure 14.2
Supine hamstring stretch with ankle DF

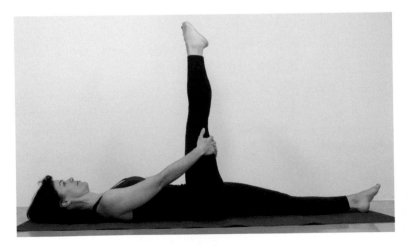

Figure 14.3
Supine hamstring stretch with ankle PF/Inv

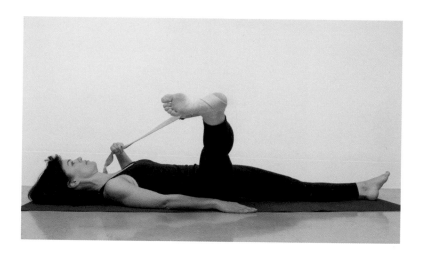

Figure 14.4
Supine hamstring stretch with abduction

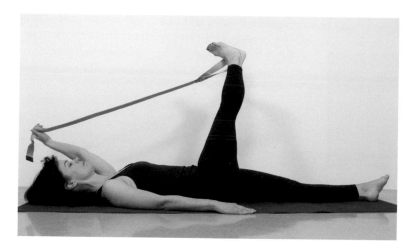

Figure 14.5
Supine hamstring stretch with adduction

As with the technique above, active plantarflexion/inversion may be added in an on/off fashion (especially if mobility of the nerve is a problem) or in a sustained fashion.Supine hamstring stretches with abduction, adduction (yoga strap assisted):

1. The spine is neutral, ASISs are level, the right leg is guided into abduction (Figure 14.4). This pose stretches the medial line, Spiral Line and (because of the adductors), the DFL of fascia.

2. As above, but the right leg is guided into adduction, which also stretches the Lateral Line and Spiral Line (Figure 14.5). For a variation, hip external rotation may also be added.

Superficial Back Line yoga poses

Cat part of cat/cow (Figure 14.6)

This pose is focal to the part of the SBL that involves the trunk, head, and neck. It also affects the posterior spiral and posterior arm lines. The pose begins in a four-point kneel position, with the hands spread wide underneath the shoulders, and the knees under the pelvis. The spine is flexed, beginning with the coccyx, producing posterior pelvic tilt and moving gradually up the kinetic chain to include cervical flexion. It is generally done with exhalation. This pose may be progressed by adding slight hip flexion, as this maneuver specifically targets the lumbosacral fascia.

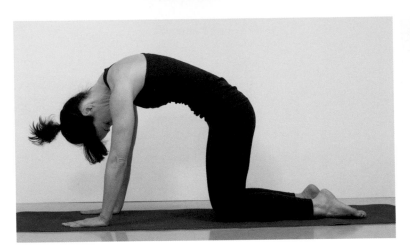

Figure 14.6
SBL yoga pose – cat part of cat/cow

Child pose (Figure 14.7)

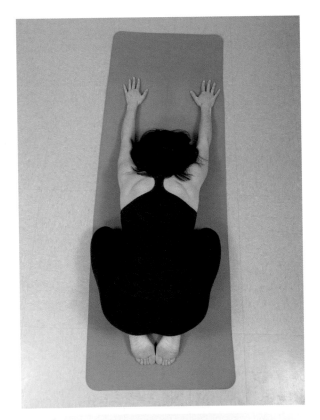

Figure 14.7
SBL yoga pose – child pose

This pose also affects the trunk, head and neck portions of the SBL, as well as the posterior functional line. It requires optimal mechanics of the hip and knee and should not reproduce pain in either of these areas. The pose begins in a four-point kneel position as above, but the pose may also be done with the knees apart. The movement is one of leaning back toward full flexion of the hips and knees, as well as reaching forward with the arms in scaption (midway between shoulder flexion and abduction). The forehead may rest on the floor or on a yoga block. The breath is directed toward the back body and/or the shoulders. If the pose is done with the heels apart and intentional imaging of creating a sense of space between the ischial tuberosities, this pose may also help maintain mobility of the pelvic floor muscles (including obturator internus), especially if the lumbar spine is in a lordotic position. This then becomes a useful pose for maintaining mobility of the pelvic floor portion of the DFL of fascia.

Lateral child pose (Figure 14.8)

This is a variation of the child pose, in which the thoracolumbar fascia and latissmus dorsi can be put on stretch (especially if the arm is in a "thumbs up" position, which externally rotates the arm). This pose affects the posterior functional line of fascia, which, if tight, can tug on the sacroiliac area as the patient attempts to do activities involving shoulder flexion. This pose is also useful to stretch the quadratus lumborum, psoas, and iliacus, which are part of the DFL of fascia.

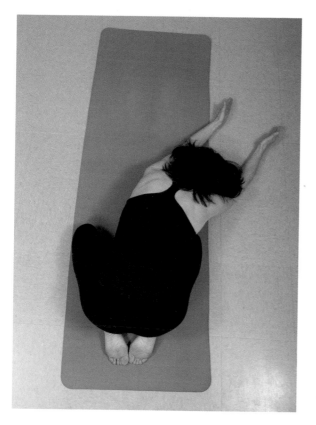

Figure 14.8
Lateral child pose

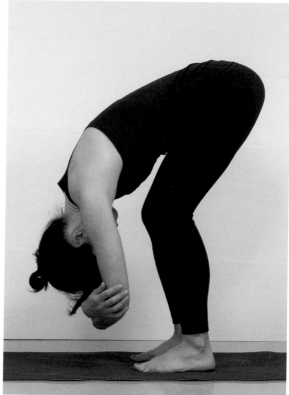

Figure 14.9
SBL yoga pose – standing forward bend

Standing forward bend (Figure 14.9)

This pose is done in a standing position, with the trunk folded forward at the hips so that the belly rests on the thighs. The knees are slightly bent and the elbows are cupped by the hands so that the arms "hang loose" to produce distraction of the trunk. The buttocks reach long towards the ceiling. The neck and head also hang loose. Breath is directed toward areas of tension. The pose may be altered by adding micro-movements into shoulder flexion/extension, abduction/adduction ("rock the baby"). The standing forward bend pose is a stretch for the SBL, but it is also particularly useful as a way to create length and space between the thoracic rings.

Pigeon pose for buttocks (Figure 14.10)

This pose is useful for stretching the gluteal muscles as well as a number of myofascial lines because of the asymmetrical nature of the pose. To stretch the right side, the right leg is bent and placed so that the right heel rests near the groin. The left leg is positioned in hip extension, behind the trunk. The practitioner reaches forward toward the floor with the trunk. The elbows may be bent or straight. The stretch can be modified by adding micro-movements of the pelvis to the right or the left and by varying the degree of right knee flexion. It can also be done with spinal extension, which emphasizes a stretch on the DFL of fascia. This pose may also be repeated for the other side.

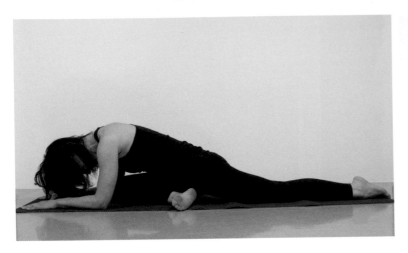

Figure 14.10
SBL yoga pose – pigeon pose

Seated toe flexor stretch (Figure 14.11)

This is a variation of the thunderbolt pose, in that the toes are in dorsiflexion instead of plantarflexion. The pose starts from a four-point kneel position. The toes are in full dorsiflexion, taking care to keep a neutral position for the rest of the foot; that is, weight-bearing equally on the first and fifth metatarsals. The pelvis rocks back towards the heels until a stretch is felt in the plantar aspect of the feet. Progressing towards the kneeling position increases the stretch. This stretch is particularly good for the foot portion of the SBL as well as the DFL of fascia.

Downward-facing dog (Figure 14.12)

This pose is an advanced posture that stretches the whole SBL. It requires full glenohumeral flexion as well as good hip flexion. The spinal curves should remain in neutral, especially the lower lumbar and upper thoracic curves, which tend toward excessive flexion in this pose. The head should hang down completely in this pose, with no active contraction of the cervical extensors. If spinal curves are maintained, the heels may or may not reach the floor and the knees may or may not achieve full extension, depending on the extensibility of this SBL of fascia. This pose should be avoided in those with acute sciatic nerve irritation.

Walk the dog (Figure 14.13)

This pose is a variation of the downward-facing dog, which focuses on the lower part of the SBL. The pose is frequently used as a "warm-up" to the full downward-facing dog pose.

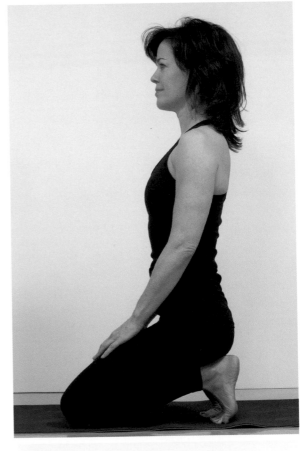

Figure 14.11
SBL yoga pose – seated toe flexor stretch

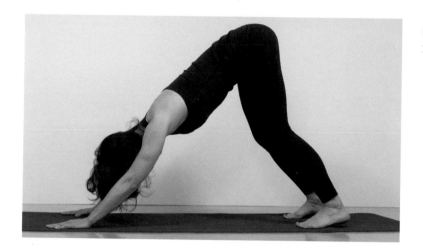

Figure 14.12

SBL yoga pose – downward facing dog

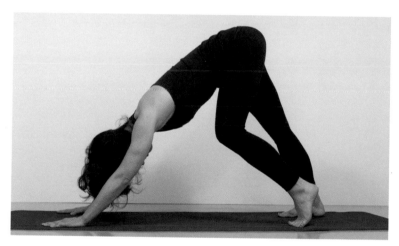

Figure 14.13

SBL yoga pose – walk the dog

From the position of downward-facing dog, one knee is flexed as the other remains extended. The pose requires slow, alternating movement from one leg to the other, with emphasis on the leg that is in dorsiflexion, heel toward the floor.

Downward-facing dog for soleus stretch (Figure 14.14)

This pose is also a variation of the downward-facing dog. The main difference is that the knees are deliberately flexed so as to stretch the soleus muscle and its fascia.

Deep Front Line stretches

Prone extension breathing (Figure 14.15)

This exercise is one of my "go to" exercises, frequently prescribed for those patients with decreased mobility of the DFL. It is simple to do and can be done first thing in the morning and/or just before bedtime. The patient is in a prone position, with the lumbar spine in extension, elbows underneath the shoulders, hands supporting the chin. The patient is asked to breathe deeply, with the emphasis on expiration (small breath in, long, slow breath out). The umbilicus is encouraged to sink toward the floor on expiration. It is recommended to maintain the position and the breathing for approximately two minutes. This exercise may reproduce low back pain on expiration. This is acceptable, as long as the pain resolves within a few minutes after the exercise. Even in those patients with hypermobile lower lumbar spines, this exercise is a safe way to regain upper lumbar and thoracolumbar extension without irritating the lower lumbar spine.

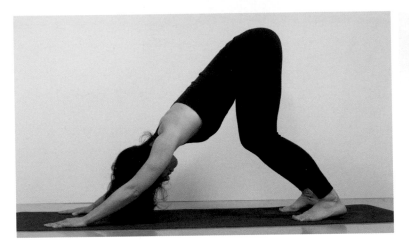

Figure 14.14
SBL yoga pose – downward facing dog for soleus stretch

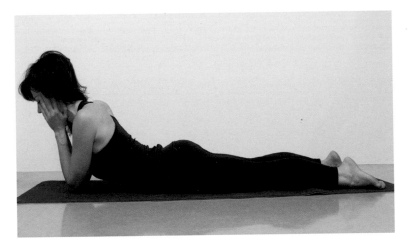

Figure 14.15
Prone extension breathing exercise for DFL

Progression of prone extension breathing exercise (Figure 14.16)

The exercise above is progressed by adding bilateral knee flexion and ankle dorsiflexion/eversion, either on the breath out or sustained throughout the two-minute exercise.

Upper quadrant Deep Front Line stretch (Figures 14.17, 14.18)

This exercise is a very good stretch for the upper quadrant part of the front lines, whether the SFL or the DFL. The patient's hands are crossed and placed over the manubrial/sternal area centrally. A posterior and caudal pressure of the hands is applied to stabilize this area. The patient's tongue touches the roof of the mouth, as if to say the letter "N". The cervical spine slowly extends back, with care, to perform the movement segmentally and not shear forward at the mid-cervical spine. The patient should feel a stretch in the front of the cervical/throat area. The stretch is maintained for 10–20 seconds and normal breathing is encouraged. A variation of this exercise is to stabilize one side of the upper thorax/subclavicular area with both hands and perform cervical extension and side-flexion to the right or left. (Figure 14.18 shows this exercise for the right side of the DFL of fascia.)

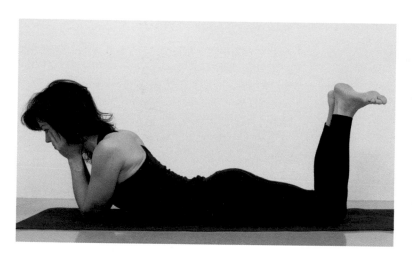

Figure 14.16
Progression of prone extension breathing exercise for DFL

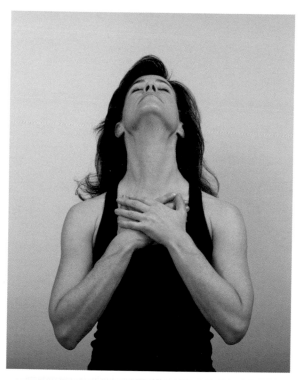

Figure 14.17
Upper quadrant DFL stretch exercise

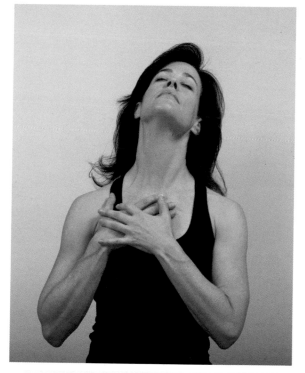

Figure 14.18
Modification for right side of DFL

Deep Front Line yoga poses

Cow part of cat/cow pose (Figure 14.19)

This variation produces myofascial tensile force through the SFL, anterior functional, anterior arm and DFL of fascia. The pose begins in a four-point kneel position, with the hands spread wide underneath the shoulders, and the knees positioned under the pelvis. The spine is extended, beginning with the coccyx, producing an anterior pelvic tilt and gradually moving up the kinetic chain to include cervical extension. It is generally done on the inhale. Patients with spinal stenosis and spondylolysthesis should be careful not to reproduce pain in the trunk or extremities with this pose.

Cobra pose (Figure 14.20)

This pose begins in a prone position, with the hands and wrists directly beneath the shoulders. Keeping the cervical spine neutral, the arms are used to extend the thoracic and lumbar spine. The transversus abdominis is contracted to dynamically stabilize the trunk during this pose. The pelvis should not rise from the floor.

Sphinx pose (Figure 14.21)

This pose is considered a variation of the cobra pose and is done in a prone position, with the body propped up on the forearms. This pose is particularly helpful to stretch the fascia of the mid-thoracic region. The pose is done with isometric shoulder flexion so as to move the body away

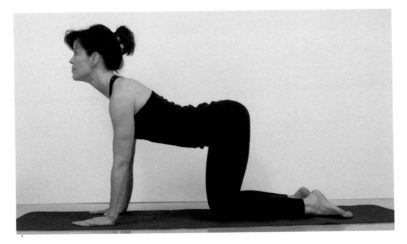

Figure 14.19
DFL yoga pose – cow part of cat/cow

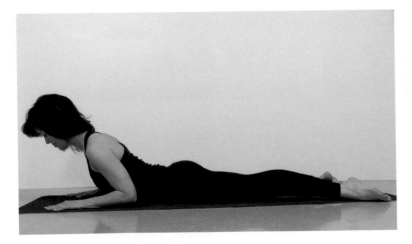

Figure 14.20
DFL yoga pose – cobra pose

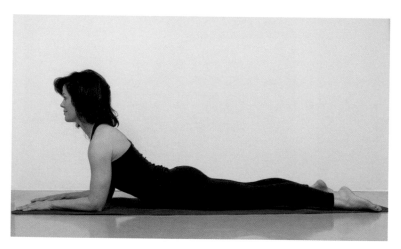

Figure 14.21
DFL yoga pose – Sphinx pose

from the forearms, and the breath may be used to further extend the mid-thoracic region in this position.

Upward-facing dog (Figure 14.22)

This is an advanced pose that emphasizes spinal extension. It affects both the SFL and DFL of fascia, as well as the anterior functional line and the anterior arm lines. The beginner may find it easier to initiate the movement through thoracic extension first, followed by lumbar extension. The beginner may also leave the pelvis and lower extremities in contact with the floor, as in cobra. The advanced practitioner may clear the knees off the floor in this position.

The cervical spine may stay in a neutral position, but adding cervical extension while maintaining the tongue

on the roof of the mouth will add further stretch to the DFL of fascia.

Lunge (Figure 14.23)

This pose is a pre-requisite for the Sun Salutations in yoga. It stretches both the SFL and DFL of fascia on the side of the straight leg and the SBL of the bent leg. It may be done with the hands on the floor or on yoga blocks, or with the arms in shoulder flexion and the chest lifted, as pictured. The knee of the front leg stays over the ankle, the front foot is in neutral position and the patella is aligned over the second metatarsal. If more stretch is required, then the practitioner should extend the straight leg farther back. Care is taken to keep the pelvis level in the transverse plane (facing forward) and to control the position of the

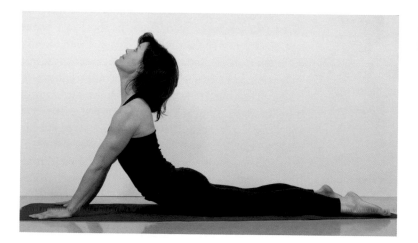

Figure 14.22
DFL yoga pose – upward facing dog

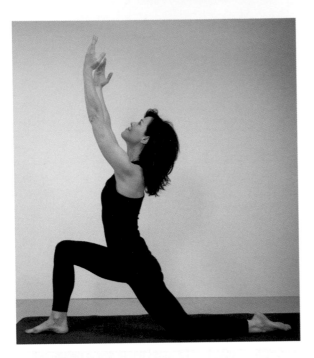

Figure 14.23
DFL yoga pose – lunge

spine and pelvis using the dynamic stabilizers of the trunk (transversus abdominis, deep multifidus).

Warrior 1 pose (Figures 14.24, 14.25)

This pose is similar to the lunge except that it is done standing, which requires more dynamic stabilization and proprioception. In this position, the foot of the back leg can be placed either in dorsiflexion/eversion (Figure 14.24) or in plantarflexion with the toes extended (Figure 14.25). The arms are in full flexion, with the forearms supinated so that the thumbs face backwards. If more stretch is required, then the practitioner should extend the straight leg farther back and/or lower the body towards the floor. This pose may also be repeated for the other side.

Warrior 2 pose (Figure 14.26)

Warrior 2 pose strengthens both the upper and lower extremities and stretches the adductors of the back leg. As with warrior 1 pose, warrior 2 also improves stamina, endurance, balance and concentration. In this picture,

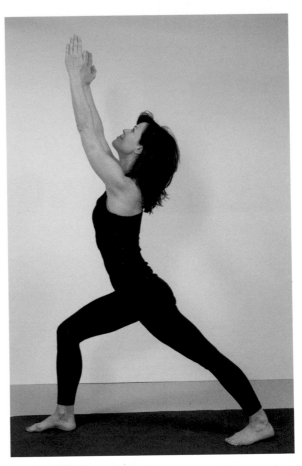

Figure 14.24
DFL yoga pose – warrior 1 with DF/Ev

the left leg is straight and the right hip and knee are flexed. The left foot is parallel to the short edge of the mat, and the heel of the right foot is in line with the heel of the left foot. The right foot faces the corner of the mat and maintains a neutral position (not collapsed into pronation). The arms are extended out into abduction with the palms facing down. The head is turned to the right and the gaze is forward. The right knee is stacked directly over the right ankle and the shin is perpendicular to the floor. The patella is aligned over the second metatarsal. If more stretch is required, then the practitioner should extend the straight leg farther back. The pelvis faces the left side of the mat. This pose may also be repeated for the other side.

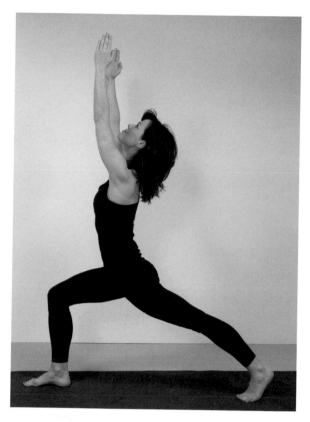

Figure 14.25
DFL yoga pose – warrior 1 with PF

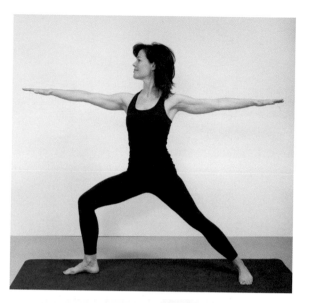

Figure 14.26
DFL yoga pose – warrior 2

pelvic region. A yoga block is placed under the sacrum, with the cranial edge of the block placed at the base of the sacrum (S1). The arms are by the side or may be positioned at 90 degrees of abduction in order to open up the anterior arm lines. The cervical spine is in neutral position (avoid chin poking). One or two legs can be extended, depending on comfort. Deep breaths are encouraged in this position.

Supported bridge with yoga block at sacrum (Figure 14.27)

The anterior sacral fascia may be accessed with this pose, so this is particularly useful for DFL restrictions of the

Supine with yoga block at mid-thorax +/− frog position (Figure 14.28)

The DFL of the mid-thoracic region is accessed with this pose. A yoga block is placed under the mid-thoracic region,

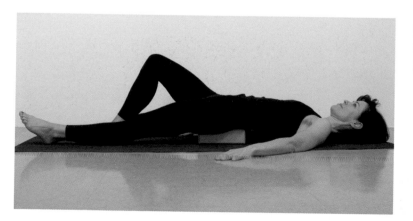

Figure 14.27
DFL yoga pose – supported bridge with yoga block at sacrum

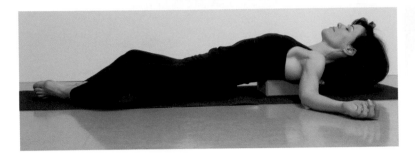

Figure 14.28
DFL yoga pose – yoga block at mid-thorax

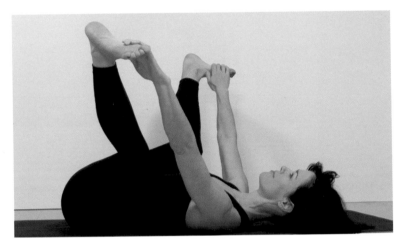

Figure 14.29
Happy baby pose

with the caudal edge of the block placed at about the T7 level. The arms are at 90 degrees of abduction in order to open up the anterior arm lines. The cervical spine is in neutral position – the head may need support of a second yoga block or a folded towel under the occiput in order to maintain a neutral cervical spine. The legs can be extended, as above, or placed in a "frog" position, with the soles of the feet together and the hips abducted and externally rotated. This position adds tension to the adductors of the hip, also part of the DFL. Various angles of hip flexion in this position may be explored to find the areas of most restriction. Deep breathing is encouraged.

Happy baby pose (pelvic floor, adductors) (Figure 14.29)

This pose promotes mobility of the hips in FABER (flexion/abduction/external rotation) as well as spinal flexion and sacral counternutation. The medial arches of both feet are grasped by the hands and the hips open so that the knees are directed toward the floor. The cervical spine maintains a

neutral position. Experimenting with small rocking motions into lumbopelvic flexion/extension or rotations is encouraged.

Windshield wiper (Figure 14.30)

This pose improves mobility in the Spiral Line and arm lines but is particularly good for DFL restrictions, if done with certain modifications. The pose begins in a crook-lying position, with the arms placed at 90 degrees of abduction in order to open up the anterior arm lines. The feet are on the outside edge of the mat or even off the mat, if more stretch is required. In Figure 14.30, the right knee moves medially toward the floor within available FADDIR (flexion/adduction/internal rotation) as the left knee moves toward FABER (flexion/abduction/external rotation). The neck rotates toward the right side. The opposite windshield wiper movement can also be performed, as the practitioner alternates from one side to the other. If a deeper stretch for the DFL is desired, the knees may be fully flexed, with the heels closer to the buttocks. As the right leg moves into

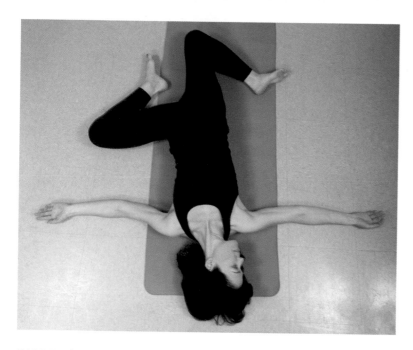

Figure 14.30
DFL yoga pose – windshield wiper

FADDIR, the right ilium may reach anteriorly and caudally ("reach long towards the knee") to deepen the stretch. Deep breathing in this position is encouraged in order to activate the diaphragmatic portion of the DFL.

Superficial Front Line stretches

Clavicular opening stretch (Figure 14.31)

This exercise is indicated for patients who show signs of ISGT (intra-shoulder girdle torsion (see Chapter 12). The intention of the exercise is to create a sense of space between the two clavicles and the front body and to minimize the excessive medial compression at the sternoclavicular joints. The fingers are loosely placed on both clavicles and the cervical spine is in a neutral position. The patient feels the motion of the clavicles coming apart slightly on inspiration and coming back together on expiration. Once that sensory experience is understood, the patient is asked to maintain the sense of space between the two clavicles on expiration as well as inspiration and to repeat this three to five times. Creating the sense of space between the clavicles comes "from within" and not from using the hands to do the motion. This exercise may be progressed by adding other movements (such as axial extension or thoracic rotation) as the practitioner maintains the sense of space between the clavicles.

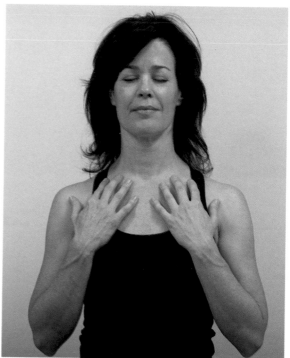

Figure 14.31
Clavicular opening stretch exercise

Quads in side-lying with plantarflexion of foot and toes (Figure 14.32)

The stretch is a variation of the standard quadriceps stretch exercise that is performed in a side-lying position. In Figure 14.32, the right hip is flexed and supported by the arm so as to protect the lumbar spine from excessive extension. The top (left) knee is fully flexed and the practitioner grasps the leg by the toes, to gently pull toward hip extension. The fact that ankle and toe plantarflexion has been added makes this more of a SFL stretch than a simple quadriceps stretch exercise. Care is taken to keep the left knee in line with the hip. This pose may also be repeated for the right side.

Superficial Front Line yoga poses

Seated toe extensor stretch (Figure 14.33)

The thunderbolt pose starts from a four-point kneel position. The toes are in full plantarflexion, taking care to keep a neutral position for the rest of the foot; that is, avoiding placing the foot in plantarflexion/inversion. The pelvis rocks back toward heel sitting until a stretch is felt in the dorsal aspect of the feet and/or toes. Care must be taken to avoid knee pain with this pose. Progressing toward the kneeling position increases the stretch. This stretch is particularly good for the toe extensors that are at the tail end of the SFL of fascia. Tension in this area can contribute to the development of hammer toes.

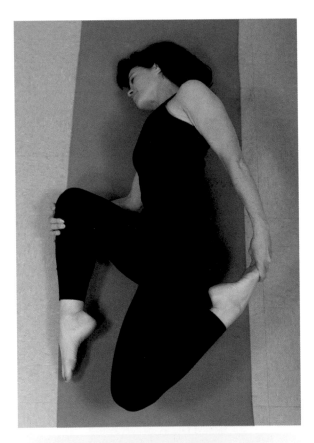

Figure 14.32
SFL stretch – quadriceps with ankle and toe PF

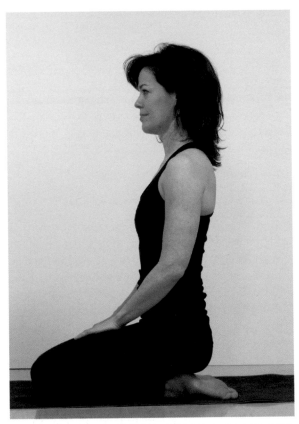

Figure 14.33
SFL yoga pose – seated toe extensor stretch

Spiral Line yoga poses

Pectoralis stretch with lumbar rotation (Figure 14.34)

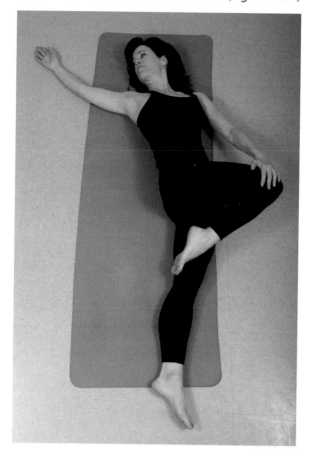

Figure 14.34

Spiral Line yoga poses – pectoralis stretch with lumbar rotation

This position is particularly useful to stretch the pectoralis major and minor muscles, muscles that are frequently shortened in those patients whose work or sports require much pectoral work (such as computer work or manual therapy!).

It is also a good stretch for the buttock muscles, as well as the posterior and the anterior functional lines. The pose is begun in the crook-lying position. To stretch the right pectoral muscles, the pelvis is displaced slightly toward the right. The right arm is placed in a combined position of flexion/abduction. The knees drop to the left side, which puts the Spiral Line and anterior functional line under tension, deepening the stretch of the pectoral muscles. This position also stretches the right buttock muscles and the posterior functional line of fascia. If additional stretch of the lower quadrant is desired, the left hand can rest on top of the right distal thigh. The patient is encouraged to breathe into the chest, torso, and hips and allow gravity to do the work. Experimenting with the angle of flexion/abduction of the shoulder is suggested in order to find those "delicious" places where most tension is felt.

Thinking about keeping the clavicles open, turning the head towards the right side, and thinking of letting the right pelvis "reach long" toward the knee all help to deepen the stretch. This pose may also be repeated for the left side.

Lord of the fishes (seated spinal twist) (Figure 14.35)

This pose stretches multiple myofascial lines, especially the Spiral and Functional lines. In the sitting position, the right leg rests, foot flat and knee flexed, on the outside of the left knee. The left leg is straight, but may be placed in FABER for a more advanced pose. The lumbar spine maintains a neutral position and the weight of the practitioner is equally distributed between the two ischial tuberosities. The right arm reaches back to provide stability and a lever arm so that the thorax rotates to the right as the right leg is gently pulled into further FADDIR (flexion/adduction/internal rotation). The thorax "reaches long" toward axial extension, in order to encourage optimal biomechanics of the thoracic rings (i.e., the thoracic rings should stack up underneath each other, like a stack of dinner plates). This pose may also be repeated for the left side.

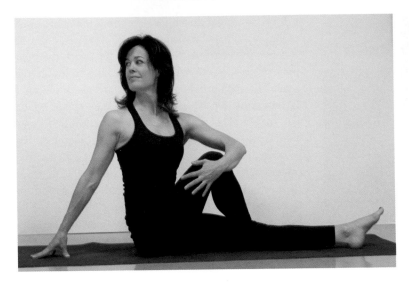

Figure 14.35

Spiral Line yoga pose – lord of the fishes

Threading the needle(Figure 14.36)

This position is particularly useful to stretch the scapular muscles and the thoracolumbar fascia in relation to a spinal twist. In Figure 14.36, the pose begins in a four-point kneel position. For thoracic right rotation, the practitioner reaches forward with the left arm "underneath the trunk" until the left scapula is anchored to the floor. With the left scapula anchored, the right hand pushes into the floor to create maximum pull in the left thoracic/scapular area. The practitioner is encouraged to breathe into the area of perceived tightness to create more space.

Triangle pose (Figure 14.37)

This pose is an advanced triplanar pose (frontal, sagittal, and transverse) that stretches all myofascial lines. Because it is an advanced pose, there are many elements that must

be taken into consideration in order for this pose to be done safely. Please refer to Ginger Garner's book *Medical Therapeutic Yoga: Biopsychosocial Rehabilitation and Wellness Care* (Handspring Publishing), for details on proper execution of this pose (Garner 2016).

Lunge/twist (Figure 14.38)

This pose combines a lunge with thoracic rotation and is particularly useful to stretch the anterior functional line, as well as the DFL of fascia. From the standing position, with the right foot parallel to the edge of the mat and the left foot angled to the corner of the mat, the practitioner flexes the left hip and knee, making sure that the patella is aligned with the second metatarsal. The left forearm may be used to support the body on the left thigh. In order to encourage optimal biomechanics of the thoracic rings, the

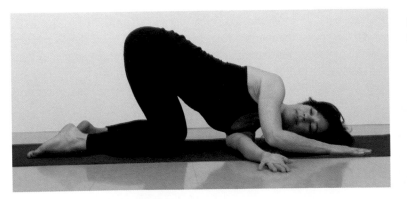

Figure 14.36

Spiral Line yoga pose – thread the needle

thorax "reaches long" toward axial extension at the same time as the thorax rotates to the right. The cervical spine also rotates right. The right arm may be placed in flexion so that it is in line with the body or with the hand behind the back (as pictured). This pose may also be repeated for the other side.

Lateral Line stretches

"C" exercise supine with breath (Figure 14.39)

This exercise is a relatively easy exercise that helps to improve the mobility of the Lateral Line of fascia. It is done in a supine position and requires no props, so it can easily

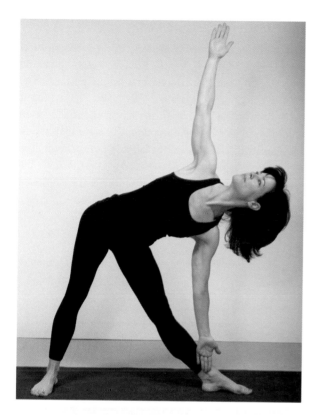

Figure 14.37 Triangle yoga pose

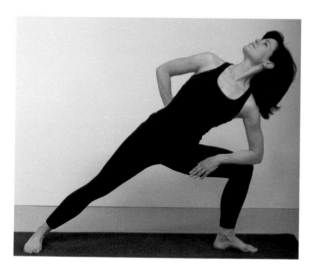

Figure 14.38 Lunge/rotation yoga pose

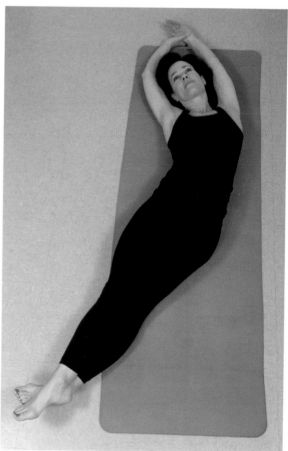

Figure 14.39 Lateral Line stretch – "C" exercise

be done in bed. To stretch the left side, the pelvis is shifted to the left; both legs are extended and shifted to the right. The legs may be crossed at the ankles to further the stretch. The arms are flexed overhead, with the right hand clasping the left wrist to pull the left arm towards the right side and encourage thoracic right-side-flexion. The practitioner is encouraged to breathe into the area of perceived tightness to create more space.

Cross leg sitting Lateral Line stretch (Figure 14.40)

This more advanced stretch is done in sitting, with the right leg under the left leg, the left ankle over the right distal thigh. Note that the right hip is not in an abducted position – it is in slight adduction and full available external rotation. The practitioner sits upright, careful to maintain lumbar lordosis. The left hand grasps the right flexed elbow to encourage side-bending of the trunk to the left.

Shirley's exercise (Figure 14.41)

This pose was described to me by a colleague (physiotherapist Shirley Kushner). It is a combined Lateral Line and DFL stretch pose that is done in a supine position. The picture depicts a stretch for the left side. The left leg is tucked under the right, with the hip in slight adduction and full available external rotation. The right foot lies on the anterior distal aspect of the left thigh to anchor it. The right hand grasps the left wrist to create side-flexion of the trunk to the right. As usual, the practitioner is encouraged to breathe into the area of perceived tightness to create more space.

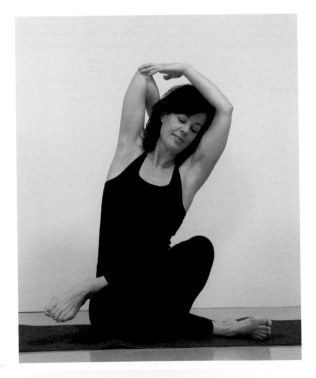

Figure 14.40
Cross leg sitting Lateral Line stretch

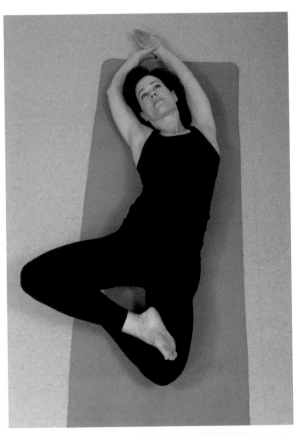

Figure 14.41
Shirley's exercise

Lateral Line yoga poses

Standing side-bend (Figure 14.42)

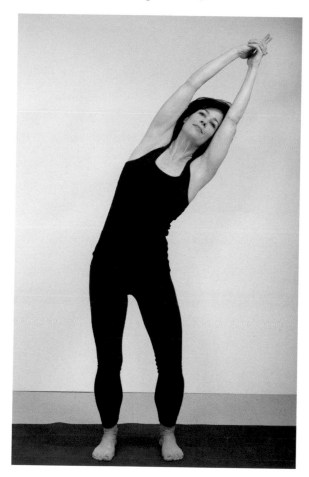

Figure 14.42
Lateral Line yoga pose – standing side-bend

This yoga pose is done in standing. The feet are shoulder-width apart and the knees slightly flexed. The hands are clasped together in prayer position, with the index fingers in "steeple" position. Imagining that the body is like a piece of bread in a toaster, the practitioner is encouraged to reach long toward the tips of the index fingers as the trunk side-bends to the right or left. The image of a piece of bread in a toaster encourages the body to stay in the frontal plane, allowing little movement into flexion/extension or rotation.

As usual, the practitioner is encouraged to breathe into the area of perceived tightness to create more space.

Later, micro-movements into rotation or flexion/extension may be added.

Gate pose (Figure 14.43)

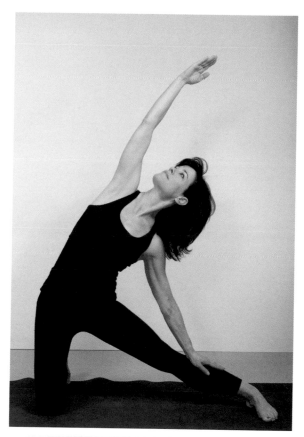

Figure 14.43
Lateral Line yoga pose – gate pose

This pose is particularly useful to stretch the Lateral Line of fascia (the right Lateral Line in Figure 14.43) as well as the adductors of the other leg. Starting from a kneeling position, the practitioner straightens the left leg into available abduction, with the left foot parallel to the edge of the mat. The practitioner uses the left arm and rests it against the left lateral leg (avoiding the knee). He/she uses the right arm to reach upward to produce left side-bending of the torso without rotation or flexion, always sending breath into the side body. This pose may also be repeated for the other side.

Sitting Lateral Line stretch (Figure 14.44)

To stretch the left lateral body in the sitting position, the practitioner sits with the right leg extended out to the side and the left leg flexed and externally rotated at the hip. The right forearm drops down and rests on the right thigh, as the left arm reaches overhead to side-bend the trunk to the

right. The spine stays long in this pose, as the lumbar spine maintains a neutral position. The thorax actively rotates to the left throughout this pose in order to keep the thorax facing forward. This pose is more about creating space in the body rather than getting low. It may also be repeated for the other side.

Variation for thoracolumbar fascia (Figure 14.45)

The pose above may be adjusted to produce a stretch for the thoracolumbar fascia. In the same seated position as above, the practitioner uses the left arm to reach forward as far

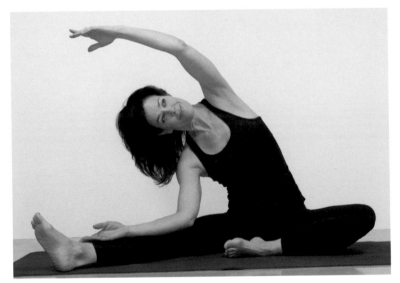

Figure 14.44
Lateral Line yoga pose – sitting

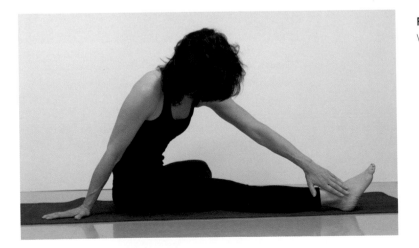

Figure 14.45
Variation – thoracolumbar fascia stretch

down as possible the lateral aspect of the right leg. This will produce a stretch in the right hamstring area. However, if the practitioner uses their right hand to push against the floor and create a "C" position of the thoracolumbar area (side-bending to the right) this provides a nice stretch to the left thoracolumbar fascia. As usual, the breath is used to accentuate the stretch.

Front Arm Line yoga poses

Shoulder opener with belt (Figure 14.46)

This pose is useful to stretch the anterior lines of the arms as well as to open up the chest area. The pose may be done with the hands clasped behind the back or by using a yoga strap (as pictured). The practitioner grasps the belt with both arms pronated and the hands placed apart, shoulder-width distance. Keeping a neutral spine throughout, the arms are gently pulled up to the ceiling to produce bilateral shoulder extension. The pose may be progressed by maintaining the shoulders in the extended position as the practitioner leans forward over the thighs, with full hip flexion and the knees slightly flexed.

Eagle pose (Figure 14.47)

This pose stretches the posterior arm lines (including the rotator cuff muscles) and the posterior spiral and functional

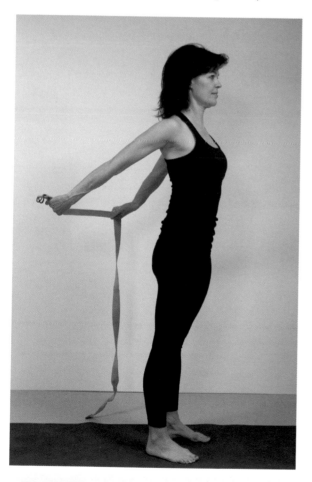

Figure 14.46
Front Arm Line yoga poses – belt shoulder opener

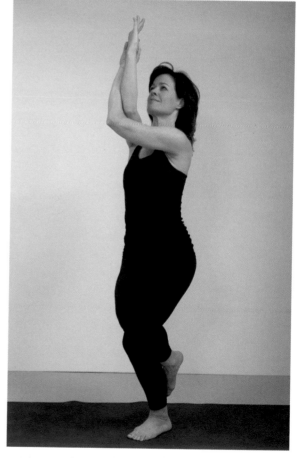

Figure 14.47
Eagle pose

lines. It is also used to work hip and knee stability and balance. The shoulders and elbows are flexed to 90 degrees, with the scapulae engaged to prevent excessive protraction. The right elbow is placed in the bend of the left elbow and the arms are intertwined until the palms touch. The right leg crosses over the left leg and, if possible, hooks around the left calf. If not, the right toes may gently rest on the floor. The arms are gently lifted towards the ceiling. Balance is maintained in this position.

The above list of yoga poses is simply a suggestion and by no means exhaustive. A regular practice of yoga (and there are many kinds), guided by a good teacher, is a way to maintain overall flexibility, strength, and balance. Other practices (mentioned in the list of other integrative movement therapies) also achieve similar goals. The point is to find a regular activity that challenges the body to move in "out-of-the-ordinary" ways and that promotes mind–body–spirit health.

Chelsea Lee, a yoga therapist from Vancouver, British Columbia, sums it up well:

While yoga postures can help one to lengthen, strengthen and align the body so that it can move more optimally, the internal alchemy that occurs through this process is really what will make the most meaningful change in the experience off of the mat and in life. It's more than stretching the hamstrings and improving thoracic rotation. You will discover a heightened awareness of your body, breath and mind while generating healthy stress in a safe and contained space, so that when the pressure is on outside of the studio, you have tools to help you show up as your best self.

Optimizing therapeutic outcomes

There was a time when I debated whether this chapter should be included in this book. My left brain certainly could agree with the concept of including discussion of the effects of nutrition, hydration, and hormone health on treatment outcomes. However, I would be remiss if I did not include the more nebulous, right brain approach to treatment, which includes information not only about creating an optimal therapeutic environment for the patient, but just as importantly, about creating an optimal therapeutic environment for the therapist. Treating from the "whole" brain, allows for more "holistic" approaches to treatment and more fulfilling outcomes for both therapist and patient.

It is important for physiotherapists to be aware of "out of scope" information, as nothing is separate in the body. We must consider the whole body/whole person that stands before us in our treatment room and recognize that there are other systems, such as the gut, that may influence musculoskeletal and brain health. Our clients may need a different health professional to help "clean up their physiology," preventing them from wasting time and money on some of our treatments, especially if they are not responding as expected.

Effect of nutrition on the body's tissues

Have you ever been in a situation where your patient's tissues feel like dried-up leather? Certainly not like the juicy fascia that Dr Jean-Claude Guimberteau has demonstrated in his *in vivo* videos. One common reason why certain people tend to develop dense, tight fascia is due to their dietary habits. According to a study by Pavan and colleagues, diet, exercise, and overuse syndromes can modify the viscosity of loose connective tissue within fascia, causing densification (Pavan et al. 2014). It is important to note that an acidic diet can lead to systemic issues that maintain an inflammatory environment and thus lead to the densification of fascia. The common culprits in the average North American diet include:

- high blood glucose levels (sugar)
- alcohol
- hydrogenated oils
- aspartame.

High blood glucose levels (sugar)

Dr Christiane Northrup, board certified Ob/Gyn (obstetrics/gynaecology) and author of several books on women's health, recommends an anti-inflammatory alkaline diet for optimal function of the connective tissue matrix. She sums up the effect of a high sugar diet as follows:

Sugars affect your body at a cellular level, even whole grains. The genetically altered grains of today are very different from those our grandparents enjoyed. They have a much higher gluten content. That causes cellular inflammation, because the cells don't know what these particles are and they want to neutralize them by surrounding them with fluid. Your hormonal system responds to all the sugars by having your pancreas pump out more insulin to get the extra sugar in your blood to go into cells, where it can be used. The inflammation causes oxidative stress, destabilizing the cells. This may show up as physical discomfort, aching muscles, bloating, headache, insomnia and weight gain. Over time, chronic degenerative disease such as heart disease, arthritis, high blood pressure, Alzheimer's, diabetes, and cancer are a result. Fortunately, this domino effect of sugar / inflammation / disease can be counteracted and reversed by lowering blood sugar intake and paying attention to the types and forms of sugars you eat. (Northrup 2015)

Tom Myers also advocates cutting out sugars and other acid-producing foods: "Sugar is sticky, and that's what it does in the body. It's hard to force water into sticky areas. Depending on your constitution, cheese or meat or peanuts or other allergens could be causing this stickiness. Not my area of expertise, but a good nutritionist can advise you."

In his talk about "Food Pain and Dietary Effects of Inflammation", Dr Hal Blatman (Blatman 2016) advocates avoiding inflammatory foods, including white sugar, white flour, potatoes and fruit juices. He also includes in this list bread, pasta, cereal and wheat grain (often used as a thickener in processed soups and sauces). He quotes a study in which sugar-sweetened beverage consumption was shown to promote inflammation in healthy young men (Aeberli et al. 2011).

Alcohol

Alcohol of any kind is a sugar and so is metabolized similarly. Again, moderation is the key.

Hydrogenated oils/trans fats

When we think of hydrogenated fat, margarine comes to mind. When margarine was first formulated, hydrogenated gas was put into vegetable oil in an attempt to stop it from growing mold, thereby improving shelf life. Today, all partially hydrogenated vegetables oils and most processed foods contain trans fats. One major reason that trans fats have been allowed to persist is that food additives, in use before the US FDA enacted the Food Additive Amendment in 1958, did not require FDA approval. In other words, trans fats were grandfathered in as acceptable because they were in use as of 1958 (Kaslow 2018).

Dr Kaslow sums up the effect of trans fats hydrogenated oils on the cell membrane:

Hydrogenated trans fats affect the cell membrane and so govern their function and communication with other cells. Trans fats are absorbed into the cell membrane, where healthy essential fats should be integrated. The human lipase enzyme is ineffective with the trans configuration, so trans fat remains in the blood stream for a much longer period of time and is more prone to arterial deposition and subsequent plaque formation. Trans fats raise LDL cholesterol and lower HDL cholesterol levels in your blood, which is the opposite of the ideal cardiovascular ratio. Thus the very basic and crucial actions of cells and the proper functioning of your body are to a great extent dependent on the oils you consume every day.

Dr Blatman also mentions the many negative side effects of hydrogenated oil. More notably, hydrogenated oils have been associated with rising cholesterol levels (Sartika 2011), an increase in incidence of diabetes (Chartrand et al. 2003), and a change in cell membrane composition (Clandinin et al. 1991). In addition, saturated fatty acids have been shown to activate skeletal muscle cells to release inflammatory mediators that trigger macrophages (Pillon et al. 2012).

Here is an interesting fact that resonated with me from listening to Dr Blatman's Food and Pain lecture. If one eats a bag of Cheezies, or some French fries, the trans fats that are ingested will be used to form the cell wall of hemoglobin. Trans fats render the red blood cell useless for binding to oxygen, which ultimately affects delivery of oxygen to our muscles and our brain, contributing to increased pain. The cell life of a red blood cell is four months. This means that there are useless cells remaining in the body for four months resulting from eating one bag of Cheezies! Imagine the hemoglobin cellular function of the person who eats a bag of these daily. It is not "Oh well, its just one bag and only today." No, it lasts four months.

Aside from dietary changes, there are ways that we can enhance the composition of the cell membrane and minimize the development of inflammation and pain. Dr Blatman advocates the use of fish oil supplements. This recommendation is backed by a number of studies that show improvement in joint tenderness and swelling in patients with rheumatoid arthritis (Kremer et al. 1990), prevention of atherosclerosis (Shewale et al. 2015), and cancer (Hardman et al. 1999).

Aspartame

This common sugar substitute is widely used in processed foods, including baked goods, soft drinks, canned foods, dairy products, and scores of other foods and beverages. While the sweetener remains popular, it has also triggered controversy in recent years. Critics have claimed that aspartame has long-term repercussions on the body. When the body processes aspartame, part of it is broken down into methanol, which can then break down into formaldehyde (Hertelendy et al. 1993; Trocho et al. 1998). Clearly not a desirable substance to ingest! Another study noted an increased risk of non-Hodgkin's lymphoma and leukemia with drinking more than one can of diet soda or a high consumption of regular soda per day (Schernhammer et al. 2012).

Balancing the gut microbiome

The gut microbiome is essential for human health and physiology. It is defined as the collective genomes of the microbes (composed of bacteria, bacteriophage, fungi, protozoa and viruses) that live inside and on the human body. We have about ten times as many microbial cells as human cells. Microbes can be categorized as symbiotic (healthy flora) or dysbiotic (toxic flora). Toxic flora thrive on white flour, sugar, and the residue of red meat. Healthy flora thrive on green leafy vegetables. We all have a mixture of both kinds of flora and ideally, our immune system keeps the toxic flora under control. However, triggers such as viral or bacterial infections, fungal/yeast infections, NSAIDs, and radiation/chemotherapy can induce what is called a "leaky gut syndrome," where intestinal permeability is altered. This can lead to hypersensitivity responses to foods, inflammatory bowel disease (Crohn's), irritable bowel syndrome, chronic inflammatory joint disease, eczema, and chronic fatigue syndrome (Blatman 2016). Animal studies show that different microbial populations can dramatically affect susceptibility to chronic inflammation (Ferreira et al. 2011; Willing et al. 2011; Wlodarska et al. 2011). This dynamic may also have repercussions in relation to obesity, atherosclerosis, autism, and allergies, as well as asthma and celiac disease. Knowing what we currently know about the pathophysiology of fascial dysfunction and the effect of chronic inflammation on fascia, we can also add fascial dysfunction to the list of repercussions possible when the gut microbiome is not balanced.

Michael Pollan, author of *Food Rules: An Eater's Manual*, distills 64 food rules to guide Americans away from the Western diet of processed "edible food-like substances" and toward diets that originated in traditional food cultures. He sums up his philosophy nicely with three short instructions," Eat food, not very much, mostly plants" (Pollan 2009).

Hydration

The human body is 75 percent water. Two-thirds of the body's water is contained in the fascia. Hence the importance of drinking water for optimal fascial health and, especially, when working with the fascial system. Fascia has less blood supply than muscles, so structures such as ligaments, tendons, and cartilage have a more difficult time healing as a result of injury. Fascia relies on water seeping into the area in order to stimulate the repair process. Tom Myers notes that it is important to MOVE in order to get water into fascial tissues, preferably in patterns differing from our usual habits. "If you do the same exercise or movement routine all the time, the water will be driven down familiar pathways, and will end up in your bladder. What movements can you do that are unusual? Take a belly dance class, learn tumbling, try contact improv – do something unusual to push the water into these dry and sticky places." An appropriate amount of rest time is also important, in order to allow fascial tissues to re-hydrate (Myers 2017).

Hormone health

Menopause in women brings about hormonal changes that can affect the soft tissues of the body. The perimenopausal stage begins around age 45 and can last a decade or more. Initially, progesterone levels decline, which may manifest in feelings of sadness, as progesterone acts like a natural valium. In the early 50's, the ovaries shut down, which then affects the level of estrogen in the body. The brain does not react as quickly (producing "memory burps") and women become thicker in the middle of the body. This thickening is the body's attempt to compensate for the loss of estrogen, as breast tissue and abdominal fat produce estrogen.

Christiane Northrup points out that, in an attempt to deal with menopausal symptoms, medicine turned to synthetic hormone replacement therapy (HRT). This trend abruptly reversed in 2002, when the Women's Health Initiative study showed higher rates of breast cancer and heart disease in thousands of women who were given HRT in the form of Prempro (a combination of Premarin, which is horse urine, and Provera, which is synthetic progestin). Thankfully, Dr Northrup states that there are other options for relief from menopausal symptoms, with bio-identical hormones, such as bioidentical estrogen gel applied to the skin along with oral bioidentical progesterone.

Northrup notes that males also undergo hormonal changes with *andropause*, as their testosterone levels drop. This shift causes muscle tone to decrease and it makes it more difficult to build healthy muscle. There is also an effect on bone health, with an increase in osteopenia /osteoporosis. Women too have similar symptoms, as their testosterone levels (although lower than males) also decrease.

A functional medicine doctor is best trained to recommend what approaches may be best for optimal hormone health.

Stress hormones

Dr Northrup suggests that in perimenopause or menopause, the number one hormone to be concerned about is cortisol. This stress hormone is designed to be released in the body in situations of acute stress, in order to help us deal with physical danger quickly. It also temporarily activates the immune system in the case where a bacteria or virus has entered the system. An inflammatory response then occurs; white blood cells gather around the pathogen to isolate it before attacking it. The problem is that if the cortisol and its partner, epinephrine (adrenaline) are not cleared from the system quickly and, instead, linger for days, weeks, or even months, they have the opposite effect of lowering your immunity and energy. According to Dr Northrup,

> *Stress – mental, physical, emotional, or spiritual – creates inflammatory chemicals in the brain and body and may lead to cellular degeneration. This response may occur in the brain and manifest as memory deterioration. It may also occur in the fascia, where we store all of our traumas, whether physical, mental, or spiritual. These traumas create thickened, dense fascia, which eventually leads to pain and limited range of motion. Chronic fear, anger, sadness and resentment keep stress hormones in your system, setting the stage for poor health, including depression, cancer and heart disease. (Northrup 2015)*

The mechanism by which trauma can create densification of fascia is unknown. Perhaps there is a link between stress, hormonal changes and inflammation. Although inflammation is critical for normal healing processes, too much or prolonged inflammation may lead to binding down of fascia and fibrosis, or, as the Stecco's call it, densification of fascia.

In summary, what we put into our bodies, how we move, how we manage hormonal changes and stress – all these factors play a role and impact the health of the fascial system. If our patients have difficulty with maintaining effects of treatment with any kind of manual therapy, or if they plateau with treatment, it is wise to consider appropriate professional help to address these additional dimensions of health.

Creating an optimal therapeutic environment for the patient

It is important for the patient to receive treatment in an environment that optimizes the therapeutic outcome. The following are a few suggestions to consider:

- Treat in private spaces when possible. This privacy not only helps control the level of noise, but also allows for confidential and safe conversations between therapist and patient.

- Use ambient lighting (preferably natural).

- Ensure neutral to warm room temperature (it stimulates the parasympathetic nervous system).

- Consider the whole person – bio-psycho-social model – energetic and spiritual dimensions (more on this below).

- In addition to treating with manual therapy and exercise, the therapist may also consider educating the patient on ways to desensitize the sympathetic nervous system (SNS). These tools can help to tone down the vagus nerve, decrease anxiety, and deal with negative thoughts:
  - slow, rhythmic, diaphragmatic breathing. Breathing from the diaphragm and into the pelvic floor and sacrum, rather than shallowly from the top of the lungs, stimulates and tones the vagus nerve.
  - alternate nostril breathing
  - humming
  - Mindfulness Meditation

– MUSE – a brain sensing headband that helps one to focus during meditation as it gently guides a meditation session through changing sounds of weather, based on the real-time state of the brain.

Creating an optimal therapeutic environment for the therapist

Creating an optimal environment also applies to the therapist. A number of issues come to mind here, gleaned not only from my past 40 year experience as a physiotherapist, but also from the insights of many other therapists, whose opinions and reflections I value.

Accessing both sides of the brain

I believe that the best treatment approach is a combined approach, one that appreciates the importance of sound assessment, based on a left-brain, linear, structured approach but that also makes room for another element, the right-brain, creative, intuitive approach. Unfortunately, many physiotherapists are either left-brain thinkers or right-brain thinkers. A few state their views passionately on social media, dismissing or even vilifying the approaches of fellow therapists who think differently than they do.

Therapists who rely solely on the intuitive, creative aspects of the brain tend to "go with the flow" often not explaining what they are doing for the patient. This approach unwittingly creates a more passive role for the patient, and frames treatment as a process in which the therapist alone does the "healing". Few objective tests are used to evaluate the effects of their treatments. Diagnosis is based mainly on palpatory findings and clinical reasoning is often lacking.

By contrast, left-brained, analytical minds may be great at creating structure, using a test/retest approach to see if they are on the right track with their therapies, but they may have difficulty thinking "outside of the box" when their standard tools are not working for the patient. Such an approach may lead the therapist to conclude that the patient must have a central pain component to their problem. Admittedly, many chronic conditions do have a mixture of both primary nociceptive and central pain phenomena, but my personal experience, based on treating mostly chronic conditions, is that the pendulum has swung too far to the side of believing that all pain is of central origin.

In reality, "The magic happens in the middle" (Peter O'Sullivan). The optimal therapeutic intervention involves accessing both the scientific literature and structured learning in the classroom in order to create a solid base from which to begin the clinical reasoning process as well as tapping into the resources of intuition, deep wisdom and creativity. Working with the fascial system is a great way to combine both perspectives.

Heather Williamson-Vint, a physiotherapist from British Columbia, Canada, sums it up well:

Our ego serves us well in life. It allows us to conquer fears, attend school and grind out papers and acquire knowledge. Our ego can also get in the way of the "art" of healing. If we learn to lead with the heart as well as the mind, then intuition can play a role in our treatments, rather than reason alone. Ego is our link to control. It is cultivated by fear, whereupon many of us diminish this sense of fear through developing our egos, our inner "control freaks" that sadly, when put in the lead, can take us down paths that aren't our ultimate best routes. The art of letting go, physically and subconsciously, isn't taught in physiotherapy programs but can be cultivated with experience.

The importance of a good subjective exam

"Listen to your patients. Not only will they tell you what the problem is but also how to treat it." This was the single most important take-home message I received from Geoffrey Maitland's presentation on the subjective exam at the IFOMPT Conference in Vail, Colorado, in 1992. In particular, I remember a slide in which he demonstrated the use of P/A pressures on the upper lumbar spine with the patient in a prone position, his lumbar spine extended and the ipsilateral knee flexed. At the time, there was very little discussion in the world of manual physiotherapy about the importance of maintaining mobility of the nerves, but essentially, Maitland was a depicting a technique that later came to be described as a way to improve mobility of the femoral nerve. Maitland had offered no explanation for why he used this technique, except to say that it corresponded with the patient's subjective complaints and brought about positive treatment outcomes. He was certainly ahead of his time! Maitland's message has served me well throughout my career. Patients live in their body and have a sense of what is going on, even if it is subconscious. They can convey important cues to the therapist if the therapist pays careful attention to what they are saying.

Manual therapy

The fact is that any time we skillfully lay our hands on a patient, we are performing manual therapy. The idea that there is a dichotomy between "hands on" or "hands off" is essentially saying that we give up what makes us truly physiotherapists. For too long, certain people have looked at manual therapy as a purely passive treatment; clearly, it is not. We touch people when they are moving. We touch people to facilitate moving. We touch people to enhance movement. This is manual therapy. (Diane Lee)

Dialoguing with the tissues

- When using any manual therapy, it is important to "dialogue with the tissues". When we move any tissue of any kind, we must connect to the resistance in the tissues between our hands. Maitland's movement diagram helps put on paper what we are feeling in terms of early or late resistance, and the end-feel.

- "Rather than forcing a tissue to do something, pull a certain way, trying to mold it physiologically to respond, we must *listen* to the tissue, our own intuition, as to line of pull, tolerance of tissue to handling, load, stress and stretch. Once the listening element is put into practice regularly, it becomes instinctual, just like noting anteriorly tipped scapula or asymmetric load bearing." (Heather Williamson-Vint)

- Patients can feel threat in their bodies when your hands produce a movement that is interpreted as "unsafe". This "unsafe" interpretation may be due to the following:
  - the maneuver is being performed too quickly, without waiting for "permission" from the patient's tissues

- the therapist is producing a movement that is too deep or a grade of movement that is too high for the state of the irritability of the tissues
- the maneuver is done automatically, the therapist not "tuning in" to what they are sensing under their hands.

- "Seduce the tissues" rather than imposing a certain direction and force into the patient's tissues. Knock on the door and ask to be "let in." Wait for the body's response. When wondering if the patient can tolerate a certain maneuver, use the "listening" approach (see Chapter 4). In doing so, we can be reassured that the body will not allow any changes that it is not ready to receive.

- Trust your hands. They never lie. Listen to the body's response – a system-wide response in the parasympathetic direction, much like a system "sigh," is a sign that you are moving in the right direction. Increased sweating, anxiety, and a shallow, apical breathing pattern are all signs of a sympathetic reaction, and signal that we must change something in our treatment approach.

Art and science

- What we do in healthcare is both an art and a science. One cannot exist without the other. Art and science butt heads beginning in elementary school, where oftentimes physical education and art are abandoned as unnecessary topics expendable in the face of such subjects such as math and reading. However, art allows our species to learn. Art makes sense of the unspeakable, and gives us insight when there are no words. (Dr Ginger Garner)

- Manual therapy is an art form. We have to work at it in order to improve. The brain map for a new manual approach is initially small. Practice and the neuroplastic changes in the brain will make the brain map for this experience larger. Subtle changes then become huge. (Diane Lee)

Research

- Clearly, there is a need for ongoing research in every field of manual therapy and the MMS approach is no exception.

- However, we cannot expect for there to be evidence for every patient we see. RCT's are not the best way to measure optimal treatment options – individual programs that follow a clinical reasoning approach are the way to go (Gwen Jull, keynote address, IFOMPT, Québec City, 2012).

- There are many variables that we must consider in a treatment session and these variables make the clinician's daily experience with patients difficult to research. Your treatment room is your research lab (Diane Lee and Gregory Grieves – first edition of *Modern Manual Therapy*).

Psycho-socio-emotional vs physical

- "As physiotherapists, we get to work on the physical body, which I think of as a membrane between the external world all around us, and each individual's own internal world. Their perceptions of pain, health, stress, life fulfilment, and general day-to-day thoughts and emotions, can influence this physical vessel. We would be remiss as clinicians to not fully embrace the psycho social and spiritual elements in the process of healing from injury." (Heather Williamson-Vint).

- "As we plod along in our human journeys through life, we can't help but spend a bit of time at "the bottom of the barrel." We experience challenges, tragedies, and difficult situations aplenty. A lot of how we navigate this and come out the other side, for worse or for better, comes down to socio-emotional resilience: "An ability to recover from or adjust easily to misfortune or change." Our own tissues also experience resilience: "The capability of a strained body to recover its size and shape after deformation." Using this comparison, our physical body is the barrier between our internal and our external worlds. Basically, how we cope with our external environment displays itself in our physical self. We can come out of a difficult experience jaded, distrustful and at the same time, stooped, dehydrated and poorly oxidized. Or we emerge more knowledgeable of our physical, emotional and mental limits and can redirect ourselves with our tools, avoiding some major health challenges." (Heather Williamson-Vint)

Things I wish I knew as a young therapist

- We do not "fix" or heal patients. In reality we function more as a coach – helping to bring awareness to our patient's mind/body. Only they can make a difference in their brain map. (Diane Lee)

- There is no such thing as a cure in the body. We only help the patient manage it better by helping them understand their condition and by empowering them to take charge of their healing.

- Education is a large part of what we do for a patient, whether that is teaching them how to position their back to safely brush their teeth or simply de-escalating their fear. Don't underestimate education.

- Part of the education piece for our patients is to watch for their "languaging" of their painful experience. For example, "I'm falling apart", "My body is killing me" or "I have to expect this at my age". Our reality is shaped by our thoughts. Negative thought patterns adversely affect the experience of pain as they contribute to the DIM'S (Danger in Me) neurotags. Instead, we can empower our patients with messages like "You can be sore but safe. Your hurts won't harm you". (NOI notes, 2017)

- Ageism is a negative perception of getting older and of older people. It is a really big personal and societal DIM (Danger in Me neurotag) and it needs to be challenged. Young and old people can be ageist. Older people can be ageist about themselves. Health professionals and sometimes government departments and companies are ageist. Let us challenge it, first by obliterating some myths about pain and ageing. (NOI notes, 2018)

- Even though X-rays and scans may show things such as narrowing of joint spaces, such alterations have NO relation to increased pain. These are age changes and more age does not equal more pain. (NOI notes, 2018) (APTEI, VOMIT: Victim of Medical Imaging Technology, 2014)

- "We are what we focus on. As therapists, we all have the "pain chasers" that try to relocate the pain as soon as their treatment is finished. That pain pathway is so etched into their nociceptive memory banks (especially those with more chronic pain) that it is easy enough to find. I tell clients to trust in their body's potential to heal. Once they "buy in" to this process, the rest follows fairly smoothly. Giving a gentle nudge of self-responsibility and self-management to people is both worthwhile and empowering. As a clinician, I find it most rewarding to see the evolution of body and thought awareness take place in some patients. Once a client becomes aware of the stretches, exercises, breathing patterns, postures, imagery and/or mantras that they find useful for self-care, they can use these to pre-empt old pain patterns or toxic thoughts before they take hold of the whole person. Being able to control our thoughts and re-align our bodies consciously is a huge part of living a life in balance and wellness". (Heather Williamson-Vint).

- Look out for patients who may feel that they are victims of their pain. Perhaps they feel that their workplace or their family dynamic is the *perpetrator*. The corollary to this is that we, as physiotherapists and body workers, can become the *rescuer*. "Be careful of this triangle. We are none of these things. These are simply a perception of our reality that plays out in our physical world. We can change all this with a perspective shift and the right encouragement. Patients with healthier perspectives and the ability to change a negative internal script to a more positive one have better results, regardless of what tricks are up the therapist's sleeve." (Heather Williamson-Vint)

- Nurture compassion, both for your patients and, perhaps more importantly, for yourself. Therapists tend to have perfectionist traits. Developing compassion for yourself and your imperfections is vital to your well-being.

- Don't be so hard on yourself. We cannot help everyone. We can only facilitate the path for the patient but it is up to him/her to choose the path.

- Don't compare yourself to any of your colleagues. Only compete with yourself – are you a better therapist than you were last year?

- Follow your intuition. Don't suppress it because it isn't "scientific". But back it up with critical thinking and clinical reasoning.

- Be willing to shift your beliefs and paradigms as data and clinical experience guides us. (Peter O'Sullivan)

- Stay curious and hungry for knowledge. I frequently end the fascia courses that I teach with a quote from Tom Myers: "The more I learn, the farther the horizon of my ignorance extends." I hope I never get to the point where I feel that I have all of the answers. Then there would be no more room to grow.

- Value intellectual humility. (Peter O'Sullivan)

- What you have learned at university is just the tip of the iceberg. You learn from treating your patients, especially the more challenging cases. You learn through taking postgraduate courses. You learn through asking questions. You learn by teaching. Don't stop.

- Take as many postgrad courses as you possibly can – they stimulate your brain and keep challenging your paradigms. A word of caution, however; don't get hung up on any one approach to treatment and believe that it will solve all your patients' problems. It is best to have many tools in your clinician's toolbox. Pull out what you need for the right patient at the right time. Good clinical reasoning will help you sort out which tool(s) you will need for your particular client.

- Find yourself a mentor who can facilitate your learning. I have had many mentors in my career and I learned a great deal from each of them. In turn, I hope and believe that I have "given back" by mentoring another generation of skilled clinicians.

- Embrace social support. Cultivate friendships that will feed your mind, body, and soul.

- Deepen your spiritual connection.

Spirit

Connect to your purpose / meaning.

Spirit is not necessarily about religion (although it can be). Some people see it as connecting to purpose, meaning, to true essence of self and the world around. As Shelley Prosko, PT, explains in her WOW chat with Diane Lee, "Everything is impermanent except for Essence." Lao Tzu, an ancient a Chinese philosopher credited with founding the philosophical system of Taoism, states, "Care about what other people think and you will always be a prisoner."

So what is reality? Reality will often differ, depending on how we sense, perceive, and interpret information. Learn to witness yourself and get to know your own personal biases and filters from which we observe the world.

Learn how to "step away" and witness yourself reacting to a certain situation. "Hmmm, I'm doing this again". Not in a judgemental away – just an awareness of your tendencies and patterns playing themselves out. Our biases and personal beliefs contribute to how we react to situations. Be mindful of the "reactive" state. We are never in our power there and cannot be effective healers.

Use your gifts – Kelly's story

Our children are some of our greatest teachers.

Their demands on our time are a gift, since they force us to develop a better work-life balance. If it wasn't for my two children, I would be much more of a workaholic than I already am! Kelly and Michael are now grown adults and they continue to inspire me, using their gifts in their own special way to make the world a better place.

This lesson was brought home for me when Kelly was five years old. I had opted to stay home for one year when she was born and then went back to work. Technically, it was a part-time job at the clinic, but with administrative tasks of managing a clinic, teaching manual therapy courses for the Orthopaedic Division of the Canadian Physiotherapy Association, and working as an Examiner (and later, Chief Examiner) for that same Association, it became clear to my daughter that I had other responsibilities aside from being her Mom. She was in a home daycare for a couple of years, and then a more structured educational daycare. By the time she was five years old, she was in kindergarten and came to realize that some mothers stayed home with their children and did not work. One night, in the process of being tucked into bed after reading stories, she asked

me, "Mommy, why do you work?" I thought about it for a moment and replied, "Well, if I didn't work, then we wouldn't live in a home with a pool in the backyard". "I don't care", she replied. "We would have to live in a smaller house", I countered. Once again, she replied, "I don't care." What she was really trying to tell me is that my work had taken up too much time and that she needed more of me. Evidently, although we had quality time, the quantity was insufficient for her. I went to bed that night, thinking about our conversation and started to reflect on why I really worked. Of course, the money allowed the family to enjoy a certain quality of life, but then I thought, "What if I won the lottery tomorrow? Would I still continue to work?" The answer was a resounding "YES". The next evening, at Kelly's bedtime ritual, I brought up the topic once again. "I thought about what you asked me last night, Kelly, and I realized something. Do you see these hands of mine? They are God's gift to me and I use them to help make people feel better. Now your job is to find out what your gift or gifts are and use them to make the world a better place. But I hear you. I have been working too much and need to cut down some of my teaching so we can have more time together." Her response was simply "OK – sounds good", but the lessons we both learned from that conversation stayed with us. In future conversations, she would often bring up the topic of "using our gifts to share with the world".

My story

My story about learning to connect to Spirit is more difficult for me to share than Kelly's story, as it forces me go to that vulnerable place, where I know I will be opening myself up to criticism. But I choose not to let fear dictate my life, so here goes.

I grew up in a family of five children, where education was of primary importance. The emphasis in school in those days was science, and my left-brain resonated with this approach. My parents helped encourage my development in the arts through dance and piano lessons, and gymnastics was my sport of choice throughout high school. We all trotted off to church on Sundays and religion to me was a bunch of "shoulds" and "should-nots". There was little talk in those days of developing a personal relationship with God. Going through adolescence and early adulthood brought with it a certain "disillusionment" with the Church, although I still believed in God or a higher source and I still appreciated the traditions associated with Christian holidays, such as Christmas and Easter.

Moving forward through my middle years, I was busy establishing a clinic and raising young children and gave little thought to all things Spirit. I have always had a sense, however, that something very important would happen to me when I was 38 years old.

My father's health crisis precipitated a spiritual crisis within me. At the time, I was seeing a patient who insisted that she needed to speak to me about my Dad – that she had information that I needed to know so that I could help him. I had not told her anything about my father's health issues. He had been diagnosed with prostate cancer a few months back and had undergone radiotherapy treatments. Finally, I took some time to hear my patient out. She told me that she had spirit guides who told her that my father was ill with prostate cancer and that it had spread to his back (all true). Her spirit guides wanted to let me know that, I, too, had spirit guides, and I could learn to use them to help treat my Dad. "But I don't treat cancer – I treat musculo-skeletal conditions!" I exclaimed. You can imagine how my left-brain, logical mind reacted to this information! It was a struggle that took some time to work through.

In the end, I suspended my beliefs in an attempt to try to help my father. This decision led to the development of a personal relationship with God / Higher power/ Universe – call it what you will. It opened up a whole new world of energy, as my hands learned to feel things on a whole other (energetic) level. I also came to recognize that I too, had spirit guides, some to help me personally in my life and others, specifically to guide me in my treatment sessions with my patients. I had to learn how to communicate with them and to invite them when I was unsure how to proceed with a particular patient. I have learned to listen to their advice. When my mind decides otherwise, the results are never as good, so I have learned to listen, and to trust. My guides never cease to surprise me. I also must give credit where credit is due. Much of the MMS treatment approach that I use with my patients, and that I teach throughout Canada and Europe, is actually information that has

gradually been downloaded "from above" throughout the past 20 years. My only "job" before I start my workday is to do a quick meditation to clear my energies, so that I can "get myself out of the way" to be able to hear the messages from above without having to filter through my own issues. When I spend a few minutes in the morning at the start of my workday, the day generally runs smoothly and with ease. This personal connection to the Universe has also helped me immensely with personal life challenges. I truly do not know how I would have handled certain situations without the tools I had developed to connect to Spirit.

So how does one recognize that our Spirit guides are communicating with us? Initially, I would ask a question in a "yes" or "no" format. I could not "hear" an answer but it would come to me in a guttural, kinesthetic way, an almost imperceptible nodding motion of the head for "yes" and a gentle side-to-side shaking for a "no". The first time I experienced this, I thought I was making it up, but I have learned to discern true communication from wishful thinking on my part. Sometimes, I do not get an answer, as if Spirit is trying to tell me "it's not yet time". Another way to differentiate wishful thinking from Spirit communication is that the answer comes to you even before you have finished formulating the question! It is as if they are a step ahead of you and know what you will be asking! Certainly, not left-brain thinking.

Ultimately, I was able to learn to communicate beyond ways that require a yes or no response. In many ways, it is like an idea that pops into your brain from nowhere. This is how many of the MMS techniques came about. I stored the information I read about the Anatomy Trains Lines in my "left-brain" all the while, keeping the patient's subjective and functional complaints in mind, along with the information gleaned from my assessments and using a clinical reasoning approach. I then learned to combine it with the creative, intuitive workings of the right brain. Such moments are when work becomes play. "It's OK to make things up – as long as it's helping people feel better and move better. Just play. Just play." (Diane Lee)

I believe that Spirit guides us and encourages us to use all of the resources we have at our disposal as therapists – mind, body and soul.

Connecting to Spirit for help with my challenging patients has become a regular habit. I don't do this for every patient, of course, but if I question what my next step should be, or even how much treatment a certain patient can tolerate within one treatment session, I ask. And I always get the appropriate answer. Some answers do not come but if you invite the divine to come and be a part of your healing space, miracles really can happen. The trick is in the asking – Spirit will never impose itself. It must be invited in.

Fascia in the Fifth Dimension

This brings us to muse about fascia in the fifth dimension. Heather Williamson-Vint summarizes her perspective: "Bodies are more than cells, and organ systems, obviously. They tell a wonderful story of where the client has been in their lives, not just physically but mentally as well. Their beliefs also affect the physical system and its chemical constituents. Is the world a trustful, safe place? Or is the world one best trod upon carefully, with held breath, in subconscious fascial tension?

When someone comes for treatment, we have the privilege of working directly with someone's "life script". The fascia is a structure that holds this information. It also serves as a wonderful literal metaphor for how someone is "metabolizing life". It has inert and contractile components, responds over time to habitual posturing and chronic stress. Are they adequately oxidized (think rib expansion, how much lung capacity is used due to posture of the thorax), are their tissues adequately hydrated, or acidic, stiff and painful to touch? All these physical issues have other layers to them. Nutrition is very influential, and the gut and its relationship to mood is now a topic being increasingly researched. What about the effectiveness of gut peristalsis and general well being if its suspension among the fascia in the peritoneal cavity is compromised? These thoughts convey the far-reaching impacts of fascia and its overall influence on our holistic well-being. I see fascia as a five-dimensional tool to gain access to the individual in all their planes of existence."

My hope is that the reader will take on this world of fascia, as they accompany their patients through their healing journeys, using both sides of the brain to access logic and science as well as creativity and intuition. There are a number of fascial approaches to treatment and all have value. I have simply shared my own approach to treatment, based on my background as a physiotherapist. My wish is that my contribution to the paradigm shift in rehabilitative care brings about interdisciplinary education and research, so that therapists and patients alike can benefit.

REFERENCES

Chapter 1

Axer H, Keyserlingk DG and Prescher A (2001a) Collagen fibers in linea alba and rectus sheaths. I. General scheme and morphological aspects. Journal of Surgical Research 96 (1) 127–134.

Axer H, Keyserlingk DG and Prescher A (2001b) Collagen fibers in linea alba and rectus sheaths. Journal of Surgical Research 96 (2) 239–245.

Bois D (2013) About DBM and the CSBMT [online] Available: http://thecsbmt.com/aboutdanisbois.html [20 May 2018].

Butler D and Mosely L (2013) Explain pain, 2nd edn, Adelaide, Australia Noigroup Publications.

Chaitow L and Delany J (2000) Clinical applications of neuromuscular techniques, vols 1–2, Edinburgh: Churchill Livingstone.

Deising S, Weinkauf B, Blunk J, Obreja O, Schmelz M and Rukwied R (2012) NGF-evoked sensitization of muscle fascia nociceptors in humans. Pain 153 (8) 1673–1679.

Findley TW and Shalwala M (2013) Fascia Research Congress: Evidence from the 100 year perspective of Andrew Taylor Still. Journal of Bodywork and Movement Therapies 17 (3) 356–364.

Gautschi RU (2012) Trigger points as a fascia-related disorder, in Schleip R, Findley TW, Chaitow L and Huijing PJ (eds), Fascia: The Tensional Network of the Human Body, Edinburgh: Churchill Livingstone/Elsevier, ch 5.7.

Gibson W, Arendt-Nielsen L, Taguchi T, Mizumura K and Graven-Nielsen T (2009) Increased pain from muscle fascia following eccentric exercise: Animal and human findings. Experimental Brain Research 194 (2) 299–308.

Guimberteau J-C (2015) Architecture of human living fascia: The extracellular matrix and cells revealed through endoscopy, Pencaitland UK: Handspring Publishing.

Huijing PA (2012) Myofascial force transmission: An introduction, in Schleip R, Findley T, Chaitow L and Huijing P (eds) Fascia: The tensional network of the human body, Edinburgh: Churchill Livingstone/Elsevier, ch 3.2.

Huijing PA and Baan GC (2003) Myofascial force transmission: Muscle relative position and length determine agonist and synergist muscle force. Journal of Applied Physiology 94 1092–1107.

Ingber DE (2003) Tensegrity I. Cell structure and hierarchical systems biology. Journal of Cell Science 116 (7) 1157–1173.

Juhan D (1998) Job's Body: A Handbook for Bodywork, Barrytown, NY: Station Hill Press.

Klinger W, Schleip R and Zorn A (2004) European Fascia Research Project Report, Fifth World Congress on Low Back and Pelvic Pain, Melbourne.

Langevin HM (2006) Connective tissue: a body-wide signalling network? Medical Hypotheses 66 1074–1077.

Langevin HM, Keely P, Mao J, Hodge LM, Schleip R, Deng G, Hinz B, Swartz MA, de Valois BA, Zick S and Findley T (2016) Connecting (t)issues: How research in fascia biology can impact integrative oncology. Cancer Research 76 (21) 6159–6162.

Lee L-J and Lee D (2011) Clinical practice – the reality for clinicians, in Lee D, The Pelvic Girdle: An Integration of Clinical Expertise and Research, 4th edn, Edinburgh: Elsevier, pp 147–171.

Mense S (2007) Presentation on neuroanatomy and neurophysiology of low back pain, First International Fascia Research Congress, Boston.

Myers T (2011) Massage Magazine [online] Available: https://www.massagemag.com, pp 58–61.

Myers T (2014) Anatomy Trains: Myofascial meridians for manual and movement therapists, 3rd edn, Edinburgh: Churchill Livingstone/Elsevier.

Myers T (March 2017) How to train fascia. Tip 3: Hydration [online] Available: https://www.anatomytrains.com/blog/2017/03/14/train-fascia-tip-3-hydration/ [20 May 2018].

Northrup C (2016) Making life easy: A simple guide to a divinely inspired life, Carlsbad, CA: Hay House Inc.

Oschman JL (2000) Energy medicine: The scientific basis, Edinburgh: Churchill Livingstone.

Paoletti S (2006) The fasciae: Anatomy, dysfunction and treatment, Seattle, WA:Eastland Press.

Pipelzadeh MH and Naylor IL (1998) The in vitro enhancement of rat myofibroblast contractility by alterations to the pH of the physiological solution. European Journal of Pharmacology 357 (2–3) 257–259.

Reed R, Lidén A and Rubin K (2010) Edema and fluid dynamics in connective tissue remodelling. Journal of Molecular and Cellular Cardiology 48 (3) 518–523.

Scheunke M (2015) Presentation. Fourth International Fascia Research Conference, Washington DC.

Schierling R (2017) Fascia [online] Available: http://www.doctorschierling.com/fascia.html [20 May 2018].

Schleip R (2003) Fascial plasticity – a new neurological explanation: Part 1. Journal of Bodywork and Movement Therapies 7 11–19.

Schleip R (2012) Fascia as an organ of communication, in Schleip R, Findley T, Chaitow L and Huijing P (eds) Fascia: The tensional network of the human body, Edinburgh: Churchill Livingstone/Elsevier, pp 77–79.

Schleip R, Klinger W and Lehmann-Horn F (2007) Fascia is able to contract in a smooth muscle-like manner and thereby influence musculoskeletal mechanics. Paper presented at the Sixth Interdisciplinary World Congress on Low Back and Pelvic Pain, Barcelona, Spain, November 7–10, 2007.

Schleip R, Findley T, Chaitow L and Huijing P (eds) (2012a) Fascia: The tensional network of the human body, Edinburgh: Churchill Livingstone/Elsevier, ch 2.5, pp 103–112.

Schleip R, Jäger H and Klingler W (2012b) What is "fascia"? A review of different terminologies, Journal of Bodywork and Movement Therapies 16 496–502.

Schultz RL and Feitis R (1996) The endless web: Fascial anatomy and physical reality, Berkeley, CA: North Atlantic Books.

Schwind P (2006) Fascial and membrane technique: A manual for comprehensive treatment of the connective tissue system, Edinburgh: Churchill Livingstone/Elsevier.

Shah JP, Phillips TM, Danoff JV and Gerber LH (2005) An in vivo microanalytical technique for measuring the local biochemical milieu of human skeletal muscle. Journal of Applied Physiology 99 (5) 1977–1984.

Shah JP, Danoff JV, Desai MJ, Parikh S, Nakamura LY, Phillips TM and Gerber LH (2008) Biochemicals associated with pain and inflammation are elevated in sites near to and remote from active myofascial trigger points. Archives of Physical Medicine and Rehabilitation 89 (1) 16–23.

Stecco C (2015a) Arriving at a definition of fascia: Findings of the Fascial Nomenclature Commmittee. Fourth International Fascia Research Conference, Washington DC.

Stecco C (2015b) Functional atlas of the human fascial system, Edinburgh: Churchill Livingston.

Stecco L (2004) Fascial manipulation for musculoskeletal pain, Padua, Italy: Piccin Nuova Libraria.

Tajik A, Zhang Y, Wei F, Sun J, Jia Q, Zhou W, Singh R, Khanna N, Belmont AS and Wang N (2016) Transcription upregulation via force-induced direct stretching of chromatin. Nature Materials 15 (12) 1287–1296.

Tesarz J, Hoheisel U, Wiedenhöfer B and Mense S (2011) Sensory innervation of the thoracolumbar fascia in rats and humans. Neuroscience 194 302–308.

Utting B (2013) Bindegewebsmassage. Washington Massage Journal 24–25.

Van den Berg F (2007) Angewandte Physiologie. Band 3: Therapie training and Tests Kapitel 1 – 1, Stuttgart: Thieme Verlag.

Van der Wal J (2009) The architecture of the connective tissue in the musculoskeletal system – an often overlooked functional parameter as to proprioception in the locomotor apparatus. International Journal of Therapeutic Massage and Bodywork 2 (4) 9–23.

Willard FH, Vleeming A, Schuenke MD, Danneels L and Schleip R (2012) The thoracolumbar fascia: Anatomy function and clinical considerations. Journal of Anatomy 221 (6) 507–536.

Chapter 2

Keown D (2014) The spark in the machine: How the science of acupuncture explains the mysteries of western medicine, London: Singing Dragon.

Langevin HM and Yandow JA (2002) Relationship of acupuncture points and meridians to connective tissue planes. Anatomical Record 269 (6) 257–265.

Lee L-J and Lee D (2011) Clinical practice – the reality for clinicians, in Lee D, The Pelvic Girdle: An Integration of Clinical Expertise and Research, 4th edn, Edinburgh: Elsevier, pp 147–171.

Myers T (2014) Anatomy Trains: Myofascial meridians for manual and movement therapists, 3rd edn, Edinburgh: Churchill Livingstone/Elsevier.

Uridel M (2015) Advanced anatomy: Myofascial meridians [online] Available: http://www.healingartscontinuingeducation.com

Wilke J, Krause F, Vogt L and Banzer W (2016) What is evidence-based about myofascial chains: A systematic review. Archives of Physical Medicine and Rehabilitation 97 (3) 454–461.

Chapter 3

Canadian Physiotherapy Association, Level IV/V Manual [online] Available: http://www.orthodiv.org/education/documents/contra-indications to manual therapy

Lee L-J and Lee D (2011) Techniques and tools for addressing barriers in the lumbopelvic–hip complex, in Lee D, The Pelvic Girdle: An Integration of Clinical Expertise and Research, 4th edn, Edinburgh: Elsevier.

Chapter 4

Butler D (1991) Mobilisation of the nervous system, Edinburgh: Churchill Livingstone.

Currier DP and Nelson RM (1992) Dynamics of human biologic tissues, Philadelphia: FA Davis.

Guimberteau J-C (2015) architecture of human living fascia: The extracellular matrix and cells revealed through endoscopy, Pencaitland, UK: Handspring Publishing.

Kaltenborn F (2014) Manual mobilization of the joints. Vol 1: The extremities, 8th edn, Orthopedic Physical Therapy and Rehabilitation.

Keown D (2014) The spark in the machine: How the science of acupuncture explains the mysteries of western medicine, London: Singing Dragon.

Lee L-J and Lee D (2011) Techniques and tools for addressing barriers in the lumbopelvic–hip complex, in Lee D, The Pelvic Girdle: An Integration of Clinical Expertise and Research, 4th edn, Edinburgh: Elsevier, p 287.

Hartman L (1997) Handbook of osteopathic technique, 3rd edn, Dordrecht: Springer Science Business Media BV.

Maheu E (2007) Grades of passive movement, Orthopaedic Division Review, Canadian Physiotherapy Association [online] Available: http://www.orthodiv.org/education/documents/contra-indications to manual therapy

Maitland G (2005) Maitland's vertebral manipulation, 7th edn, Churchill Livingston/Elsevier.

Myers T (2014) Anatomy Trains: Myofascial meridians for manual and movement therapists, 3rd edn, Edinburgh: Churchill Livingstone/Elsevier.

Orthopaedic Division Review Canadian Physiotherapy Association [online] Available: http://www.orthodiv.org/education/documents/contra-indications to manual therapy

Paoletti S (2006) The fasciae: Anatomy dysfunction and treatment, Seattle: Eastland Press.

Schleip R (2003) Fascial plasticity – a new neurobiological explanation: Part 1. Journal of Bodywork and Movement Therapies 7 (1) 11–19.

Shacklock M (2005) Clinical neurodynamics: A new system of neuromusculoskeletal treatment, Edinburgh: Elsevier/Butterworth-Heinemann.

Chapter 5

Lee D (2003) The thorax: An integrated approach, Diane G Lee, Physiotherapist Corporation, p 77.

Mens JM et al. (1999) Active straight leg raising test: A clinical approach to the load transfer function of the pelvic girdle, in Vleeming A, Mooney V, Snijders CJ, Dorman TA, Stoeckart R, Movement stability and low back pain, Edinburgh: Churchill Livingstone.

Mens JM, Vleeming A, Snijders CJ, Koes BW and Stam HJ (2001) Reliability and validity of the active straight leg raise test in posterior pelvic pain since pregnancy. Spine 26 (10) 1167–1171.

Chapter 6

Paoletti S (2006) The fasciae: Anatomy dysfunction and treatment, Seattle: Eastland Press.

Chapter 7

Adams C and Logue V (1971) Studies in cervical spondylotic myelopathy: Movement of cervical roots dura and cord and their relation to the course of the extrathecal roots. Brain 94 557–568.

Breig A and Troup T (1979) Biomechanical considerations in the SLR test: Cadaveric and clinical studies of medial hip rotation. Spine 4 (3) 242–250.

Butler D (2000) The sensitive nervous system. Adelaide, Australia: NOI Group Publications.

Goddard M and Reid J (1965) Movements induced by straight leg raising in the lumbo-sacral roots, nerves and plexus, and in the intrapelvic section of the sciatic nerve. Journal of Neurology Neurosurgery and Psychiatry 28 (12) 12–18.

Liem T (2004) Cranial osteopathy: Principles and practice, 2nd edn, Edinburgh: Elsevier Churchill Livingstone.

Louis R (1981) Vertebroradicular and vertebromedullar dynamics. Anatomica Clinica 3 1–11.

Magoun HI (1976) Osteopathy in the cranial field, 3rd edn, Boise, ID: Cranial Academy.

Shacklock M (2005) Clinical neurodynamics: A new system of neuromusculoskeletal treatment, Edinburgh: Elsevier/Butterworth-Heinemann.

Chapter 8

Butler D (2000) The sensitive nervous system, Adelaide, Australia: NOI Group Publications.

Clifton-Smith T and Rowley J (2011) Breathing pattern disorders and physiotherapy. Physical Therapy Reviews 16 (1) 75–86.

Lee L-J and Lee D (2011) Techniques and tools for addressing barriers in the lumbopelvic–hip complex, in Lee D, The Pelvic Girdle: An Integration of Clinical Expertise and Research, 4th edn, Edinburgh: Elsevier, p 287.

Chapter 9

Butler D (1991) Mobilisation of the nervous system, Edinburgh: Churchill Livingstone.

Lee L-J and Lee D (2011) Techniques and tools for assessing the lumbopelvic–hip complex, in Lee D, The Pelvic Girdle: An Integration of Clinical Expertise and Research, 4th edn, Edinburgh: Elsevier, pp 173–254.

Myers T (2014) Anatomy Trains: Myofascial meridians for manual and movement therapists, 3rd edn, Edinburgh: Churchill Livingstone/Elsevier.

Vleeming A, Stoeckart R and Snijders C (1989) The sacrotuberous ligament: A conceptual approach to its dynamic role in stabilizing the sacro-iliac joint. Clinical Biomechanics 4 201–203.

Chapter 10

Clifton-Smith T and Rowley J (2011) Breathing pattern disorders and physiotherapy. Physical Therapy Reviews 16 (1) 75–86.

Hodges PW, Sapsford R and Pengel LH (2007) Postural and respiratory functions of the pelvic floor muscles. Neurourology and Urodynamics 26 (3) 362–371.

Lee L-J and Lee D (2011a) Clinical practice – the reality for clinicians, in Lee D, The Pelvic Girdle: An Integration of Clinical Expertise and Research, 4th edn, Edinburgh: Elsevier, pp 147–171.

Lee L-J and Lee D (2011b) Techniques and tools for addressing barriers in the lumbopelvic–hip complex, in Lee D, The Pelvic Girdle: An Integration of Clinical Expertise and Research, 4th edn, Edinburgh: Elsevier, pp 173–254.

Myers T (2014) Anatomy Trains: Myofascial meridians for manual and movement therapists, 3rd edn, Edinburgh: Churchill Livingstone/Elsevier.

Stecco C, Macchi V, Porzionato A, Tiengo C, Parenti A, Gardi M, Artibani W and De Caro R (2005) Histotopographic study of the rectovaginal septum. Italian Journal of Anatomy and Embryology 110 (4) 247–254.

Chapter 11

Aguilar N (2015) Functional Patterns. Posture correction techniques: How to address duck feet [online] YouTube.

Bolivar VA, Munuera PV and Padillo P (2013) Relationship between tightness of the posterior muscles of the lower limb and plantar fasciitis. Foot and Ankle International 34 (1) 42–48.

Chen H, Ho HM, Ying M and Fu SN (2013) Association between plantar fascia vascularity and morphology and foot dysfunction in individuals with chronic plantar fasciitis. Journal of Sports and Orthopaedic Physical Therapy 43 (10) 727–734.

Khan KM, Cook JL, Bonar DF, Harcourt P and Astrom M (1999) Histopatholgy of common tendinopathies: Update and implications for clinical management. Sports Medicine 27 (6) 393–408.

Khan KM, Cook JL, Kamus P, Maffuli N and Bonar DF (2002) Time to abandon the "tendinitis" myth. British Medical Journal 324 (7338) 626–627.

Lee L-J, Lee D (2011) Techniques and tools for addressing barriers in the lumbopelvic–hip complex, in Lee D, The Pelvic Girdle: An Integration of Clinical Expertise and Research, 4th edn, Edinburgh: Elsevier, pp 173–254.

Myers T (May 2015) Plantar fasciitis [online] Available: http://wwwanatomytrains.com/blog [20 May 2018].

Young C (November 2016) [online] Available: Medscape/Sports Medicine Plantar Fasciitis https://www.emedicine.medscape.com/article/86143-overview

Chapter 12

Green RA, Taylor NF, Watson L and Ardern C (2013) Altered scapula position in elite young cricketers with shoulder problems. Journal of Science and Medicine in Sport 16 (1) 22–27.

KenHub November (2017) Clavipectoral fascia – anatomy components and function [online] Available: https://www.kenhub.com/en/library/anatomy/the-clavipectoral-fascia [8 Nov 2017].

Konieczka C, Gibson C, Russett L, Dlot L, MacDermid J, Watson L and Sadi J (2017) What is the reliability of clinical measurement tests for humeral head position? A systematic review. Journal of Hand Therapy 30 (4) 420–431.

Lee D (2003) The thorax: An integrated approach, Diane G Lee Physiotherapist Corporation, p 77.

Lee D (2018) The thorax: An integrated approach, Edinburgh: Handspring Publishing (in press).

Volker JH (November 2017) Clavi-pectoral fascia [online] Available: https://www.earthslab.com/anatomy/deep-cervical-fascia-fascia-colli/

Watson L (2013) Level 1 Shoulder Physiotherapy Course Manual, Lyn Watson Shoulder Physio, p 44.

Chapter 14

Garner G (2016) Medical therapeutic yoga: Biopsychosocial rehabilitation and wellness care, Edinburgh: Handspring Publishing.

Hebb D (1949) The organization of behavior (Hebbian theory), New York: John Wiley and Sons.

Herbert RD, de Noronha M and Kamper SJ (2011) Stretching to prevent or reduce muscle soreness after exercise. Cochrane Database of Systematic Reviews Jul 6;(7):CD004577.

Kreiger M (2018) DoYogaWithMe Bend and stretch class [online] Available: https://www.doyogawithme.com/content/stretch-and-bend [20 May 2018].

Larkam E (2017) Fascia in motion: Fascia-focused movement for Pilates. Edinburgh: Handspring Publishing.

Myers T (April 2015) Foam rolling and self-myofascial release [online] http://www.anatomytrains.com/blog

Myers T (May 2015) Pre and post exercise stretching: Pros and cons [online] http://www.anatomytrains.com/blog.

Myers T (September 2016) Optimal time to hold a yoga pose? [online] http://www.anatomytrains.com/blog

Schleip R and Bayer J (2017) Fascial fitness: How to be vital, elastic AND dynamic in everyday life and sport. Chichester: Lotus Publishing.

Chapter 15

Aeberli I, Gerber PA, Hochuli M, Kohler S, Haile SR, Gouni-Berthold I, Berthold HK, Spinas GA and Berneis K (2011) Low to moderate sugar-sweetened beverage consumption impairs glucose and lipid metabolism and promotes inflammation in health young men: A randomized controlled trial. American Journal of Clinical Nutrition 94 (2) 479–485.

APTEI (2014) VOMIT: Victim of medical imaging technology [online] http://www.aptei.ca/library-article/vomit-victim-of-medical-imaging-technology/ [20 May 2018].

Blatman H (2016) Food pain and dietary effects of inflammation, December 2016, 24th Annual World Congress on Anti-Aging Medicine, Las Vegas.

Chartrand R, Matte JJ, Lessard M, Chouinard PY, Giguère A and Laforest JP (2003) Effect of dietary fat sources on systemic and intrauterine synthesis of prostaglandins during early pregnancy in gilts. Journal of Animal Science 81 (3) 726–734.

Clandinin J, Cheema S, Field CJ, Garg ML, Venkatraman J and Clandinin TR (1991) Dietary fat: Exogenous determination of membrane structures and cell function. FASEB Journal 5 (13) 2761–2769.

Ferreira AV, Mario EG, Porto LC, Andrade SP and Botion LM (2011) High-carbohydrate diet selectively induces tumor necrosis factor-α production in mice liver. Inflammation 34 (2) 139–145

Garner G (2016) Medical therapeutic yoga: Biopsychosocial rehabilitation and wellness care, Edinburgh: Handspring Publishing.

Hardman WE, Moyer MP and Cameron IL (1999) Fish oil supplementation enhanced CPT-11 (irinotecan) efficacy against MCF7 breast carcinoma xenografts and ameliorated intestinal side-effects. British Journal of Cancer 81 (3) 440–448.

Hertelendy ZI, Mendenhall CL, Rouster SD, Marshall L and Weesner R (1993) Biochemical and clinical effects of aspartame in patients with chronic, stable alcoholic liver disease. American Journal of Gastroenterology 88 (5) 737–743.

Kaslow JE (2018) Trans Fats [online] www.drkaslow.com/html/trans_fats.html [20 May 2018]

Kremer JM, Lawrence DA, Jubiz W, DiGiacomo R, Rynes R, Bartholomew LE and Sherman M (1990) Dietary fish oil and olive oil supplementation in patients with rheumatoid arthritis: Clinical and immunologic effects. Arthritis and Rheumatism 33 (6) 810–820.

Myers T (March 2017) How to train fascia. Tip 3: Hydration [online] Available: https://www.anatomytrains.com/blog/2017/03/14/train-fascia-tip-3-hydration/ [20 May 2018].

NOI notes (Neuro Orthopaedic Institute) December (2017) Metaphors we feel by.

NOI notes (Neuro Orthopaedic Institute) February (2018) Oldies are goldies.

Northrup C (2015) Goddesses savor the pleasure of food, in Goddesses Never Age, Carlsbad, CA: Hayhouse, pp 243–245.

Pavan PG, Stecco A, Stern R and Stecco C (2014) Painful connections: Densification versus fibrosis of fascia. Current Pain and Headache Reports 18 (8) 441.

Pillon NJ, Arane K, Bilan PJ, Chiu TT and Klip A (2012) Muscle cells challenged with saturated fatty acids mount an autonomous inflammatory response that activates macrophages. Cell Communication and Signaling 10 (1) 30.

Pollan M (2009) Food rules: An eater's manual, New York: Penguin Books.

Sartika RA (2011) Effect of trans fatty acids intake on blood lipid profile of workers in East Kalimantan, Indonesia. Malaysian Journal of Nutrition 17 (1) 119–127.

Schernhammer ES, Bertrand KA, Birmann BM, Sampson L, Willett WC and Feskanich D (2012) Consumption of artificial sweetener and sugar-containing soda and risk of lymphoma and leukemia in men and women. American Journal of Clinical Nutrition 96 (6) 1419–1428.

Shewale SV, Boudyguina E, Zhu X, Shen L, Hutchins PM, Barkley RM, Murphy RC and Parks JS (2015) Botanical oils enriched in n-6 and n-3 FADS2 products are equally effective in preventing atherosclerosis and fatty liver. Journal of Lipid Research 56 (6) 1191–1205.

Trocho C, Pardo R, Rafecas I, Virgili J, Remesar X, Fernández-López JA and Alemany M (1998) Formaldehyde derived from dietary aspartame binds to tissue components in vivo. Life Sciences 63 (5) 337–349.

Willing BP, Antunes LC, Keeney KM, Ferreira RB and Finlay BB (2011) Harvesting the biological potential of the human gut microbiome. Bioessays 33 (6) 414–418.

Wlodarska M, Willing B, Keeney KM, Menendez A, Bergstrom KS, Gill N, Russell SL, Vallance BA and Finlay BB (2011) Antibiotic treatment alters the colonic mucus layer and predisposes the host to exacerbated Citrobacteria rodentium-induced colitis. Infection and Immunity 79 (4) 1536–1545.

INDEX